Evidence-Based Practices in Behavioral Health

Series Editor
Nirbhay N. Singh
Department of Psychiatry and Health Behavior
Medical College of Georgia
Augusta University
Augusta, USA

More information about this series at http://www.springer.com/series/11863

Russell Lang • Terry B. Hancock
Nirbhay N. Singh
Editors

Early Intervention for Young Children with Autism Spectrum Disorder

Springer

Editors
Russell Lang
Texas State University Clinic for Autism Research Evaluation and Support
San Marcos, TX, USA

Terry B. Hancock
Texas State University Clinic for Autism Research Evaluation and Support
San Marcos, TX, USA

Nirbhay N. Singh
Department of Psychiatry and Health Behavior
Medical College of Georgia
Augusta University
Augusta, GA, USA

ISSN 2366-6013 ISSN 2366-6021 (electronic)
Evidence-Based Practices in Behavioral Health
ISBN 978-3-319-30923-1 ISBN 978-3-319-30925-5 (eBook)
DOI 10.1007/978-3-319-30925-5

Library of Congress Control Number: 2016938681

Printed on acid-free paper

This Springer imprint is published by Springer Nature
The registered company is Springer International Publishing AG Switzerland

For our children and grandchildren:
Emerson Lang, Lindsey Hancock Williamson,
William Hancock, Hunter Hancock,
McClain Williamson, Ashvind Singh,
Subhashni Joy, Astarko Joy, Priya Joy,
Anicca Adkins Singh, Pierce Adkins Singh,
and all of the other children and families
who have taught us so much

Preface

A number of interventions designed to ameliorate the cognitive, social, language, and other behavioral deficits present in children with autism spectrum disorder (ASD) have been developed over the past 50 years. These interventions tend to be most effective when they are early, intensive, and behavioral. Understandably, parents of children with ASD, practitioners serving this population, and researchers in this area consider early intensive behavioral intervention (EIBI) to be of paramount importance for children with ASD. This book presents nine chapters focused on issues related to EIBI for children with ASD. The book begins with a brief introductory chapter that defines EIBI and summarizes research indicating that EIBI produces meaningful change in the lives of children with ASD. Next, because access to effective intervention often depends on early diagnosis, Chap. 2 covers common approaches to ASD diagnosis, recent innovations that facilitate accurate early diagnosis and directions for future research.

The next five chapters are devoted to specific EIBI approaches. The five interventions included in this text share many common core components (e.g., reinforcement), and all have been demonstrated to be effective in studies using a variety of research designs including randomized clinical trials and rigorous single case designs. Leading researchers in the field, and in some cases the creators or co-creators of specific intervention packages, authored the chapters. The five intervention approaches included in this text are Discrete Trial Training in Chap. 3, Pivotal Response Training in Chap. 4, Early Start Denver Model in Chap. 5, Prelinguistic Milieu Teaching in Chap. 6, and Enhanced Milieu Teaching in Chap. 7. These intervention chapters cover the theoretical underpinnings, specific procedures, research base, areas of future research, and considerations for practitioners for each of these evidence-based EIBI approaches. The book concludes with issues related to parent-implemented intervention in Chap. 8 and ethical issues related to fad, pseudoscientific, and controversial interventions commonly used with children with ASD in Chap. 9.

This book is unique in that it presents practical information on EIBI implementation (i.e., fidelity of implementation checklists, task analyses, and other implementation instructions) in tandem with discussion of theoretical underpinnings, analysis of research base, and directions for future research. This text is intended to serve as a resource for graduate students in clinical child, school, and developmental psychology, family studies, behavior analysis, special education, and public health interested in both the theory and practice of EIBI and for practitioners devoted to ensuring that the services they deliver are firmly rooted in research. We hope this text will provide a much needed overview of the field of EIBI for children with ASD useful to advanced practitioners, graduate students, and researchers.

San Marcos, TX, USA Russell Lang
San Marcos, TX, USA Terry B. Hancock
Augusta, GA, USA Nirbhay N. Singh

Contents

About the Editors

Russell Lang, Ph.D., B.C.B.A.-D. is an associate professor of Special Education at Texas State University and a Board Certified Behavior Analyst. Dr. Lang is also the Executive Director of Texas State University's Autism Treatment Clinic. He earned a doctoral degree in Special Education with an emphasis in Autism and Developmental Disabilities from the University of Texas at Austin and completed a postdoctoral researcher position at the University of California in Santa Barbara. His primary research interests include teaching play and leisure skills, assistive technology, and the treatment of problematic behaviors in individuals with autism spectrum disorders. He is a former Co-Editor-in-Chief of Developmental Neurorehabilitation and an Associate Editor for the *Journal of Developmental and Physical Disabilities* and the *Journal of Child and Family Studies*.

Terry B. Hancock, Ph.D., B.C.B.A.-D. is a professor of Clinical Practice in Special Education at Texas State University, a Board Certified Behavior Analyst, and a licensed psychologist. Dr. Hancock is also the Research Director at the Clinic for Autism Research, Evaluation and Support. She earned a doctoral degree in Education and Human Development with an emphasis in Early Childhood Special Education from Vanderbilt University. She has been an investigator on 12 federally funded grants related to communication and behavior interventions for young children. She was on the special education faculty at Vanderbilt University for 20 years and was the co-developer of Enhanced Milieu Teaching.

Nirbhay N. Singh, Ph.D., B.C.B.A.-D. is Clinical Professor of Psychiatry and Health Behavior at the Medical College of Georgia, Augusta University, Augusta, GA, CEO of MacTavish Behavioral Health, in Raleigh, NC, and a Board Certified Behavior Analyst. Prior to his current appointments, he was a Professor of Psychiatry, Pediatrics and Psychology at the Virginia Commonwealth University School of Medicine and Director of the Commonwealth Institute for Child and

Family Studies, Richmond, Virginia. His research interests include mindfulness, behavioral and psychopharmacological treatments of individuals with disabilities, and assistive technology for supporting individuals with diverse abilities. He is the Editor-in-Chief of two journals: *Journal of Child and Family Studies* and *Mindfulness*, and Editor of three book series: *Mindfulness in Behavioral Health*, *Evidence-Based Practice in Behavioral Health*, and *Springer Series on Children and Families*.

About the Contributors

Kristen Ashbaugh, M.A. is a doctoral student in the Counseling, Clinical, and School Psychology program at the University of California, Santa Barbara. She works under the advisement of Drs. Robert and Lynn Koegel and runs a program to provide behavioral intervention programs for college students and adults with autism spectrum disorder (ASD). Her primary research interests include increasing empathy for individuals with ASD, increasing socialization for college students on the spectrum, and improving social conversation and employment skills for adults with ASDs.

Kevin Ayers, Ph.D., B.C.B.A.-D. is a professor of Special Education at the University of Georgia and a Board Certified Behavior Analyst. Currently, Dr. Ayres coordinates the UGA Applied Behavior Analysis Support Clinic where he conducts research on skill acquisition and behavior reduction. The bulk of Ayres's research over the past decade has focused on behavioral applications of technology to help improve independent functioning of adolescents with autism and or intellectual disability. Dr. Ayres also currently serves as a co-editor for Focus on Autism and Other Developmental Disabilities.

Stephen Crutchfield, Ph.D. is an Assistant Professor of Special Education at California Polytechnic State University. He earned his doctorate from the University of Kansas and also completed a postdoctoral fellowship at Juniper Gardens Children's Project in the Life Span Institute at the University of Kansas. He is a former classroom teacher of students with autism, and his primary research focuses on how emerging technology can be leveraged to improve social skill and adaptive skill outcomes for young children and youth with autism both in and outside the classroom.

Geraldine Dawson, Ph.D. is the Director of the Duke Center for Autism and Brain Development and Professor of Psychiatry and Behavioral Sciences, Psychology and Neuroscience, and Pediatrics, at Duke University.

Robert Didden, Ph.D. is Professor of Intellectual Disability, Learning and Behaviour at the Behavioural Science Institute of the Radboud University Nijmegen, The Netherlands. As a health care psychologist he is affiliated with Trajectum, a facility for individuals with mild intellectual disability and severe behavioral disorders. His clinical and research interests include assessment and treatment of substance abuse, aggressive behaviors, sleep disorders, and trauma/PTSS in individuals with intellectual disability. He is associate editor of *Journal of Developmental and Physical Disabilities*, *Review Journal of Autism and Developmental Disorders*, and *Current Developmental Disorders Report.*

Annette Estes, Ph.D. is the Director and Susan and Richard Fade Endowed Chair of the UW Autism Center, Research Associate Professor in the Department of Speech and Hearing Sciences and Adjunct Research Associate Professor in the Department of Psychology at the University of Washington.

Rebecca Frantz, M.A. is a doctoral student in the Special Education Program at the University of Oregon. She obtained a master's degree from Teachers College, Columbia University, in Psychology in Education. Rebecca's primary research interests include early social communication intervention for young children with autism spectrum disorders and family-centered practices including parent-implemented intervention for symptoms of autism.

Terry B. Hancock Texas State University Clinic for Autism Research Evaluation and Support San Marcos, TX, USA

Sarah G. Hansen, M.A. is a doctoral candidate at the University of Oregon in Special Education with a focus on Early Intervention. Sarah received her Master's in Early Childhood Education at Mills College in Oakland, California, and her Bachelors of Science in Psychology at the University of California at Davis. Sarah's research interests focus on preparing children with developmental disabilities for success in the preschool classroom through intervention on early social skills.

Alexandria Howell, M.Ed., B.C.B.A. works for the San Antonio Independent School District. Her primary interests include early language and social skill interventions for individuals with autism spectrum disorder and issues related to implementing research-based practices in school settings.

Bibi Huskens, Ph.D. is a psychologist at the treatment center for children and a senior researcher at the Applied Behavior Analysis (ABA) research division at the Dr. Leo Kannerhuis, a center for autism spectrum disorders (ASD) in the Netherlands. She earned a doctoral degree in Social Sciences with an emphasis in ASD from the Radboud University in Nijmegen. Her research primarily focuses on staff training and parent training in ABA techniques and the effects on children with ASD.

Lynn Kern Koegel, Ph.D. the Clinical Director of Autism Services in the UCSB Autism Research Center and the Director of the Eli and Edythe L. Broad Center for Asperger's Research, has been active in the development of programs to improve communication in children with autism, including the development of first words, grammatical structures, pragmatics, and social conversation. In addition to her published books and articles in the area of communication and language development, she has developed and published procedures and field manuals in the area of self-management and functional analysis that are used in school districts and by parents throughout the United States, as well as translated in other major languages. Dr. Lynn Koegel is the author of *Overcoming Autism* and *Growing Up on the Spectrum* with parent Claire LaZebnik, published by Viking/Penguin and available in most bookstores.

Robert Koegel, Ph.D. has focused his career in the area of autism, specializing in language intervention, family support, and school inclusion. He has published over 200 articles and papers relating to the treatment of autism. Models of his procedures have been used in public schools and in parent education programs throughout California, the United States, and in other countries. Dr. Koegel has written seven books including *the PRT Pocket Guide*, *Pivotal Response Treatments*, and *Positive Behavioral Support* and is the founding Editor of the *Journal of Positive Behavior Interventions*. He has trained many top health care and special education leaders in the United States and abroad.

Sarah Kuriakose, Ph.D., B.C.B.A.-D. is a clinical assistant professor of Child and Adolescent Psychiatry at New York University Langone Medical Center (NYULMC). She is a clinical psychologist and a Board Certified Behavior Analyst. She currently serves as the Clinical Director of the Autism Spectrum Disorder Clinical and Research Program at the Child Study Center at NYULMC. Dr. Kuriakose earned a doctoral degree in Counseling, Clinical, and School Psychology with an emphasis in Clinical Psychology from the University of California in Santa Barbara. She completed her internship and fellowship at Harvard Medical School. Her primary clinical and research interests are in behavioral intervention for individuals with autism spectrum disorders and co-occurrence of psychiatric and developmental disorders.

Russell Lang Texas State University Clinic for Autism Research Evaluation and Support San Marcos, TX, USA

Linda LeBlanc, Ph.D., B.C.B.A.-D. is the Executive Director of Research and Clinical Services at Trumpet Behavioral Health and a Board Certified Behavior Analyst and Licensed Psychologist. Dr. LeBlanc earned a doctoral degree in Clinical Psychology at Louisiana State University and completed her internship and post-doctoral fellowship at the Kennedy Krieger Institute and Johns Hopkins University School of Medicine. Dr. LeBlanc has served as associate editor for *Education and Treatment of Children, The Analysis of Verbal Behavior, Journal of Applied*

Behavior Analysis, and *Behavior Analysis in Practice*. She has also served on the editorial boards of *Research in Developmental Disabilities*, *Behavioral Interventions*, *Research in Autism Spectrum Disorders*, and *The Behavior Analyst*. She has published over 85 articles and book chapters on topics such as behavioral treatment of autism, technology-based behavioral interventions, behavioral gerontology, and training and systems development in human services.

Katherine Ledbetter-Cho, M.Ed., B.C.B.A. is a doctoral student in the Autism and Developmental Disabilities program at the University of Texas at Austin and a research assistant at Texas State University's Autism Treatment Clinic. She received funding to complete her program of study as a scholar of the National Center for Leadership in Intensive Intervention. Her primary research interests include interventions to improve communication and play skills in young children with autism.

Dorothea C. Lerman, Ph.D., B.C.B.A.-D. is a Professor of Psychology at the University of Houston—Clear Lake (UHCL), where she coordinates a master's program in Behavior Analysis and serves as Director of the UHCL Center for Autism and Developmental Disabilities. She is a Board Certified Behavior Analyst and Licensed Psychologist. Dr. Lerman received her doctoral degree in Psychology from the University of Florida. Her areas of expertise include developmental disabilities, early intervention, teacher and parent training, and treatment of severe behavior disorders. Dr. Lerman has published more than 80 research articles and chapters, served as Associate Editor for *The Journal of Applied Behavior Analysis* and *Research in Developmental Disabilities*, was the founding Editor of *Behavior Analysis in Practice*, and recently completed a term as Editor-in-Chief of the *Journal of Applied Behavior Analysis*.

Wendy Machalicek, Ph.D., B.C.B.A.-D. is an Associate Professor in the Special Education and Clinical Services Department at the University of Oregon and a Board Certified Behavior Analyst. She earned a doctoral degree in Special Education with an emphasis in Autism and Developmental Disabilities from the University of Texas at Austin. Her primary research interests include three overlapping themes related to the assessment and treatment of autism spectrum disorder and related developmental disorders: systematic reviews of the intervention literature, assessment and treatment of challenging behavior, and technology-mediated teacher and parent training in evidence-based practices. She is a Co-Editor-in-Chief of Developmental Neurorehabilitation.

Larah van der Meer, Ph.D. is an Assistant Professor in the School of Education at Victoria University of Wellington, New Zealand. She received the Vice Chancellor's Strategic Research Scholarship to complete her doctoral studies in Education at Victoria University of Wellington. This research focused on enhancing communication intervention for children with autism spectrum disorders. Her primary research interests include the use of assistive technology to support the communicative functioning of children and adults with developmental and intellectual disabilities as well as early intervention for children with autism spectrum disorders. She has co-authored various peer-reviewed research articles and presented her research at international and local conferences.

Nienke C. Peters-Scheffer, Ph.D. is Assistant Professor at the Behavioural Science Institute of the Radboud University Nijmegen, The Netherlands. She combines clinical work and research at Driestroom, a facility for assessment and treatment of individuals with intellectual disabilities. Her main research interests are in autism spectrum disorder, intellectual disability, and applied behavior analysis, including early intervention and instructional procedures for individuals with developmental disabilities.

Tracy Raulston, M.Ed., B.C.B.A. is a doctoral student in the Special Education Program at the University of Oregon and a Board Certified Behavior Analyst. She obtained a master's degree from Texas State University concentrating in autism, developmental disabilities, and applied behavior analysis. She has experience as a public school special education teacher, clinical and home-based ABA therapist, and district-level behavioral specialist. Her scholarship focuses on the implementation and sustainability of evidence-based practices for children with autism spectrum disorders and other related developmental delays/disabilities in schools and homes.

Sally J. Rogers, Ph.D. is a Professor of Psychiatry and the Director of the Early Start Laboratory at the UC Davis MIND Institute and one of the original developers of the Early Start Denver Model.

Traci Ruppert, M.S., B.C.B.A. is a doctoral candidate in the Special Education and Clinical Services Department at the University of Oregon and a Board Certified Behavior Analyst. Her primary research interests include family–school partnerships, behavioral parent training, positive behavior interventions and supports, and low-incidence disabilities.

Rebecca Shalev, Ph.D. is a postdoctoral fellow and clinical instructor of Child and Adolescent Psychiatry at New York University Langone Medical Center. Dr. Shalev earned a doctoral degree in School Psychology from the University of Wisconsin in Madison. She completed her predoctoral internship at the University of Nebraska Medical Center's Munroe-Meyer Institute. Her primary clinical and research interests include assessment and treatment of autism spectrum disorders.

Richard Simpson, Ph.D. is Professor of Special Education at the University of Kansas. Dr. Simpson has directed numerous University of Kansas and University of Kansas Medical Center demonstration programs for students with autism spectrum disorders and other disabilities and coordinated a variety of federal grant programs related to students with autism spectrum disorders and other disabilities. He has also worked as a special education teacher, school psychologist, and coordinator of a community mental health outreach program. He has authored numerous books, articles, and tests on a variety of topics connected to students with disabilities. Simpson is the former senior editor of the professional journal *Focus on Autism and Other Developmental Disabilities*.

Nirbhay N. Singh Department of Psychiatry and Health Behavior, Medical College of Georgia Augusta University Augusta , GA , USA

Meagan R. Talbott, Ph.D. is a Postdoctoral Fellow at the UC Davis MIND Institute. She earned her doctoral degree in Psychology from Boston University, where she investigated the early language and communication development of infant siblings of children with ASD using home-based diary measures. Her research interests are in the early identification and treatment of autism, and in the development of language and social communication within everyday parent-child interactions.

Jason Travers, Ph.D., B.C.B.A.-D. is an assistant professor of special education at the University of Kansas and a Board Certified Behavior Analyst. Dr. Travers earned his doctoral degree at the University of Nevada Las Vegas while working as a special education teacher for a self-contained autism program the nation's fifth largest school district. He has published articles and book chapters on a variety of topics related to autism and special education, including the efficacy of technology-based interventions, disproportionate representation in administrative autism, evidence-based and pseudoscientific practices, and sexuality education. He currently co-directs two federally funded doctoral training grants, has presented at numerous conferences, and serves on editorial boards for five leading autism and special education journals.

Amber Valentino, Psy.D., B.C.B.A.-D. serves as the Clinical Director for the San Jose Division of Trumpet Behavioral Health in San Jose, California. Dr. Valentino earned a doctoral degree in Clinical Psychology from Xavier University in Cincinnati, OH. She completed a predoctoral internship and postdoctoral fellowship at the Marcus Autism Center/Children's Healthcare of Atlanta. Her training focused on early intensive behavioral intervention for children with autism and other developmental disabilities with a particular focus on verbal behavior. Dr. Valentino's clinical and research interests include the assessment and treatment of language deficits, primarily in children with autism. Dr. Valentino has served as a guest reviewer for the *Journal of Applied Behavior Analysis* and currently serves on the editorial board of *The Analysis of Verbal Behavior*. She has also had recent peer-reviewed publications in the *Journal of Behavioral Education*, *Research in Autism Spectrum Disorders*, *Behavior Modification*, *The Analysis of Verbal Behavior*, and the *Journal of Applied Behavior Analysis*.

Cynthia Zierhut, Ph.D. is a developmental and licensed clinical psychologist, and the Program Manager for the Early Start Denver Model Training Program at the UC Davis MIND Institute.

Contributors

Kristen Ashbaugh, M.A. UCSB Koegel Autism Center, Graduate School of Education, University of California, Santa Barbara, Santa Barbara, CA, USA

Kevin Ayers, Ph.D., B.C.B.A.-D. Department of Communication Services and Special Education, University of Georgia, Athens, GA, USA

Stephen Crutchfield, Ph.D. Special Education, California Polytechnic University, Kansas City, KS, USA

Geraldine Dawson, Ph.D. Duke Center for Autism and Brain Development, Duke University, Durham, NC, USA

Robert Didden, Ph.D. Behavioural Science Institute, Radboud University Nijmegen, Nijmegen, The Netherlands

Annette Estes, Ph.D. UW Autism Center, University of Washington, Seattle, WA, USA

Rebecca Frantz, M.A. Department of Special Education and Clinical Sciences, University of Oregon, Eugene, OR, USA

Sarah G. Hansen, M.A. Department of Special Education and Clinical Sciences, University of Oregon, Eugene, OR, USA

Alexandria Howell, M.Ed., B.C.B.A. San Antonio Independent School District, San Antonio, TX, USA

Bibi Huskens, Ph.D. Dr. Leo Kannerhuis, Center for Autism Spectrum Disorders (ASD), Doorwerth, The Netherlands

Lynn Kern Koegel, Ph.D. UCSB Autism Research Center, University of California, Santa Barbara, CA, USA

Robert L. Koegel, Ph.D. UCSB Autism Research Center, University of California, Santa Barbara, CA, USA

Sarah Kuriakose, Ph.D., B.C.B.A.-D. Department of Child and Adolescent Psychiatry, New York University Langone Medical Center (NYULMC), New York, NY, USA

Linda A. LeBlanc, Ph.D., B.C.B.A.-D. Trumpet Behavioral Health, Lakewood, CO, USA

Katherine Ledbetter-Cho, M.Ed., B.C.B.A. Department of Special Education, University of Texas at Austin, Austin, TX, USA

Dorothea C. Lerman, Ph.D., B.C.B.A.-D. Department of Psychology, University of Houston - Clear Lake (UHCL), Houston, TX, USA

Wendy Machalicek, Ph.D., B.C.B.A.-D. Department of Special Education and Clinical Sciences, University of Oregon, Eugene, OR, USA

Larah van der Meer, Ph.D. School of Education, Victoria University of Wellington, Wellington, New Zealand

Nienke C. Peters-Scheffer, Ph.D. Behavioural Science Institute, Radboud University Nijmegen, Nijmegen, The Netherlands

Tracy Raulston, M.Ed., B.C.B.A. Department of Special Education and Clinical Sciences, University of Oregon, Eugene, OR, USA

Sally J. Rogers, Ph.D. UC Davis MIND Institute, Sacramento, CA, USA

Traci Ruppert, M.S., B.C.B.A. Department of Special Education and Clinical Sciences, University of Oregon, Eugene, OR, USA

Rebecca Shalev, Ph.D. Department of Child and Adolescent Psychiatry, The Child Study Center at NYU Langone Medical Center, New York, NY, USA

Richard L. Simpson, Ph.D. Department of Special Education, University of Kansas, Lawrence, KS, USA

Meagan R. Talbott, Ph.D. UC Davis MIND Institute, Sacramento, CA, USA

Jason C. Travers, Ph.D., B.C.B.A.-D. Department of Special Education, University of Kansas, Lawrence, KS, USA

Amber L. Valentino, Psy.D., B.C.B.A.-D. Trumpet Behavioral Health, Lakewood, CO, USA

Cynthia Zierhut, Ph.D. UC Davis MIND Institute, Sacramento, CA, USA

Chapter 1
Overview of Early Intensive Behavioral Intervention for Children with Autism

Russell Lang, Terry B. Hancock, and Nirbhay N. Singh

Introduction

Child development typically occurs along a relatively predictable trajectory wherein the majority of children acquire motor skills, language and other behavioral and social competencies in approximately the same sequence and time frame. For example, typically developing children tend to imitate facial expressions in the first 2 months of life; produce babbling sounds around 3 months; and can play with other children and speak in coherent complete sentences before 3 years of age (Shelov & Altmann, 2009). In a general sense, autism is a condition wherein a child's pattern of development deviates from the typical course (e.g., Baird et al., 2000; Lang, Regester, Rispoli, & Camargo, 2010; Liu, 2012).

The diagnostic criteria for autism have changed numerous times since Infantile Autism was first included in the third edition of the Diagnostic and Statistical Manual of Mental Disorders (DSM; American Psychiatric Association [APA], 1980). Additionally, the World Health Organization (WHO) and the American Psychiatric Association (APA) both offer different diagnostic criteria and have updated their criteria at different times in different ways. Currently, the fifth edition of the DSM (DSM-5; APA, 2013) and the International Classification of Diseases and Related Health Problems (ICD-10) offer similar diagnostic criteria (WHO, 1992). The ICD-10 defines Childhood Autism as a pervasive developmental disorder

---

R. Lang (✉) • T.B. Hancock
Texas State University Clinic for Autism Research Evaluation and Support,
601 University Dr., San Marcos, TX 78666, USA
e-mail: rl30@txstate.edu

N.N. Singh
Department of Psychiatry and Health Behavior, Medical College of Georgia, Augusta University, Augusta, GA 30912, USA

R. Lang et al. (eds.), *Early Intervention for Young Children with Autism Spectrum Disorder*, Evidence-Based Practices in Behavioral Health,
DOI 10.1007/978-3-319-30925-5_1

involving abnormal functioning in reciprocal social interaction, communication, and restricted, stereotyped, repetitive behaviour. The ICD-10 further distinguishes between Childhood Autism and Atypical Autism, with the later diagnosed when abnormal functioning becomes evident after 3 years of age and/or when the child meets some but not all of the criteria for the Childhood Autism diagnosis (WHO, 1992). Comparably, the DSM-5's diagnostic criteria for Autism Spectrum Disorder (ASD) includes: (a) persistent deficits in social communication and social interaction across multiple contexts and (b) restricted, repetitive patterns of behavior, interests, or activities. However, the DSM-5 does not include diagnoses of Atypical Autism or Asperger's Syndrome (APA, 2013). Chapter 2 by Kuriakose and Shalev (2016) discusses the diagnostic criteria for ASD in detail and compares the most common assessments used to diagnosis autism in early childhood using the available psychometric data.

The DSM-5 and ICD-10 both describe a number of common comorbidities and deficits reported in samples of children with autism including intellectual disability, anxiety disorders and limited play skills and acknowledge that autism symptom severity ranges along a spectrum from mild (i.e., requiring some support to compensate for deficits) to severe (i.e., requiring a substantial amount of support) (APA, 2013; WHO, 1992). Without the proper level of support and effective intervention, children with autism may develop challenging behavior (e.g., self-injury, property destruction and aggression), experience academic failure and struggle to maintain meaningful social relationships (Lang et al., 2010, 2013; Tonge, Bull, Brereton, & Wilson, 2014; Watkins et al., 2015). Without successful intervention during childhood, adults with autism may experience difficulty finding employment, starting families and achieving a desirable quality of life (Brugha, Doos, Tempier, Einfeld, & Howlin, 2015; Taylor et al., 2012; Tobin, Drager, & Richardson, 2014; Walton & Ingersoll, 2013). In some severe cases, adults with autism are not able to live independent of intensive supports that require a substantial expenditure of resources (e.g., Chasson, Harris, & Neely, 2007; Cimera & Cowan, 2009; McGill & Poynter, 2012). Therefore, it is not surprising that a great deal of research has focused on developing effective interventions capable of addressing core symptoms and common comorbidities in ASD with the ultimate aim of enhancing quality of life and autonomy of people with autism.

Why Are Interventions for Autism Not Based on Etiology?

Biological and Nature-Based Etiological Theories

Ideally, interventions are developed to address the underlying causes of a disorder (etiology). Research has elucidated a number of biological (nature) and environmental (nurture) factors that may disrupt child development and lead to a presentation of symptoms similar to those observed in children with autism. In terms of nature, genetic abnormalities such as gene deletions, duplications, translocations, and inversions have been linked to intellectual and developmental delays (Percy, Lewkis, & Brown, 2007) comparable to characteristics observed in some people with autism. For example, Phenylketonuria (PKU) is a developmental disability also associated with intellectual disability, social deficits, comorbid psychiatric disorders and behavioral problems that is caused by a genetic abnormality that impedes the body's ability to process a specific type of protein (phenylalanine) found in many foods (Stemerdink et al., 2000). Treatment for children with PKU includes a phenylalanine-free diet and prevention of PKU is possible by strict adherence to a phenylalanine-free diet before and during pregnancy by women with PKU (Kohlschütter et al., 2009). PKU illustrates how an understanding of a disorder's etiology may guide the creation of effective intervention and even prevent some genetic disorders. In terms of autism, research has identified a number of genetic abnormalities that are more prevalent in children with autism (Richards, Jones, Groves, Moss, & Oliver, 2015). Unfortunately, no single gene, combination of genetic factors or other biomarkers (e.g., deficit of a specific neurotransmitter) can account for the majority of cases of autism and effective interventions cannot yet be derived from the genetic research related to autism to date (Minshawi, Hurwitz, Morriss, & McDougle, 2015; Richards et al., 2015; Ruggeri, Sarkans, Schumann, & Persico, 2013).

Additional biological causes for developmental delay include injury, illness and other factors that may negatively influence a child's physiological, intellectual or psychological development. For example, children without access to sufficient nutrition or health care as well as those exposed to toxins (e.g., Fetal Alcohol Spectrum Disorder) may present with symptoms comparable to what is observed in children with autism (Bishop, Gahagan, & Lord, 2007). A variety of hypotheses have been examined in an effort to identify such an etiology for autism. For example, the theory that vaccines may increase the risk of autism has been thoroughly tested and never substantiated (Fombonne, 1999; Offit, 2008). Other similar theories, such as heavy metal poisoning, gut abnormalities, gluten and casein peptides and virus-based theories, have also failed to be consistently supported by carefully controlled studies. Further, interventions derived solely from such hypotheses have not been demonstrated to be effective and, in some cases, may cause harm to the child and their family (e.g., Davis et al., 2013; Esch & Carr, 2004; Fombonne, 1999; Mulloy et al., 2010, 2011). Chapter 9 by Travers, Ayers, Simpson, and Crutchfield (2016) focuses on fad, controversial and pseudoscientific interventions. Many of the interventions discussed in that chapter are fundamentally flawed because they are derived from false etiological theories of ASD.

Environmental and Nurture-Based Etiological Theories

In terms of nurture, learning history and other environmental factors may impede children's language, social and intellectual development (Bijou & Baer, 1961, 1965) and lead to behavioral excesses and deficits similar to those in autism. For example, children living in spartan environments absent sufficient stimulation and those who suffer from neglect and/or abuse may experience a variety of developmental delays and detrimental psychological conditions (Ellenbogen, Klein, & Wekerle, 2014; Mills et al., 2011). An outdated etiological theory purported that unloving and emotionally distant mothers (callously termed "refrigerator mothers") were the cause of the social and language deficits observed in children with autism (Bettelheim, 1972), but this deeply insensitive and obviously inaccurate theory has now been entirely discredited (Silvermann, 2012). Parent involvement is considered a key element in many interventions for children autism, and parent training in intervention implementation is an effective approach to delivering higher doses of intervention across settings (Lang, Machalicek, Rispoli, & Regester, 2009; Machalicek, Lang, & Raulston, 2015; Makrygianni & Reed, 2010; Struass, Mancini, The SPC Group, & Fava, 2013; Tonge et al., 2014). However, these parent-based approaches to early intervention are in no way related to the rejected notion that mothers (or any other caregivers) are in anyway responsible for causing autism. In Chap. 8 Ruppert, Machalicek, Hansen, Raulston, and Frantz (2016) review research involving parent-implemented early interventions for children with ASD and discuss evidenced-based approaches to training parents to implement interventions accurately.

The best available evidence suggests the etiology of autism is some unknown combination of an innate genetic disposition involving multiple genes and some unknown environmental trigger (Fakhoury, 2015; Kohane, 2015; Richards et al., 2015; Ruggeri et al., 2013). In any case, research into autism's etiology has not yet been able to meaningfully guide the development of effective interventions. Despite the absence of a clear etiology, a number of interventions demonstrated to be capable of ameliorating symptom severity and potentially improving long-term outcomes for people with autism have been developed. These interventions tend to be most effective when they are early, intensive and behavioral (Granpeesheh, Dixon, Tarbox, Kaplan, & Wilkc, 2009; Ramey & Ramey, 1998; Reichow, 2012).

Early Intervention

Results from some studies suggest that outcomes tend to be better the earlier in a child's life intervention is initiated (e.g., Bradshaw, Steiner, Gengoux, & Koegel, 2015; Harris & Handleman, 2000; Smith, Klorman, & Mruzek, 2015). However, results of other studies suggest that the child's age may not be of particular importance (e.g., Makrygianni & Reed, 2010; Virués-Ortega, 2010). The differences in conclusions regarding the significance of age may be due to (a) the large range of symptom severity inherent to the autism spectrum; (b) differences in research designs; (c) differences in setting (e.g., home or clinic-based); and/or (d) different types of outcome measures (e.g., school placement, target skill mastery, parent report, and standardized assessments) across intervention studies (Fava & Strauss, 2014; Virués-Ortega, 2010; Warren et al., 2011).

Although the debate regarding child characteristics (e.g., age, language proficiency and IQ) that can predict response to intervention continues (Camarata, 2014; Charman, 2014), there are a number of reasons why interventions may be more efficient or effective early in life that can be discussed. From a biological perspective, it is possible that the rapid and radical brain development that occurs during the first years of a child's life offers a window of opportunity for optimal intervention timing (Pickles, Anderson, & Lord, 2014; Webb, Jones, Kelly, & Dawson, 2014). Specifically, the brain's ability to change (plasticity) in terms of how it responds to environmental stimuli appears to be greatest in most individuals early in life (Holland et al., 2014). For example, ongoing brain development may account, at least in part, for the relative ease with which children of typical development acquire a staggering amount of language during early childhood (Ambridge, Kidd, Rowland, & Theakston, 2015).

Another complimentary explanation for increased efficiency and effectiveness of early intervention relative to intervention delivered later in life is that learning new skills may allow children to experience a wider variety of learning opportunities and more complex environmental contingencies. For example, a child with autism who learns to play with toys in a way that looks like the way a child of typical development plays with toys (e.g., rolling a car along the ground as opposed to spinning and staring at a wheel) may be more often approached by other children to play, creating more opportunities for social interaction (Hine & Wolery, 2006; Lang et al., 2014). Similarly, a child who learns to ask for a drink during early intervention would seem more likely to be asked by caregivers whether or not they would prefer water or milk. Exposure to more questions may facilitate acquisition of question-asking skills and the ability to ask questions could assist with learning even more skills (Raulston et al., 2013). If acquiring these types of pivotal skills results in increased opportunities for learning and, if at least some of those opportunities eventual facilitate the acquisition of even more skills and so on, it stands to reason that this process should begin during the period of time associated with the greatest plasticity (Webb et al., 2014) and before decisions determining future environments that will influence learning opportunity (e.g., school placement) are made.

In the same way that changing the angle of a projectile's trajectory only slightly makes a large difference in where the projectile lands after traveling a long distance; acquiring fundamental skills at an early age may result in greater outcomes when considered across a lifespan. Figure 1.1 visually represents the potential for a small change to result in a large difference in outcome. However, the stylized figure represents the rate of development as a straight line and, of course, the actual rate of human development is far more variable (Klintwall, Eldevik, & Eikeseth, 2015; Mawhood, Howlin, & Rutter, 2000; Webb et al., 2014).

Likely, nature (e.g., genetics and brain development) and nurture (e.g., learning history) interact in a variety of ways to account for any increased effectiveness of interventions delivered early in life (e.g., Kok et al., 2015; Webb et al., 2014). However, whatever the reasons, the impact of the environment on early child development is undeniable. For example, in a seminal study, Hart and Risely (1995) measured the occurrence of spoken language in the homes of 42 families with

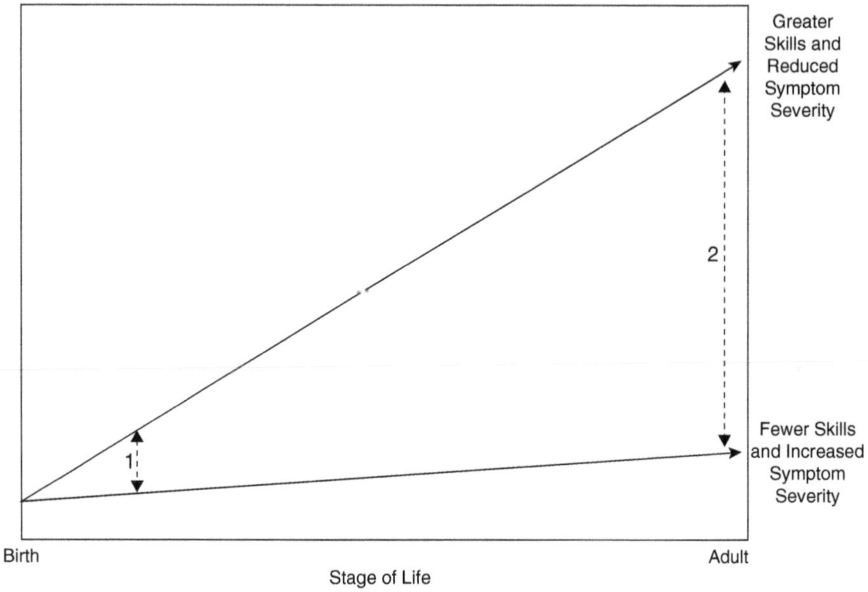

Fig. 1.1 Stylistic representation of a small change in developmental trajectory early in life (point 1) may result in a big difference in outcomes later in life (point 2)

children of typical development between the ages of 7 months and 3 years. The researchers then followed-up when the same group of children were 9 years old and found that the more language a child was exposed to before 3 years of age, the better their academic achievement. Further, and perhaps more relevant to early intervention in ASD, more exposure to language (i.e., more talking around the child) during early childhood was strongly associated with better receptive and expressive vocabularies later in life.

Comparable evidence involving language acquisition has also been reported in more recent research involving children referred for autism. For example, Pickles et al. (2014) administered multiple standardized assessments of expressive and receptive language at six time points between the ages of 2 and 19 years with 192 children initially referred for autism diagnostic evaluation. Although a notable amount of variation was reported within the sample of children, the results suggest a "greater sensitivity in the early years to environments that are more or less supportive of language development" (pp. 1354). Ultimately, their results buttress previous research suggesting that children with autism may experience the same period of sensitivity to language rich environments as children of typical development. These findings have clear implications regarding the timing of intervention initiation as well as the use of strategies designed to increase exposure to language during early interventions for children with autism (e.g., Hancock, Ledbetter-Cho, & Lang, 2016; Peters-Scheffer, Huskens, Didden, & van der Meer, 2016).

Intensive Intervention

Interventions for children with autism tend to be more effective when they are intensive (Howard, Stainslaw, Green, Sparkman, & Cohen, 2014; Klintwall et al., 2015; Virués-Ortega, 2010). Intensity is usually discussed in terms of the number of hours per week intervention is delivered and an intervention is usually considered intense when it is delivered for 20 h per week or more (Matson & Konst, 2014). In a pioneering study investigating early intensive behavioral intervention (EIBI) for children with autism, Lovaas (1987) included a comparison of outcomes when intervention was implemented 10 h or 40 h per week. The 40 h group experienced significantly more improvement in IQ than the lower-intensity 10 h group. The results of Lovaas' comparison of treatment intensity have been replicated in a number of more recent studies involving different intervention dosages, for example: (a) 30 h per week was found to yield statistically better outcomes than 12 h per week (Reed, Osborne, & Corness, 2007); (b) 16–40 h of intervention was better than 1–15 h in parent-implemented interventions by parents with low levels of stress (Osborne, McHugh, Sounders, & Reed, 2008); and (c) approximately 25 h of direct intervention was found to be better than a less intense parent training control (Smith, Groen, & Wynn, 2000).

In an innovative study involving a database populated from previous intervention studies, Klintwall et al. (2015) graphed the developmental trajectories (i.e., change in age-equivalent scores over time) of 453 children 5 years of age or younger with autism who had received either EIBI, a comparable intervention, or were in a control group. For every hour the children in the EIBI group received intervention their developmental trajectories improved (see also Eldevik et al., 2010). Klintwall et al. pointed out that this relationship between dosage of intervention and outcome is comparable to the dose-response concept prevalent in medical research. Specifically, the existence of such a relationship increases certainty regarding influence of the intervention on the dependent variables. In other words, if outcomes are better when more intervention is provided, there is more certainty that it is the intervention, and not some other factor, that is responsible for the improvements (Virués-Ortega, 2010).

There is some debate regarding the seemingly obvious conclusion that the more intervention a child receives the better off the child will be. First, there is likely a point at which an additional hour per week could be counter-productive. Matson and Smith (2008) suggest children could "burn out", that is become too fatigued as a result of the intervention procedures or lose interest in the programmed contingencies intended to reinforce target behaviors. Further, parents are often asked to implement intervention as a means to increase the number of hours the child receives intervention. Osborne et al. (2008) reported an interaction between parent stress level and intervention intensity wherein more hours of parent-implemented intervention by parents with low levels of stress resulted in better child outcomes, however; child outcomes were not better when intervention implemented by parents with high levels of stress was delivered for more hours per week. Finally, Fava and

Strauss (2014) raise several important points that arise from the consideration of intervention intensity only in terms of hours per week. Specifically, they summarized findings from a number of recent meta-analyses and intervention studies and suggest that, in addition to hours per week, intervention intensity should also be considered in terms of (a) active involvement of child and implementer (therapist or parent); (b) setting (e.g., home and community); and (c) treatment fidelity variables (e.g., supervision of implementation to ensure adherence to intervention protocols).

Behavioral Intervention

An intervention can be considered behavioral when it involves the intentional use of operant principles (Skinner, 1988) via applied behavior analysis (ABA) in an effort to improve observable and measureable skills (Baer, Wolf, & Risely, 1968). In a broad sense, behavioral interventions focus on altering the interaction between the child and the child's immediate environment in order to provide specific types of learning experiences. Interventions that (a) involve only medication (e.g., secretin), diet manipulations (e.g., gluten- and casein-free diet) or medical procedures (e.g., chelation) or (b) fail to acknowledge the influence of embedded reinforcement, stimulus control and other behavioral mechanisms (e.g., Sensory Integration Therapy) would not be considered behavioral (Davis et al., 2013; Esch & Carr, 2004; Lang et al., 2012).

Lovaas' (1987) study is widely recognized as the first EIBI applied to a group of children diagnosed with autism. Prior to treatment, children in that study suffered from speech delays, intellectual disability, stereotypy, social deficits and challenging behavior (e.g., aggression and self-injury). Nineteen children received 40 h per week of EIBI for approximately 2 years. Following intervention, 47 % of those children achieved normal intellectual functioning resulting in placement in typical first grade classrooms. Of the 40 children serving as the control group, only 2 % obtained IQs in the typical range and the remainder had intellectual disability and were placed in more restrictive settings. Lovaas' (1987) study is seminal because it challenged that decade's paradigm regarding the nature of disability and the extent to which children with autism could be successfully treated.

A number of attempts to replicate the findings of Lovaas (1987) have been included in meta-analyses and systematic reviews of the literature (e.g., Eldevik et al., 2009; Makrygianni & Reed, 2010). Five or those meta-analytic reviews containing a total of 26 EIBI studies were then summarized by Reichow (2012). Reichow reported that four of the five meta-analyses concluded that EIBI was an effective approach to the treatment of children with autism. Using a variety of different definitions for what constitutes an evidenced-based practice (e.g., Silverman & Hinshaw, 2008), Riechow then concluded that EIBI could be considered an evidence-based practice for children with autism. Riechow also noted that the meta-analysis that did not report EIBI to be effective incorrectly interpreted the results of one of the included studies. The results of Riechow's overview of meta-analyses supported the findings of other systematic reviews focused EIBI research that utilized different approaches in summarizing the research base but also found EIBI to be effective (e.g., Kuppens & Onghena, 2012; Matson & Smith, 2008; Peters-Scheffer et al., 2011; Rogers & Vismara, 2008).

There are at least two notable reviews that concluded there was insufficient evidence to consider EIBI empirically-validated (i.e., Camarata, 2014; Warren et al., 2011). However, Warren et al. (2011) excluded a very large body of research involving experimental single-case designs (SCD) and Camarata (2014) built from the findings of Warren et al. and used a less systematic qualitative approach to review. Koegel, Koegel, Ashbaugh, and Bradshaw (2014) pointed out that SCDs are the most common approach used to evaluate intervention effects with children with autism and that SCDs have more internal validity than randomized clinical trials (RCT) where individual differences in response to intervention may be masked. Although one SCD study may not have the external validity (certainty effects will apply to people not involved in the study) that is obtained via one RCT, replications of effects across numerous SCDs studies does provide certainty regarding the generalizability of findings; leading some to argue that the SCD approach is preferable to RCTs given the heterogeneity of the autism population (Keenan & Dillenburger, 2011). Regardless, no other intervention approach for young children with autism has produced as much supporting research as EIBI (Howard et al., 2014; Klintwall et al., 2015; Koegel et al., 2014; Matson, Tureck, Turygin, Beighley, & Rieske, 2012).

A number of variations in EIBI have emerged since Lovaas (1987) and, although these approaches involve ABA (e.g., environmental arrangement, prompting and reinforcement), they can be distinguished by the degree to which they emphasize: (a) natural environments and routines; (b) involve parents as interventionists; (c) focus on specific target behaviors (e.g., pivotal responses and prelinguistic communications); and (d) following the child's lead as opposed to being adult-directed.

The five specific interventions included in the remainder of this book share many common core components (e.g., reinforcement) and all have been demonstrated to be effective in a variety of research designs including both RCTs and SCDs. Leading researchers in the field and, in some cases the creators or co-creators of specific intervention packages, authored the chapters. The five intervention approaches included in this text are Discrete Trial Training in Chap. 3 (Lerman, Valentino, & LeBlanc, 2016), Pivotal Response Training in Chap. 4 (Koegel, Ashbaugh, & Koegel, 2016), Early Start Denver Model in Chap. 5 (Talbot, Estes, Zierhut, Dawson, & Rogers, 2016), Prelinguistic Milieu Teaching in Chap. 6 (Peters-Scheffer et al., 2016), and Enhanced Milieu Teaching in Chap. 7 (Hancock et al., 2016). These chapters cover the theoretical underpinnings, specific procedures, research base, directions for future research, and considerations for practitioners for each of these evidenced-based EIBI approaches. The book concludes with issues related to parent-implemented intervention in Chap. 8 (Ruppert et al., 2016) and ethical issues related to fad, pseudoscientific and controversial interventions commonly used with children with ASD in Chap. 9 (Travers et al., 2016).

References

Ambridge, B., Kidd, E., Rowland, C. F., & Theakston, A. L. (2015). The ubiquity of frequency effects in first language acquisition. *Journal of Child Language, 42*, 239–273.

American Psychiatric Association. (1980). *Diagnostic and statistical manual of mental disorders: DSM-III*. Washington, DC: American Psychiatric Association.

American Psychiatric Association. (2013). *Diagnostic and statistical manual of mental disorders: DSM-5*. Washington, DC: American Psychiatric Association.

Baer, D., Wolf, M., & Risely, R. (1968). Some current dimensions of applied behavior analysis. *Journal of Applied Behavior Analysis, 1*, 91–97.

Baird, G., Charman, T., Baron-Cohen, S., Cox, A., Swettenham, J., Wheelwright, S., & Drew, A. (2000). A screening instrument for autism at 18 months of age: A 6-year follow-up study. *Journal of the American Academy of Child and Adolescent Psychiatry, 39*, 694–702.

Bettelheim, B. (1972). *The empty fortress: Infantile autism and the birth of the self*. New York, NY: The Free Press.

Bijou, S. W., & Baer, D. M. (1961). *Child development. Vol. I: A systematic and empirical theory*. New York, NY: Appleton-Century-Crofts.

Bijou, S. W., & Baer, D. M. (1965). *Child development. Vol. II: Universal stage of infancy*. Oxford, England: Appleton-Century-Crofts.

Bishop, S., Gahagan, S., & Lord, C. (2007). Re-examining the core features of autism: A comparison of autism spectrum disorder and fetal alcohol spectrum disorder. *Journal of Child Psychology and Psychiatry, 48*, 1111–1121.

Bradshaw, J., Steiner, A. M., Gengoux, G., & Koegel, L. K. (2015). Feasibility and effectiveness of very early intervention for infants at-risk for autism spectrum disorder: A systematic review. *Journal of Autism and Developmental Disorders, 45*, 778–794.

Brugha, T. S., Doos, L., Tempier, A., Einfeld, S., & Howlin, P. (2015). Outcome measures in intervention trials for adults with autism spectrum disorders: A systematic review of assessments of core autism features and associated emotional and behavioural problems. *International Journal of Methods in Psychiatric Research, 24*, 99–115.

Camarata, S. (2014). Early identification and early intervention in autism spectrum disorders: Accurate and effective? *International Journal of Speech-Language Pathology, 16*, 1–10.

Charman, T. (2014). Early identification and intervention in autism spectrum disorders: Some progress but not as much as we hoped. *International Journal of Speech-Language Pathology, 16*, 15–18.

Chasson, G. S., Harris, G. E., & Neely, W. J. (2007). Cost comparison of early intensive behavioral intervention and special education for children with autism. *Journal of Child and Family Studies, 16*, 401–413.

Cimera, R. E., & Cowan, R. J. (2009). The costs of services and employment outcomes achieved by adults with autism in the US. *Autism: The International Journal of Research and Practice, 13*, 285–302.

Davis, T. N., O'Reilly, M., Kang, S., Lang, R., Rispoli, M., Sigafoos, J., … Mulloy, A. (2013). Chelation treatment for autism spectrum disorders: A systematic review. *Research in Autism Spectrum Disorders, 7*, 49–55.

Eldevik, S., Hastings, R. P., Hughes, C. J., Jahr, E., Eikeseth, S., & Cross, S. (2009). Meta-analyses of early intensive behavioral intervention for children with autism. *Journal of Clinical and Child Adolescent Psychology, 38*, 439–450.

Eldevik, S., Hastings, R. P., Hughes, C. J., Jahr, E., Eikeseth, S., & Cross, S. (2010). Using participant data to extend the evidence base for intensive behavioral intervention for children with autism. *American Journal on Intellectual and Developmental Disabilities, 115*, 381–405.

Ellenbogen, S., Klein, B., & Wekerle, C. (2014). Early education as a resilience intervention for maltreated children. *Early Child Development and Care, 184*, 1364–1377.

Esch, B., & Carr, J. E. (2004). Secretin as a treatment for autism: A review of the evidence. *Journal of Autism and Developmental Disorders, 34*, 543–556.

Fakhoury, M. (2015). Autistic spectrum disorders: A review of clinical features, theories and diagnosis. *International Journal of Developmental Neuroscience, 43*, 70–77.

Fava, L., & Strauss, K. (2014). Response to early intensive behavioral intervention for autism—An umbrella approach to issues critical to treatment individualization. *International Journal of Developmental Neuroscience, 39*, 49–58.

Fombonne, E. (1999). Are measles infections or measles immunizations linked to autism? *Journal of Autism and Developmental Disorders, 29*, 349–350.

Granpeesheh, D., Dixon, D. R., Tarbox, J., Kaplan, A. M., & Wilke, A. E. (2009). The effects of age and treatment intensity in behavioral intervention outcomes for children with autism spectrum disorders. *Research in Autism Spectrum Disorders, 3*, 1014–1022.

Hancock, T. B., Ledbetter-Cho, K., & Lang, R. (2016). Enhanced milieu teaching. In R. L. Lang, T. Hancock, & N. N. Singh (Eds.), *Early intervention for young children with autism spectrum disorder*. New York, NY: Springer.

Harris, S., & Handleman, J. (2000). Age and IQ at intake as predictors of placement for young children with autism: A four- to six-year follow-up. *Journal of Autism and Developmental Disorders, 30*, 137–142.

Hart, B., & Risely, T. R. (1995). *Meaningful difference in the everyday experiences of young American children*. Baltimore, MA: Paul Brookes.

Hine, J. F., & Wolery, M. (2006). Using point-of-view video modeling to teach play to preschoolers with autism. *Topics in Early Childhood Special Education, 26*, 83–93.

Holland, D., Chang, L., Ernst, T. M., Curran, M., Buchthal, S. D., Alicata, D., … Dale, A. M. (2014). Structural growth trajectories and rates of change in the first 3 months of infant brain development. *Journal of American Medical Association Neurology, 10*, 1266–1274.

Howard, J. S., Stainslaw, H., Green, G., Sparkman, C. R., & Cohen, H. G. (2014). Comparison of behavior analytic and eclectic early interventions for children with autism after three years. *Research in Developmental Disabilities, 35*, 3326–3344.

Keenan, M., & Dillenburger, K. (2011). When all you have is a hammer…: RCTs and hegemony in science. *Research in Autism Spectrum Disorders, 5*, 1–13.

Klintwall, L., Eldevik, S., & Eikeseth, S. (2015). Narrowing the gap: Effects of intervention on developmental trajectories in autism. *Autism: The International Journal of Research and Practice, 19*, 53–63.

Koegel, L. K., Ashbaugh, K., & Koegel, R. (2016). Pivotal response treatment. In R. L. Lang, T. Hancock, & N. N. Singh (Eds.), *Early intervention for young children with autism spectrum disorder*. New York, NY: Springer.

Koegel, L. K., Koegel, R. L., Ashbaugh, K., & Bradshaw, J. (2014). The importance of early identification and intervention for children with or at risk for autism spectrum disorders. *International Journal of Speech-Language Pathology, 16*, 50–56.

Kok, R., Thijssen, S., Bakermans-Kranenburg, M. J., Jaddoe, V. W. V., Verhulst, F. C., White, T., … Tiemeier, H. (2015). Normal variation in early parental sensitivity predicts child structural brain development. *Journal of American Academy of Child and Adolescent Psychiatry, 54*, 824–831.

Kohane, I. S. (2015). An autism case history to review the systematic analysis of large-scale data to refine the diagnosis and treatment of neuropsychiatric disorders. *Biological Psychiatry, 77*, 59–65.

Kohlschütter, N., Ellerbrok, M., Merkel, M., Tchirikov, M., Zschocke, J., Santer, R., & Ullrich, K. (2009). Phenylalanine tolerance in three phenylketonuric women pregnant with fetuses of different genetic PKU status. *Journal Of Inherited Metabolic Disease, 32*, 1–4.

Kuppens, S., & Onghena, P. (2012). Sequential meta-analysis to determine the sufficiency of cumulative knowledge: The case of early intensive behavioral intervention for children with autism spectrum disorders. *Research in Autism Spectrum Disorder, 6*, 168–176.

Kuriakose, S., & Shalev, R. (2016). Early diagnostic assessment in autism spectrum disorder. In R. L. Lang, T. Hancock, & N. N. Singh (Eds.), *Early intervention for young children with autism spectrum disorder*. New York, NY: Springer.

Lang, R., Machalicek, W., Rispoli, M., O'Reilly, M., Sigafoos, J., Lancioni, G., … Didden, R. (2014). Play skills taught via behavioral intervention generalize, maintain, and persist in the absence of socially-mediated reinforcement in children with autism. *Research in Autism Spectrum Disorders, 8*, 860–872.

Lang, R., Machalicek, W., Rispoli, M. J., & Regester, A. (2009). Training parents to implement communication interventions for children with autism spectrum disorders: A systematic review of training procedures. *Evidenced Based Communication Assessment and Intervention, 3*, 174–190.

Lang, R., O'Reilly, M., Healy, O., Rispoli, M., Lydon, H., Streusand, W., … Giesbers, S. (2012). Sensory integration therapy for autism spectrum disorders: A systematic review. *Research in Autism Spectrum Disorders, 6*, 1004–1018.

Lang, R., Regester, A., Rispoli, M., & Camargo, S. P. H. (2010). Rehabilitation issues for children with autism spectrum disorders. *Developmental Neurorehabilitation, 13*, 153–155.

Lang, R., Sigafoos, J., van der Meer, L., O'Reilly, M. F., Lancioni, G. E., & Didden, R. (2013). Early signs and early behavioral intervention of challenging behavior. In R. Hastings & J. Rojahn (Eds.), *Challenging behavior. International review of research in developmental disability* (44th ed., pp. 1–35). London: Elsevier Inc. Academic Press.

Lerman, D., Valentino, A. L., & LeBlanc, L. A. (2016). Discrete trial training. In R. L. Lang, T. Hancock, & N. N. Singh (Eds.), *Early intervention for young children with autism spectrum disorder*. New York, NY: Springer.

Liu, T. (2012). Motor milestone development in young children with autism spectrum disorders: An exploratory study. *Educational Psychology in Practice, 28*, 315–326.

Lovaas, O. I. (1987). Behavioral treatment and normal educational and intellectual functioning in young autistic children. *Journal of Consulting and Clinical Psychology, 55*, 3–9.

Machalicek, W., Lang, R., & Raulston, T. J. (2015). Training parents of children with intellectual disabilities: Trends, issues, and future directions. *Current Developmental Disorders Report, 2*, 110–118.

Makrygianni, M. K., & Reed, P. (2010). A meta-analytic review of the effectiveness of behavioral early intervention programs for children with autistic spectrum disorders. *Research in Autism Spectrum Disorders, 4*, 577–593.

Matson, J. L., & Konst, M. J. (2014). Early intervention for autism: Who provides treatment and in what settings? *Research in Autism Spectrum Disorders, 8*, 1585–1590.

Matson, J. L., & Smith, R. M. (2008). Current status of intensive behavioral interventions for young children with autism and PDD-NOS. *Research in Autism Spectrum Disorders, 2*, 60–74.

Matson, J. L., Tureck, K., Turygin, N., Beighley, J., & Rieske, R. (2012). Trends and topics in early intensive behavioral interventions for toddlers with autism. *Research in Autism Spectrum Disorders, 6*, 1412–1417.

Mawhood, L., Howlin, P., & Rutter, M. (2000). Autism and developmental receptive language disorder: A comparative follow-up in early adult life. I. Cognitive and language outcomes. *Journal of Child Psychology and Psychiatry, 41*, 547–559.

McGill, P., & Poynter, J. (2012). High cost residential placements for adults with intellectual disabilities. *Journal of Applied Research in Intellectual Disabilities, 25*, 584–587.

Mills, R., Alati, R., O'Callaghan, M., Najman, J. M., Williams, G. M., Bor, W., & Strathearn, L. (2011). Child abuse and neglect and cognitive function at 14 years of age: Findings from a birth cohort. *Pediatrics, 127*, 4–10.

Minshawi, N. F., Hurwitz, S., Morriss, D., & McDougle, C. J. (2015). Multidisciplinary assessment and treatment of self-injurious behavior in autism spectrum disorder and intellectual disability: Integration of psychological and biological theory and approach. *Journal of Autism and Developmental Disorders, 45*, 1541–1568.

Mulloy, A., Lang, R., O'Reilly, M., Sigafoos, J., Lancioni, G., & Rispoli, M. (2010). Gluten-free and casein-free diets in the treatment of autism spectrum disorders: A systematic review. *Research in Autism Spectrum Disorders, 4*, 328–339.

Mulloy, A., Lang, R., O'Reilly, M., Sigafoos, J., Lancioni, G., & Rispoli, M. (2011). Addendum to "Gluten-free and casein-free diets in the treatment of autism spectrum disorders: A systematic review.". *Research in Autism Spectrum Disorders, 5*, 86–88.

Offit, P. A. (2008). *Autism's false prophets: Bad science, risky medicine, and the search for a cure*. New York, NY: Columbia University Press.

Osborne, L. A., McHugh, L., Sounders, J., & Reed, P. (2008). Parenting stress reduces the effectiveness of early teaching interventions for autistic spectrum disorders. *Journal of Autism and Developmental Disorders, 24*, 247–257.

Percy, M., Lewkis, S. Z., & Brown, I. (2007). Introduction to genetics and development. In I. Brown & M. Percy (Eds.), *A comprehensive guide to intellectual and developmental disabilities*. Baltimore, MD: Brookes.

Peters-Scheffer, N., Didden, R., Korzilius, H., & Sturmey, P. (2011). A meta-analytic study on the effectiveness of comprehensive ABA-based early intervention programs for children with autism spectrum disorders. *Research in Autism Spectrum Disorders, 5*, 60–69

Peters-Scheffer, N., Huskens, B., Didden, R., & van der Meer, L. (2016). Prelinguistic milieu teaching. In R. L. Lang, T. Hancock, & N. N. Singh (Eds.), *Early intervention for young children with autism spectrum disorder*. New York, NY: Springer.

Pickles, A., Anderson, D. K., & Lord, C. (2014). Heterogeneity and plasticity in the development of language: A 17-year follow-up of children referred early for possible autism. *Journal of Child Psychology and Psychiatry, 55*, 1354–1362.

Ramey, C. T., & Ramey, S. L. (1998). Early intervention and early experience. *American Psychologist, 53*, 109–120.

Raulston, T. Carnett, A., Lang, R. Tostanoski, A., Lee, A., Machalicek, W., ... Didden, R. (2013). Teaching individuals with autism spectrum disorder to ask questions: A systematic review. *Research in Autism Spectrum Disorders, 7*, 866–878.

Reed, P., Osborne, L. A., & Corness, M. (2007). Brief report: Relative effectiveness of different home-based behavioural approaches to early teaching intervention. *Journal of Autism and Developmental Disorder, 37*, 1815–1821.

Reichow, B. (2012). Overview of meta-analyses on early intensive behavioral intervention for young children with autism spectrum disorders. *Journal of Autism and Developmental Disorders, 42*, 512–520.

Richards, C., Jones, C., Groves, L., Moss, J., & Oliver, C. (2015). Prevalence of autism spectrum disorder phenomenology in genetic disorders: A systematic review and meta-analysis. *Lancet Psychiatry, 2*, 909–916.

Rogers, S. J., & Vismara, L. A. (2008). Evidence-based comprehensive treatments for early autism. *Journal of Clinical Child and Adolescent Psychology, 37*, 8–38.

Shelov, S., & Altmann, T. R. (2009). *Caring for your baby and young child: Birth to age 5* (5th ed.). New York, NY: Bantam Books.

Silverman, W. K., & Hinshaw, S. P. (2008). The second special issue on evidence-based psychosocial treatments for children and adolescents: A 10 year update. *Journal of Clinical Child and Adolescent Psychology, 37*, 1–7.

Skinner, B. F. (1988). The operant side of behavior therapy. *Journal of Behavior Therapy and Experimental Psychiatry, 19*, 171–179.

Silvermann, C. (2012). *Understanding autism: Parents, doctors, and the history of a disorder*. Princeton, NJ: Princeton University Press.

Smith, T., Groen, A. D., & Wynn, J. W. (2000). Randomized trial of intensive early intervention for children with pervasive developmental disorder. *American Journal of Mental Retardation, 105*, 269–285.

Smith, T., Klorman, R., & Mruzek, D. W. (2015). Predicting outcome of a community-based early intensive behavioral intervention for children with autism. *Journal of Abnormal Child Psychology, 43*(7), 1271–1282.

Struass, K., Mancini, F., The SPC Group, & Fava, L. (2013). Parent inclusion in early intensive behavior interventions for young children with ASD: A synthesis of meta-analyses from 2009 to 2011. *Research in Developmental Disabilities, 34*, 2967–2985.

Taylor, J., McPheeters, M. L., Sathe, N. A., Dove, D., Veenstra-Vanderwele, J., & Warren, Z. (2012). A systematic review of vocational interventions for young adults with autism spectrum disorders. *Pediatrics, 103*, 531–538.

Tobin, M. C., Drager, K. D. R., & Richardson, L. F. (2014). A systematic review of social participation for adults with autism spectrum disorders: Support, social functioning, and quality of life. *Research in Autism Spectrum Disorders, 8*, 214–229.

Ruggeri, B., Sarkans, U., Schumann, G., & Persico, A. (2013). Biomarkers in autism spectrum disorder: The old and the new. *Psychopharmacology, 231*, 1201–1206.

Ruppert, T., Machalicek, W., Hansen, S., Raulston, T., & Frantz, R. (2016). Training parents to implement early intervention for children with autism spectrum disorders. In R. L. Lang, T. Hancock, & N. N. Singh (Eds.), *Early intervention for young children with autism spectrum disorder*. New York, NY: Springer.

Stemerdink, B. A., Kalverboer, A. F., van der Meere, J. J., van der Molen, M. W., Huisman, J., de Jong, L. W., … van Spronsen, F. J. (2000). Behaviour and school achievement in patients with early and continuously treated phenylketonuria. *Journal of Inherited Metabolic Disease, 23*, 548–562.

Talbot, M. R., Estes, A., Zierhut, C., Dawson, G., & Rogers, S. J. (2016). Early start Denver model. In R. R. Lang, T. Hancock, & N. N. Singh (Eds.), *Early intervention for young children with autism spectrum disorder*. New York, NY: Springer.

Tonge, B. J., Bull, K., Brereton, A., & Wilson, R. (2014). A review of evidence-based early intervention for behavioural problems in children with autism spectrum disorder: The core components of effective programs, child focused interventions and comprehensive treatment models. *Current Opinion in Psychiatry, 27*, 158–165.

Travers, J., Ayers, K., Simpson, R. L., & Crutchfield, S. (2016). Fad, pseudoscientific and controversial interventions for children with autism spectrum disorder. In R. L. Lang, T. Hancock, & N. N. Singh (Eds.), *Early intervention for young children with autism spectrum disorder*. New York, NY: Springer.

Virués-Ortega, J. (2010). Applied behavior analytic intervention for autism in early childhood: Meta-analysis, meta-regression and dose-response meta-analysis of multiple outcomes. *Clinical Psychology Review, 30*, 387–399.

Walton, K., & Ingersoll, B. R. (2013). Improving social skills in adolescents and adults with autism and severe to profound intellectual disability: A review of the literature. *Journal of Autism and Developmental Disorders, 43*, 594–615.

Warren, Z., McPheeters, M. L., Sathe, N., Foss-Feif, J. H., Glasser, A., & Veenstra-Vanderweele, J. (2011). A systematic review of early intensive intervention for autism spectrum disorders. *Pediatrics, 127*, 1303–1311.

Watkins, L., O'Reilly, M., Kuhn, M., Gevarter, C., Lancioni, G., Sigafoos, J., & Lang, R. (2015). A review of peer-mediated social interaction interventions for students with autism in inclusive settings. *Journal of Autism and Developmental Disorders, 45*, 1070–1083.

Webb, S. J., Jones, E. J., Kelly, J., & Dawson, G. (2014). The motivation for very early intervention for infants at high risk for autism spectrum disorders. *International Journal of Speech-Language Pathology, 16*, 36–42.

World Health Organization. (1992). *International classification of diseases: Diagnostic criteria for research* (10th ed.). Geneva, Switzerland: Author.

Chapter 2
Early Diagnostic Assessment

Sarah Kuriakose and Rebecca Shalev

Introduction

Access to early intervention services often depends on early in life diagnosis. The average age a child receives an ASD diagnosis varies widely internationally and nationally. A number of obstacles often dissuade or preclude an accurate ASD diagnosis and current research-based approaches capable of diagnosing ASD very early in life (i.e., less than 18 months old) are rarely available. This chapter first presents the diagnostic characteristics of ASD per the DSM-5, briefly discusses the factors hypothesized to be contributing to the rising ASD prevalence and obstacles to obtaining an accurate ASD diagnosis (e.g., access to services, pediatricians without necessary experience, etc). The most common ASD diagnostic procedures are then described and the pros and cons as well as the available psychometric data are presented in a table that enables comparison across approaches. Recent research investigating novel approaches that facilitate earlier in life diagnosis is then reviewed. The chapter concludes with suggestions for future research and guidance for practitioners.

DSM-5 Diagnostic Criteria for ASD

The Diagnostic and Statistical Manual of Mental Disorders (5th ed.; DSM-5; American Psychiatric Association, 2013) gives the comprehensive diagnostic criteria for Autism Spectrum Disorder (ASD). The DSM-5 introduced substantive

S. Kuriakose (✉) • R. Shalev
Department of Child and Adolescent Psychiatry, The Child Study Center at NYU Langone Medical Center, One Park Avenue, 7th Floor, New York, NY 10016, USA
e-mail: sarah.kuriakose@nyumc.org

R. Lang et al. (eds.), *Early Intervention for Young Children with Autism Spectrum Disorder*, Evidence-Based Practices in Behavioral Health,
DOI 10.1007/978-3-319-30925-5_2

changes in the diagnosis of ASD from previous editions. Previously, Autistic Disorder was one of five Pervasive Developmental Disorders (Autistic Disorder, Rett's Disorder, Childhood Disintegrative Disorder, Asperger's Disorder, Pervasive Developmental Disorder—Not Otherwise Specified [PDD-NOS]) under the umbrella category of Disorders Usually First Diagnosed in Infancy, Childhood, or Adolescence. The DSM-5 removed the Pervasive Developmental Disorder nomenclature entirely and classifies ASD under Neurodevelopmental Disorders. The DSM-5 also conceptualizes the clinical heterogeneity of ASD as dimensional rather than categorical, with Autism Spectrum Disorder representing Autistic Disorder, Asperger's Disorder, and PDD-NOS. Finally, ASD is now a dyad of symptom clusters rather than a triad (Social Interaction, Communication, and Restricted, Repetitive, and Stereotyped Patterns of Behavior, Interests, and Activities).

The diagnosis of ASD in the DSM-5 now requires the presence of impairments in two domains: Social Communication and Interaction and Restricted, Repetitive Patterns of Behavior, Interests, or Activities. The first domain (A) specifies deficits in social communication and social interaction across settings, with three diagnostic criteria. Individuals diagnosed with ASD must display all three criteria, either currently or by history. The four criteria are: (1) deficits in social-emotional reciprocity, (2) deficits in nonverbal communicative behavior, and (3) deficits in developing, maintaining, and understanding relationships. The text of the DSM-5 provides illustrative examples for each criterion (e.g. for A1, examples include abnormal social approach and failure of normal back-and-forth conversations).

In the second domain (B), Restricted, Repetitive Patterns of Behavior, Interests, or Activities, there are four criteria. However, individuals diagnosed with ASD are required to meet only two criteria, currently or by history. These include: (1) stereotyped or repetitive motor movements, use of objects, or speech, (2) insistence on sameness, inflexible adhere to routines, or ritualized patterns of verbal or nonverbal behavior, (3) highly restricted, fixated interests that are abnormal in intensity or focus, and (4) hyper- or hyporeactivity to sensory input or unusual interest in sensory aspects of the environment. Illustrative examples are given for each criterion (e.g. for B1, examples include lining up toys, flipping objects, and echolalia).

Three additional overarching diagnostic criteria are given. The third criterion (C) notes that symptoms must be present in the early developmental period, although impairments may not become apparent until demands are increased later in life. The fourth criterion (D) states that symptoms must cause clinically significant impairment in functioning. The last criterion (E) states that deficits should not be better explained by either Intellectual Disability or Global Developmental Delay; note, however, that Intellectual Disability and ASD can co-occur. The DSM-5 specifics that all individuals with previous well-established diagnoses of Autistic Disorder, PDD-NOS, or Asperger's Disorders should now be given the diagnosis of ASD.

The diagnosis of ASD is now made with two sets of specifiers. Severity specifiers are ratings of the level of support needed for each domain of symptoms. Domains should be rated independently as Level 1 (Requiring Support), Level 2 (Requiring Substantial Support), or Level 3 (Requiring Very Substantial Support). The text provides examples of impairments that illustrate each severity level and

Table 2.1 Diagnosis of ASD in accordance with DSM-5

Example 1.	299.00 Autism Spectrum Disorder
	Requiring support for deficits in social communication and requiring very substantial support for restricted, repetitive behavior
Example 2.	299.00 Autism Spectrum Disorder Associated with a known genetic condition (Fragile X syndrome)
	Requiring very substantial support for deficits in social communication and requiring very substantial support for restricted, repetitive behavior
	With accompanying language impairment
Example 3.	299.00 Autism Spectrum Disorder Associated with an environmental factor (fetal alcohol syndrome)
	Requiring very substantial support for deficits in social communication and requiring substantial support for restricted, repetitive behavior
	With accompanying intellectual impairment

notes that severity levels will change over the individual's lifetime. While the diagnostic criteria only provides three levels, the supporting text in the DSM-5 states that severity could be below Level 1 at times in the individual's life (e.g. not requiring supports).

The second set of specifiers requires the diagnosing clinician to note whether ASD is present: With or without accompanying intellectual impairment; With or without accompanying language impairment; Associated with a known medical or genetic or environmental factor (if associated); and Associated with catatonia (if associated). Therefore, a diagnosis of ASD in accordance with DSM-5 should be written as suggested in the examples in Table 2.1.

Finally, it should be noted that the diagnosis of Social (Pragmatic) Communication Disorder is a new addition to the DSM-5. It is categorized under Communication Disorder rather than Neurodevelopmental Disorders and is suggested as a differential diagnosis for individuals with social communication impairments but with no symptoms in the restricted, repetitive behaviors domains currently or by history. It should be noted that research is not conclusive about the diagnostic validity of Social Communication Disorder (Ozonoff, 2012; Skuse, 2012) and further studies are indicated.

Prevalence of ASD

The rising prevalence of ASD has been heavily reported across scientific and popular media outlets. The majority of prevalence studies conducted internationally focus on North America and Europe, although limited literature is available representing other parts of the globe. Overall, the research consensus indicates that the prevalence of more narrowly defined classical autism and broadly defined ASD are rising in global samples, beginning in the mid-1990s (Baron-Cohen et al., 2009;

Cavagnaro, 2009; Honda, Shimizu, Imai, & Nitto, 2005; Newschaffer, Falb, & Gurney, 2005; Rice et al., 2013; Sun & Allison, 2009; Taylor, Jick, & McLaughlin, 2013; Wong & Hui, 2008).

Systematic reviews have reported an aggregate prevalence of approximately 60–70 in 10,000 for ASD across the globe (Elsabbagh et al., 2012; Fombonne, 2009). The majority of the literature is focused on the United States, where the most recently reported figure is 1 in 68 children, which is an average across sites ranging from 1 in 45 (New Jersey) to 1 in 175 (Alabama) (Centers for Disease Control (CDC), 2014). Autism was identified in 1 in 42 boys and 1 in 189 girls (CDC, 2014). This represents a 30 % increase in prevalence of ASD among 8-year-olds from the previous CDC data (CDC, 2012).

Many factors are theorized to account for the increasing prevalence of ASD. Contributors can be classified in three domains: intrinsic identification, or measurement factors involved in documenting ASD prevalence trends, extrinsic identification, or external classification and awareness factors leading to changes in case ascertainment, and risk, or possible true change in ASD symptoms in the population over time (Rice et al., 2013). In the area of intrinsic identification, study methods are frequently cited as contributing bias to the overall prevalence. Case ascertainment methods, e.g. health records vs educational records, previous vs. prospective diagnoses, parent report vs. observational diagnoses, research vs. clinical diagnoses, sampling of urban vs. rural regions, sampling of regions with free vs. paid access to screening, sampling of ages, all have systematic impacts on prevalence (e. g., Barbaresi, Colligan, Weaver, & Katusic, 2009; Baron-Cohen et al., 2009; Matson & Kozlowski, 2011; Parner et al., 2011; Williams, Higgins, & Brayne, 2006). In fact, recent global research suggests that after adjusting for systematic bias in case-finding strategies, the prevalence of ASD is actually unchanged between 1990 and 2010 (Baxter et al., 2014). The figures cited changed from 7.5 in 1000 in 1990 to 7.6 in 1000 in 2010, which approximates the global prevalence estimated by Fombonne (2009).

In the area of extrinsic identification, it is widely known that improved awareness of ASD as well as the broadening of ASD to include milder forms over time have increased prevalence rates. Studies have shown that there has been an increase in the prevalence of ASD when major changes were made to diagnostic criteria, such as when DSM-IV criteria were introduced (King & Bearman, 2009). Improved awareness has led to increased screening, with districts and countries that introduced population-level screening showing a greater prevalence (Nygren et al., 2012; Parner et al., 2011; Wing & Potter, 2002). The shift to identifying children at younger ages also explains part of the increase (Fombonne, 2009; Hertz-Picciotto & Delwiche, 2009).

Relatedly, the identification of milder forms of ASD, which is influenced by the broadening of diagnostic criteria, is associated with increasing prevalence (Hertz-Picciotto & Delwiche, 2009). Both CDC (2014) and parent-reported data (Blumberg et al., 2013) indicate that fewer children with ASD are classified as having an intellectual disability and the greatest increases in ASD report are in milder ASD (Keyes et al., 2012). Another significant factor impacting changes in prevalence is diagnostic substitution, or the switching of a previous diagnosis or class of diagnoses to the class of ASD. Administrative data show a strong correlation between decreasing rates of other disorders like mental retardation, learning disability, or developmental language disorder and increasing rates of ASD diagnoses, suggesting diagnostic substitution (Bishop, Whitehouse, Watt, & Line, 2008; Coo et al., 2008; King & Bearman, 2009; Shattuck, 2006).

Finally, it is important to consider whether, outside of these factors, the change in prevalence is impacted by a true change in the incidence of ASD owing to environmental or other risk factors. At this point, most researchers conclude that the trend in prevalence cannot be directly attributed to increased incidence, but also that the available data are not robust enough to rule out such a hypothesis (Fombonne, 2009; Rice et al., 2013). Research continues to be conducted on environmental and biological risk factors, such as the increased viability of pre-term births, a risk factor for ASD, (Johnson et al., 2010), and others (Matson & Kozlowski, 2011; Wazana, Bresnahan, & Kline, 2007).

Obstacles to Obtaining ASD Diagnostic Assessment and/or Accurate Diagnosis

ASD can be reliably diagnosed by an experienced clinician when a child is 2 years of age (Cox et al., 1999; Kleinman et al., 2008; Lord, 1995). However, population-based estimates in the United States indicate that the median age of diagnosis ranges from 48 (CDC, 2014) to 61 months (Wiggins, Baio, & Rice, 2006) or even 58 months (Shattuck et al., 2009). This signifies a gap of several years. This gap is especially problematic given that the preponderance of evidence suggests that early intervention is most effective for improved outcome in ASD. Many parents first become concerned about their child's development before the age of 24 months (Wiggins et al., 2006) and report seeing an average of four to five doctors before receiving an ASD diagnosis (Goin-Kochel, Mackintosh, & Mysters, 2006). They report overall dissatisfaction with the process of receiving an ASD diagnosis (Smith, Chung, & Vostanis, 1994) Barriers to timely diagnosis of ASD are present at the patient, family, and community level.

Research indicates that several patient-level factors impact the timing of ASD diagnosis. Boys are diagnosed on average earlier than girls (Goin-Kochel et al., 2006), even when girls had a greater degree of cognitive impairment (Shattuck et al., 2009). Children with IQs in the range of intellectual disability were diagnosed earlier, as were children who experienced a developmental regression (CDC, 2014; Shattuck et al., 2009). Children whose symptoms are on the milder end of the spectrum are diagnosed later (Goin-Kochel et al., 2006; Mandell, Novak, & Zubritsky, 2005; Thomas, Ellis, McLaurin, Daniels, & Morrissey, 2007).

At the family level, strong associations, though not always consistent across studies, have been found between timing of diagnosis and socioeconomic status and race/ethnicity. Lower age of diagnosis has been associated with higher parental education as well as higher family income (Fountain, King, & Bearman, 2011; Goin-Kochel, Mackintosh, & Mysters, 2006). The lowest rate of diagnosed ASD, as reported by parents, was in low-income families (Liptak et al., 2008) and families near the poverty level received diagnoses nearly a year later than those with incomes greater than 100 % of the poverty level (Mandell et al., 2005).

Although ASD does not disproportionately affect any racial or ethnic group, diagnosis rates do vary. Several studies have found that ethnic minority status is associated with lower or later diagnosis of ASD (CDC, 2014; Travers, Tincani, & Krezmien, 2011). Mandell, Listerud, Levy, and Pinto-Martin (2002) found that, of children on Medicaid, white children were diagnosed at 6.3 years of age, versus 7.9 years for African American children, and 8.8 years for Latino children. Among children who were referred to specialty care who were later diagnosed with ASD, White children were 2.6 times as likely to receive an ASD diagnosis at the first visit as African American children, who were more likely to be diagnosed with ADHD, adjustment disorder, and conduct disorder (Mandell, Ittenbach, Levy, & Pinto-Martin, 2007). The authors hypothesize that this could be related to cultural differences in how parents recognize and report symptoms, race-related differences in the clinicians' interpretation of symptoms, or a combination of the two.

Community level factors also play a role in timing of diagnosis. Children living in rural areas received diagnoses on average 0.4 years later than children living in urban areas (Mandell et al., 2005). This disparity continues to be present when accessing autism-related care, with children in nonmetropolitan areas having poorer access (Thomas et al., 2007). Proximity to a medical center is associated with earlier age of diagnosis (Kalbrenner et al., 2011). Access to specialty care improves diagnosis, with those referred to a specialist receiving a diagnosis 0.3 years earlier than those who were not (Mandell et al., 2005). Most children with ASD are identified at nonschool settings, such as hospitals and clinics (Wiggins et al., 2006), and therefore, limited access to such settings may impact diagnosis. Research conflicts on whether living in a high-income community is predictive of diagnosis; while some studies support this finding (Rosenberg, Landa, Law, Stuart, & Law, 2011; Thomas et al., 2012), others note that the effect does not remain when parental education is controlled (Fountain et al., 2011).

The first point of contact for diagnosis is typically the pediatrician or primary care physician. Many research studies have focused on barriers to accurate diagnosis in primary care settings. Primary barriers include awareness, time, cost and reimbursement, and training. Although developmental screeners have been shown to more accurately identify children at risk for ASD (Miller et al., 2011), pediatricians have reported that they trust clinical acumen over such screeners (Morelli et al., 2014). Others report that they do not know how to use screeners or which screeners to use (Dosreis, Weiner, Johnson, & Newschaffer, 2006) Over 70 % of ASD diagnoses are made without using standardized instruments (Wiggins et al., 2006). Most practices do not get reimbursed at sustainable rates for providing developmental screening (Filipek et al., 2000; Shattuck & Grosse, 2007). Patients with ASD in states with better reimbursement rates have less trouble accessing care

(Thoas, Parish, Rose, & Klany, 2011). They also report not having time to do screenings (Dosreis et al., 2006; Filipek et al., 2000; Morelli et al., 2014).

Pediatrician training has become a high-priority public policy initiative, with national campaigns through the American Academy of Pediatrics (Johnson, Meyers, & The Council on Children with Disabilities, 2007) and the Centers for Disease Control. Medical students receive little focused training about diagnosis ASDs (Shah, 2001). Pediatrician training studies are overall positive but suggest caution. Many awareness building initiatives increase pediatrician knowledge but do not necessarily lead to referrals, nor is there adequate follow-up data to understand whether the referrals were appropriate and effective (Daniels, Halladay, Shih, Elder, & Dawson, 2014). While some studies show increased identification and referral (Guevara et al., 2012; Swanson et al., 2014), others show inconsistent results. Of children who screened positive for developmental delay, only 30 % (Windham et al., 2014) to 65 % (Morelli et al., 2014), were referred to treatment and of those who were referred, only half followed through (Morelli et al., 2014; Windham et al., 2014). At least one study suggests that over identification may be an issue (Zachary, Stone, & Humberd, 2009). A study in which practice parameters were distributed and publicized showed a decrease of 1.5 years in average age of ASD diagnosis; however, results were not maintained at 2-year follow-up (Holzer et al., 2006). Therefore, sustainability of such campaigns is important to consider. Some innovative models, such as telephone screening of low-resource communities (Roux et al., 2012), and screening of children using videos uploaded to smartphones (Oberleitner, Reischel, Lacy, Goodwin, & Spitalnick, 2011) are currently being evaluated, with promising results.

Assessment Practices

In response to the increasing prevalence of ASD and in the face of obstacles to accurate diagnostic assessment, health care professionals have adopted new practices to systematically detect ASD in young children. Best-practice guidelines set by the American Academy of Pediatrics now call for routine surveillance at every well-child visit, with the use of ASD-specific screening tools at 18 and 24 months (Johnson et al., 2007). Positive screen results prompt clinicians to initiate further assessment, which may lead to a diagnosis of ASD. Effective screening practices for ASD are essential in early childhood, as the majority of parents first recognize abnormalities prior to the second birthday (Baghdadli, Picot, Pascal, Pry, & Aussilloux, 2003; Chawarska et al., 2007; De Giacomo & Fombonne, 1998; Tolbert, Brown, Fowler, & Parsons, 2001). But despite the early age of parental recognition, on average, children are not diagnosed with ASD until 48 months, well after initial concerns have been noted (Centers for Disease Control, 2012). Early diagnosis of ASD increases children's access to early intervention services, which is central to achieving positive outcomes (Lovaas, 1987; National Research Council, 2001; Rogers & Vismara, 2008).

Screening for ASD

A number of autism-specific screeners have been developed to facilitate accurate detection of ASD in young children. Some systems are designed for population-based screening and, others are designed to screen children already suspected of ASD. These types of screenings are referred to as level one and level two, respectively.

To understand the utility and efficacy of a particular screening or diagnostic instrument, it is essential to have knowledge of its psychometric properties, especially the indices of sensitivity and specificity. *Sensitivity* refers to a measure's ability to correctly identify children who are at risk for the disorder; *specificity* refers to its ability to correctly rule out children who are not at risk for the disorder. According to Coonrod and Stone (2005), acceptable levels of sensitivity are specificity are .80 and higher. Although both metrics of sensitivity and specificity are relevant to accurate diagnosis, maximum sensitivity is generally achieved at the cost of lower specificity, and vice versa. Recently, several ASD-specific screeners have been developed; however, few have been carefully evaluated. Therefore, clinicians must use be some caution when selecting instruments for routine clinical practice (Charman & Gotham, 2013).

Level One

Level one ASD screeners typically use the reports of parents and caregivers to measure broad developmental constructs suggestive of ASD. They are easy and quick to administer and interpret, and they are characterized by high sensitivity. High sensitivity is favorable in level one screeners because their purpose is to identify the maximum number of children at risk for developing the disorder. But, they also lead to over-identification (i.e., false positives) due to low specificity; many children identified as at-risk following the level one screening will be determined to be unaffected by ASD after further evaluation. However, it is likely that these children have related developmental disorders (Dietz, Swinkels, van Daalen, van Engeland, & Buitelaar, 2006; Pierce et al., 2011). When it comes to level one screeners for ASD, high sensitivity is more important than high specificity, because the consequences of missing a child with ASD are far more significant than evaluating a child who is unaffected (Barton, Dumont-Mathieu, & Fein, 2012).

Several level one screening measures for ASD have been developed for clinical use in children 18-months and older (see Table 2.2). Widespread level one tools include: (a) the Checklist for Autism in Toddlers (CHAT; Baron-Cohen et al., 1992), (b) the Modified Checklist for Autism in Toddlers (M-CHAT; Robins et al., 2001), and (c) the Early Screening for Autistic Traits (ESAT; Swinkels et al., 2006).

Baron-Cohen et al. (1992) developed and validated the first level one screener for ASD in Great Britain, called the CHAT. The 14-item CHAT was designed to identify

Table 2.2 Screening instruments for ASD

Instrument	Developers	Age	Format	Administration time (min)	Level of training	Sensitivity	Specificity
Level one							
CHAT	Baron-Cohen, Allen, and Gillberg (1992)	18–24 months and older	Parent questionnaire; clinician observation	5 Not reported	Minimal	.18–.38	.98–.1
M-CHAT	Robins, Fein, Barton, and Green (2001)	16–30 months	Parent questionnaire	10	None	.87[a]	.99[a]
ESAT	Dietz et al. (2006)	14–15 months	Parent questionnaire; clinician observation	5 Not reported	Minimal	Not reported	Not reported
Level two							
CARS2	Schopler, Van Bourgondien, Wellman, and Love (2010)	2 years and older	Clinician behavioral checklist	5–10	Minimal	.81	.87
GARS and GARS-2	Gilliam (1995) Gilliam (2006)	3–22 years	Clinician behavioral checklist	5–10	Minimal	.38–.83	.68
SCQ	Rutter, Bailey, et al. (2003)	4–18 years	Parent questionnaire	10	None	.71–.88	.54–.79
SRS-2	Constantino (2012)	4–18 years	Parent questionnaire	15	None	.23–.80	.67–.96

[a] Estimated

children who show signs of ASD at 18 months old. Items focus on the attainment of key social communication milestones, such as pretend play and two aspects of joint attention. These include protodeclarative pointing (e.g., pointing at an object for the purpose of directing another person to look at it) and gaze monitoring (e.g., looking in the same direction as another person). Nine items on the CHAT are based on parent report; the remaining five are based on in-home observations conducted by health practitioners. Validation studies with high-risk and general populations indicate that although the CHAT nearly always identifies children with ASD correctly, it also misses many children (Baird et al., 2000; Baron-Cohen et al., 1996; Scambler, Rogers, & Wehner, 2001).

The M-CHAT is an extension of the CHAT. It is in the public domain and can be accessed at https://www.m-chat.org. It includes the nine parent-rated items from the CHAT and 14 original items (Robins et al., 2001). The authors of the M-CHAT created additional items in order to assess a broader range of symptoms in children aged 16- to 30-months, and to increase the sensitivity of the measure. They included parent-rated items only to account for the absence of health visitor observations in the United States (Robins et al., 2001). The original validation sample included 1293 children who were screened at the 18- and 24-month well-child visit, 58 of whom received diagnostic evaluations, and 39 of whom were diagnosed with a spectrum disorder. Although sensitivity and specificity cannot be determined until follow-up of the initial sample is complete, estimates are very promising (e.g., .87 and .99, respectively; Robins et al., 2001).

The ESAT is a 14-item parent rating scale for children between the ages of 14- and 15-months in the general population. During development, Dietz et al. (2006) screened 31,724 children for ASD in the Netherlands using a two-pronged approach. First, parents completed a four-item prescreening questionnaire at well-child appointments. Second, children with positive results were observed in the home by a mental health professional who completed the 14-item ESAT measure. Of the children who participated, 18 were diagnosed with ASD and 55 were identified as having other developmental disorders, such as language disorder ($n = 18$) and intellectual disability ($n = 13$). Although sensitivity and specificity data are not yet available, prevalence data suggest the sensitivity of the ESAT is relatively low. Further, a large number of false-positive results were generated following the prescreening phase (Dietz et al., 2006).

The Communication and Symbolic Behavior Scales Developmental Profile (CSBS DP; Wetherby & Prizant, 2002) Infant/Toddler Checklist and Pervasive Developmental Disorders Screener Screening Test, Second Edition (PDDST-II; Siegel, 2004) are two measures that offer level one and level two screening. The CSBS DP is comprised of a 24-item parent questionnaire (level one) and follow-up behavioral observation (level 2) with the Scale of Red Flags (SORF; Wetherby & Woods, 2002). The PDDST-II contains caregiver-rating forms for three settings; primary care centers, developmental disabilities clinics, and autism clinics. While the CSBS targets very young children (6–24 months) only, the PDDST is intended for use with toddlers and children under the age of 6. The CSBS and PDDST continue to be under investigation.

Level Two

In contrast to level one, level two screeners contain high specificity. High specificity is an important quality of level two screeners because it allows practitioners to discriminate developmental disabilities from other disorders and pinpoint the specific developmental condition (Bishop, Luyster, Richler, & Lord, 2008). Commonly used level two screeners include: (a) the Social Communication Questionnaire (SCQ; Rutter, Bailey, & Lord, 2003), (b) the Social Responsiveness Scale, Second Edition (SRS-2; Constantino, 2012), (c) the Childhood Autism Rating Scale, Second Edition (CARS2; Schopler et al., 2010), and (d) the Gilliam Autism Rating Scale, Third Edition (GARS-3; Gilliam, 2014).

The SCQ is 40-item caregiver questionnaire based on, and strongly correlated with (r=.71–.73; Berument, Rutter, Lord, Pickles, & Bailey, 1999; Corsello et al., 2007), the Autism Diagnostic Interview (ADI; Lord, Rutter, & Le Couteur, 1994) and Autism Diagnostic Interview-Revised (ADI-R; Rutter, Le Couteur, & Lord, 2003). Although it was originally developed for research, the SCQ is now commonly used in both research and practice (Charman & Gotham, 2013). The initial SCQ validation study conducted by Berument et al. (1999) included 160 individuals previously diagnosed with ASD and 40 without ASD. Participants ranged from ages 4 to 40 years old and were primarily British. Sensitivity and specificity were high, with values of .85 and .75, respectively. Subsequent investigations, which focused on younger participants (2–16 years old) and included American samples, showed mixed findings. Chandler et al. (2007) reported comparable sensitivity (.88) and specificity (.72) in children between the ages of 9 and 10 years old. Eaves, Wingert, Ho, and Mickelson (2006) also reported moderate sensitivity (.71) and specificity (.79) in a study with children between ages 3 and 7 years old; however, in a related study with children between the ages 4 and 6 years old, Eaves et al. (2006) reported lower sensitivity (.74) and specificity of (.54). The work of Corsello et al. (2007) provides further evidence to suggest age plays a role in the accuracy of the measure: higher sensitivity was found when the SCQ was used to screen children 11 years and older (.80), compared to children under the age of 5 years (.68). Although the utility of the SCQ has been primarily studied in the context of at-risk populations, there is some evidence to suggest it may also be an effective population-based screening tool (Chandler et al., 2007).

The SRS-2 is a 65-item rating scale for parents and teachers. Items address characteristics of autism and total scores discriminate between people with and without ASD. Like the SCQ, the SRS is strongly correlated with validated diagnostic measures, such as the ADI-R (r=.65–.77; Constantino et al., 2003). Several studies have shown that the SRS-2 effectively discriminates between children with ASD, non-ASD disorders, and those whom are typically developing. Constantino et al. (2004) reported high sensitivity (.85) and specificity (.75) in their sample of 259 children with ASD and non-spectrum disorders. In a later study of 119 children between 9 and 13 years of age, Charman et al. (2007) reported sensitivity of .78 and specificity of .67. German and Japanese translations of the SRS-2 have also been studied

(Bölte, Westerwald, Holtmann, Freitag, & Poustka, 2011; Kamio et al., 2013). When comparing ASD and non-spectrum disorders with the German version, sensitivity was .80 and specificity was .69 (Bölte et al., 2011). For the Japanese version, indices were contrasted across girls and boys, with alternate cutoff points used for each group. The results show the measure performed equally well with girls and boys. Sensitivity for girls was .32 and specificity was .95; sensitivity for boys was .23 and specificity was .96 (Kamio et al., 2013).

The CARS2 (Schopler et al., 2010) is a clinician rating system for detecting symptoms of ASD. The CARS2 is comprised of standard (CARS2-ST) and high-functioning (CARS2-HF) forms. The CARS2-ST is for children between the ages 2 and 5 years old and older individuals with below average intellectual functioning. The CARS2-HF is for children 6 years and older who are verbally fluent and have IQ in the Low Average range, or higher. The CARS2 ratings are based on an unstructured observation session and information gathered from a caregiver (Schopler et al., 2010). The CARS2 has strong technical properties. Data obtained from the verification sample indicate the indices of sensitivity (.81) and specificity (.87) are strong. Correlations between the CARS and other autism instruments are high, and the original CARS was used extensively in clinical intervention to monitor symptom severity (Schopler et al., 2010).

The GARS-3 is a clinician-rated scale for children 3–22 years old. The GARS-3 is based on the DSM-5 criteria for ASD. Similar to the CARS2, scores are classified by likelihood of ASD and severity of symptoms. To date, no independent replication studies have been published on the sensitivity and specificity of the GARS-3. Past reports of the GARS (Gilliam, 1995) and GARS-2 (Gilliam, 2006) have generally found low sensitivity and specificity, and thus indicate limited clinical utility (Norris & Lecavalier, 2010; Pandolfi, Magyar, & Dill, 2010; Sikora, Hall, Hartley, Gerrard-Morris, & Cagle, 2008).

The Screening Test for Autism in 2-Year-Olds (STAT; Stone Coonrod, & Ousley, 2000) is a level two screener for children between the ages of 24 and 36 months. The STAT involves direct assessment by a clinician. It is comprised of 12 items that cover four domains: play, requesting, directing attention, and motor imitation. Although the STAT is completed by a clinician, it is relatively brief and does not require substantial training. Psychometric data are not widely available for the STAT.

Although they CARS and GARS are intended for screening, they are sometimes used in clinical practice as diagnostic tools (Bishop, Luyster, et al., 2008). The CARS2 and GARS-3 may be appealing to clinicians because they are time-efficient and require minimal training to administer. However, these instruments should not be used in place of robust diagnostic instruments, as described below.

Diagnosing ASD

Children who perform below an established cut-off score on a level two screening, and those who demonstrate unusual patterns of development should receive an in-depth diagnostic assessment using validated instruments (see Table 2.3). Evidence

Table 2.3 Diagnostic instruments for ASD

Instrument	Citation	Age (months)	Administration time (min)	Level of training	Strengths	Limitations
Interviews						
ADI-R	Lord et al. (1994)	12 and older	90–250	Requires substantial training	Appropriate for clinical and research purposes	Does not correspond to DSM-5
					Provides guidelines for classification	Toddler Module not yet available for clinical use
					Extensively studied	Time consuming
3di	Skuse et al. (2004)	36 and older	45–120	Requires moderate training	Appropriate for clinical purposes	Does not correspond to DSM-5
					Produces computer generated reports with algorithm scores and classification	Intended for use with individuals with average IQ
						Independent replication validity studies needed
DISCO	Wing, Leekam, Libby, Gould, and Larcombe (2002)	All ages	120–180	Not reported	Appropriate for clinical purposes	Does not correspond to DSM-5
					Provides profile of skills that directly relate to treatment planning	
					Computerized diagnostic algorithms available	Limited data on use with young children and individuals with intellectual disabilities
						Validity studies have focused on discriminations between ASD and typically developing populations

(continued)

Table 2.3 (continued)

Instrument	Citation	Age (months)	Administration time (min)	Level of training	Strengths	Limitations
Observation systems						
ADOS-2	Lord, Rutter et al. (2012), Lord, Luyster, Gotham, and Guthrie (2012)	12 and older	40–60	Requires substantial training	Appropriate for clinical and research purposes	Current version is not developmentally appropriate for older adolescents and adults with limited speech
					Corresponds to DSM-5; provides guidelines for classification and severity scores	
					Extensively studied	Severity scores have not been widely studied
AOSI	Bryson, McDermott, Rombough, Brian, and Zwaigenbaum (2000)	6–18	20	Requires moderate training	Appropriate for research purposes	Not appropriate for clinical purposes
					Measures symptoms of ASD in very young children	Limited age range

suggests clinical diagnoses of ASD can be made reliably as early as 2 years (Cox et al., 1999; Kleinman et al., 2008; Lord, 1995). Because there are not yet biological markers for ASD, the gold standard for diagnosing ASD in a child is a best-estimate clinical diagnosis, provided by qualified and experienced clinicians (Chawarska, Klin, Paul, & Volkmar, 2007; Klin, Lang, Cicchetti, & Volkmar, 2000; Stone et al., 1999). Several areas of functioning are impacted by ASD and therefore the process of diagnosing ASD is complex and requires a multidimensional approach (Lord & Corsello, 2005). The National Research Council (2001) recommends that the identification of ASD include a "multidisciplinary evaluation of social behavior, language, and nonverbal communication, adaptive behavior, motor skills, atypical behaviors, and cognitive status by a team of professionals experienced with autism spectrum disorders" (p. 214). To this end, clinicians use assessment data collected through ratings scales, semi-structured interviews, and clinical observation to make ASD diagnoses (Bishop, Luyster et al., 2008; Lord, Petkova et al., 2012). Integrating information from multiple sources (e.g., caregivers, teachers and experienced clinicians) is especially useful for complex cases (Kim & Lord, 2012a).

Autism Diagnostic Tools

The Autism Diagnostic Interview-Revised (ADI-R; Lord et al., 1994) is the most widely used instrument for making diagnoses of ASD in individuals with a nonverbal mental age above 24 months (Rutter, Le Couteur, et al., 2003). The ADI-R is comprised of 93 items that address (a) background information and early development (e.g., family, education, previous diagnoses, and medications); (b) communication; (c) reciprocal interactions; (d) restricted, repetitive behaviors and interests; and (e) general behavior. The majority of items include separate codes to account for the target behavior at different points in the child's life, such as the present time, between the child's fourth and fifth birthday, and when the behavior was regarded as most atypical. Clinicians score individual items based on their judgments about the target behavior (e.g., presence and severity). Appropriate use of the ADI-R is dependent on correct administration and accurate interpretation of informant responses. Therefore, specialized training is required to learn the administration and coding procedures (Lord et al., 1994).

In addition to scoring individual items, clinicians complete diagnostic algorithms based on the child's language level. The algorithms, which include the ADI-R items that most closely map onto the clinical descriptions and diagnostic guidelines, provide cutoff scores for determining classification (Lord et al., 1994). In order to reach the ADI-R classification of "autism," individuals must meet or exceed the algorithm thresholds in communication, social reciprocity, and restricted, repetitive behaviors and interests; they must also have evidence of onset before 36 months (Rutter, Le Couteur, et al., 2003). The algorithms for children 4 years and older have not changed since they were originally published by Western Psychological Association (WPS) in 2003; however, several investigators have proposed alternate thresholds to identify the more broadly defined ASD, rather than autism only (e.g., International Molecular Genetic Study of Autism Consortium, 2001; Risi et al., 2006; Sung et al., 2005). Adapting the original algorithm to reflect a wider range of symptoms is particularly pressing in light of the DSM-5 diagnostic criteria for ASD (De Bildt et al., 2013).

A 'Toddler' version of the ADI-R has also been developed for children 4 years and younger with a nonverbal mental age above 10 months. This version includes 32 new items that assess the onset of symptoms and the child's general development (Kim & Lord, 2012b). All other items in the Toddler ADI-R are identical to the standard ADI-R, with the exception of codes for behaviors observed between the fourth and fifth birthday (theses are omitted from the Toddler ADI-R). Although the Toddler ADI-R has been used in research for several years, it is not yet published.

Risi et al. (2006) assessed the sensitivity and specificity of the ADI-R for children 3 years and older using a sample from the U.S. (N=960) and Canada (N=232). Results indicate the ADI-R has strong sensitivity (.89–.95) and adequate specificity (.56–.59) when discriminating autism plus other spectrum disorders from non-spectrum disorders (Risi et al., 2006). De Bildt et al. (2013) found comparable results in their sample of Dutch children (N=1204). However, the ADI-R has been found to be less effective at identifying children whose mental age is below 24 months, and those with profound intellectual disability (Chawarska, Klin, et al., 2007; Cox et al., 1999; Lord, 1995; Risi et al., 2006). Although the ADI-R accurately differentiates between ASD and other developmental disorders in older preschool and school-age children, several investigators have reported lower sensitivity for toddlers, due to subthreshold scores in the area of restricted, repetitive behaviors and interests (Chawarska, Klin, et al., 2007; Cox et al., 1999; Ventola et al., 2006; Wiggins & Robins, 2008).

In response, Kim and Lord (2012b) created new diagnostic algorithms for toddlers and early preschool students using assessment data from 829 children between the ages of 12 and 47 months. These algorithms include only items represented in both standard and toddler versions (Kim & Lord, 2012b). Distinct cutoff scores for research and clinical purposes were created. While the clinical cutoffs were selected to maximize sensitivity and maintain adequate specificity (above .70) for the comparison of ASD to non-spectrum disorders, research cutoffs were selected to maximize specificity (above .80) and maintain adequate sensitivity for the comparison of a narrower definition of ASD (e.g., autism) to non-spectrum disorders. Scores on the Toddler algorithm fall into two categories, which complement the DSM-5 criteria for ASD: social communication and restricted and repetitive behaviors and interests. They also correspond to three ranges of concern based ASD symptom severity: Little-to-No Concern, Mild-to-Moderate Concern, and Moderate-to-Severe Concern.

Kim, Thurm, Shumway, and Lord (2013) confirmed the diagnostic validity of the toddler algorithms in their replication study using two large independent samples provided by research sites in the U.S. and Canada. Across both datasets, and taking into account characteristics of age and language level, when applying the clinical cutoff score, sensitivity for ASD compared to non-spectrum disorders ranged from

Table 2.4 Guidelines for selecting) ADOS-2 modules

ADOS-2 module	Chronological age range	Expressive language level
Toddler	12–30 months	No speech, single words
1	31 months and older	No speech, single words
2	Any age	Phrase speech
3	Child, young adolescent)	Fluent speech
4	Older adolescent, adult	Fluent speech

.89 to .97 and specificity ranged from .58 to .94. The research cutoff for autism yielded sensitivity and specificity ranges of .69–.97 and .64–.94, respectively.

The Autism Diagnostic Observation Schedule, Second Edition (ADOS-2) is a semi-structured observational assessment for diagnosing ASD. The ADOS-2 is a revision of the Autism Diagnostic Observation Schedule (ADOS; Lord, Rutter, DiLavore, & Risi, 1999) and is presented in two parts: ADOS-2 Modules 1–4 (Lord, Rutter, et al., 2012) and ADOS-2 Toddler Module (Lord, Luyster, et al., 2012). It includes five development and language-dependent assessment modules across both parts, which support its use with toddlers, school age children, and adults with a range of abilities (Lord, Rutter, et al., 2012). The appropriateness of a given module relies on the individual's age, verbal abilities, and interests (see Table 2.4). Currently, Lord and Hus are conducting validity testing for an adapted protocol, which is intended for use with older individuals with limited language.

The Diagnostic Interview for Social and Communication Disorders (DISCO; Wing et al., 2002) and the Development, Diagnostic and Dimensional Interview, Third Edition (3di; Skuse et al., 2004) are other interview systems used to diagnosis ASD. The DISCO (Wing et al., 2002) is a semi-structured standardized interview comprised of 362 items that target ASD and related developmental and psychiatric disorders. Administration is approximately 3 h (Wing et al., 2002). Although the DISCO was designed for the purpose of systematically collecting information about a child's presenting symptoms and informing treatment recommendations, it also contains algorithms for diagnostic classification. Studies of the DISCO conducted in the US and Sweden (Nygren et al., 2009; Wing et al., 2002) revealed robust sensitivity (.82–1) and good specificity (.55–.83) for discriminating ASD from non-spectrum disorders.

The 3di (Skuse et al., 2004) is a computer-based standardized parent interview administered face-to-face by a trained clinician. It's comprised of mandatory and optional modules, including the Pervasive Developmental Disorder (PDD) Module, which targets ASD symptoms. The PDD Module takes approximately 90 min to complete. When comorbid symptoms are present, examiners administer additional modules. Following the interview, computer-generated reports are provided to inform diagnosis (Skuse et al., 2004). In contrast to semi-structured diagnostic interviews (e.g., ADI-R, DISCO), the 3di requires minimal training to administer (Skuse et al., 2004). Further, findings from Skuse et al.'s (2004) original paper of 120 children indicate the 3di accurately discriminated between children with ASD, children with non-spectrum disorders, and typically developing children with very high sensitivity (.98) and specificity (1). Psychometric properties are also strong for the abbreviated 3di (3di-sv; Santosh et al., 2009). The DISCO and 3di show great promise however; further study is necessary to truly understand their utility for diagnosing in ASD across clinical populations and settings.

The ADOS-2 is a 40–60 min play and activity based standardized assessment for observation of social and communication behaviors relevant to the clinical diagnosis of ASD (e.g., eye contact, gestures, social overtures and responses, sensory interests, restricted and repetitive behaviors, and others). During the ADOS-2, examiners deliver structured and semi-structured presses for social interaction and then code behaviors associated with particular test items. Examiners also give ratings of their overall impressions of the child's social communication skills (Lord, Rutter, et al., 2012).

In the updated revision, the authors provide unique algorithms for each of the five modules. Each module has a new algorithm in the ADOS-2, with the exception of Module 4; the Module 4 algorithm in the ADOS-2 is identical to the Module 4 algorithm in the original ADOS. However, Hus and Lord (2014) released a revised Module 4 algorithm shortly after the ADOS-2 was published by WPS. All future mentions of the Module 4 algorithm are in reference to the Hus and Lord (2014) algorithm.

For Modules 1 through 4, the algorithms provide cutoff score for determining instrument classification. Keeping in-line with the DSM-5 diagnostic criteria, the ADOS-2 algorithms for Modules 1 through 4 provide thresholds for autism *and* ASD based on the domains of "social affect" and "restricted and repetitive behavior" (Hus & Lord, 2014; Lord, Rutter, et al., 2012). They also provide Comparison Scores, which indicate an individual's severity of autism spectrum-related symptomatology compared to children with ASD who are the same age and language level. ADOS-2 Comparison Scores range from 1 to 10 and correspond to the following interpretive categories: Minimal-to-No Evidence, Low Level, Moderate Level, and High Level. These standardized severity scores not only assist clinicians in formulating their clinical impressions, but they also afford them the opportunity to monitor changes in an individual's presentation over time (Hus & Lord, 2014; Lord, Rutter, et al., 2012).

Much like its companion measure, the Toddler ADI-R, the ADOS-2 Toddler Module algorithm takes a more cautious approach to summarizing symptoms by providing three ranges of concern, rather than diagnostic classification. This approach is ideal for the Toddler Module because it reflects the uncertainty of diagnosis in young children based on clinical observation alone (Lord, Luyster, et al., 2012).

The first step in the ADOS-2 revision process was to improve the diagnostic validity of the ADOS algorithms. Gotham, Risi, Pickles, and Lord (2007) used a large sample (N=1139) of children and adolescents aged 14 months to 16 years to update the algorithms for Modules 1 through 3. Approximately one third of the participants had enrolled in earlier studies and therefore were linked to data from multiple ADOS administrations. In total, 1630 assessments comprised of an ADOS administration, a measure of verbal IQ, and the best-estimate clinical diagnosis were reviewed. Two comparisons were conducted: autism versus non-spectrum cases ($n=1157$) and non-autism ASD versus non-spectrum cases ($n=685$). The results of Gotham et al.'s (2007) analyses indicate that across modules, for children with a nonverbal mental age above 15 months, the new algorithms demonstrated adequate sensitivity (.72–.97) for both diagnostic comparisons. Specificity was also very high for discriminating autism from non-spectrum disorders (.84–.95). Specificity was slightly lower for discriminating non-autism ASD from non-spectrum disorders, though it was still strong (.76–.83).

A replication study by Gotham et al. (2008) confirmed the predictive validity of the algorithms for Modules 1 through 3. In this multisite study, data from 1282 cases were reviewed. Sensitivity was high for autism versus non-spectrum disorders comparisons (.82–.94) though slightly lower for non-autism ASD versus non-spectrum disorders comparisons (.60–.95). As expected, specificity was very high for discriminating autism from non-spectrum disorders (.80–1) and slightly lower for discriminating non-autism ASD from non-spectrum disorders (.75–1).

Hus and Lord (2014) demonstrated strong sensitivity and specificity for the ADOS-2 Module 4 algorithm in their sample of 393 young adolescents and adults ($M=21.56$) with 437 assessments. Overall, the revised algorithm demonstrated very high sensitivity (.95) and specificity (.82) for discriminating between individuals with ASD and non-ASD disorders.

The ADOS-2 Toddler validation sample included 182 young children between the ages of 12 and 30 months. Many children were enrolled in longitudinal studies resulting in multiple assessments. In total, 360 comprehensive evaluations comprised of the ADI-R, standardized cognitive and language testing, and best-estimate clinical diagnosis were analyzed. Children were assigned to one of two developmental groups, based on their chronological age and language ability: (a) children between the ages of 12 and 30 months with few to no words and (b) children between the ages of 21 and 30 months with some words. Sensitivity and specificity were excellent for both developmental groups. For the group of children with few to words, sensitivity for contrasting ASD cases with non-spectrum plus typically developing cases was .91 and specificity was .94. For the group with some words, sensitivity for contrasting ASD cases with non-spectrum plus typically developing cases was .88 and specificity was .94.

Although the ADI-R and ADOS-2 provide some overlapping information, they lead to more accurate diagnostic formulations in young children and adolescents when used in combination, rather than individually (De Bildt et al., 2004, 2013; Kim & Lord, 2012a; Le Couteur, Haden, Hammal, & McConachie, 2008; Risi et al., 2006). In effect, the sensitivity and specificity for the combined use of the two measures is better balanced than each instrument's individual properties (Kim & Lord, 2012a; Risi et al., 2006). Consequently, experts in the field recommend the use of both the ADI-R and ADOS-2 to inform diagnostic decision-making (Kim & Lord, 2012a; Risi et al., 2006). In addition to complementing each other well, the ADI-R and ADOS-2 represent the most rigorously evaluated diagnostic tools for ASD. Although other measures show great promise, they have not undergone the same degree of testing. When selecting diagnostic instruments, clinicians should carefully review the available research, including independent replication studies, and compare findings with their goals for assessment.

Developmental Assessment

In addition to administering instruments that target ASD symptoms, clinicians should complete a developmental assessment using a core battery that includes tests of cognitive abilities, language skills, and adaptive functioning, to inform diagnosis (Ozonoff, Goodlin-Jones, & Solomon, 2005). Such measures provide a context for determining whether or not a child's social, communication and play behaviors are developmentally appropriate (Bishop, Luyster et al., 2008). They also provide information relevant to effective treatment planning. The Mullen Scales of Early Learning (MSEL; Mullen, 1995) and the Differential Ability Scales, Second Edition (DAS-II; Elliott, 2007) are two cognitive tests that are frequently used in research and clinical evaluations for children suspected of ASD (Akshoomoff, 2006; Bishop, Guthriec, Coffing, & Lord, 2011; Lord, Petkova et al., 2012). Both of these measures are ideal for testing children suspected of ASD because they involve lesser demands for language compared to cognitive tests used in typically developing populations, such as the Wechsler Preschool and Primary Scale of Intelligence, Third Edition (WPPSI-III; Wechsler, 2002) and the Wechsler Intelligence Scale for Children, Fourth Edition (WISC-IV; Wechsler, 2003).

The MSEL is a comprehensive developmental assessment for infants and preschool children from birth to 68 months (Mullen, 1995). It provides a global estimate of intellectual functioning, in addition to subtest scores in five core areas: expressive language, receptive language, visual problem solving, fine motor skills, and gross motor scores. Data from multiple studies demonstrate the MSEL has good internal, test-retest, and inter-rater reliabilities, along with adequate internal consistency (Mullen, 1995). Comparisons to other established measures, such as the Bailey Scales for Infant Development (BSID; Bayley, 2005), confirm the validity of the MSEL as an effective measure of global cognitive ability.

The DAS-II is also commonly used to assess cognitive abilities in children suspected of ASD. The DAS-II is a revision of the DAS, which was published in 1990 (Elliott, 1990). The DAS-II is appropriate for children between the ages of 2 and 17. It's comprised of two batteries, based on age: Early Years (ages 2–6) and School-Age (ages 7–17). Each battery contains ten core subtests plus ten diagnostic subtests. Data from DAS-II validity studies indicate that it has strong psychometric properties, including internal, test-retest, and interrater reliabilities (Elliott, 2007). It also demonstrates adequate convergent validity with other established measures, such as the WPPSI-III (Wechsler, 2002) and WISC-IV (Wechsler, 2003). Finally, several subtests have extended norms, which increase its application to children with a broad range of abilities (Sattler, 2008).

Assessment of adaptive functioning is also crucial during autism diagnostic assessments. Adaptive skills are defined as conceptual, social, and practical skills that children develop in order to function in everyday situations (American Association on Intellectual and Developmental Disabilities, 2013). Assessment of adaptive functioning is critical to diagnosing ASD because it allows clinicians to appraise how the children's cognitive assets translate into successful functioning in everyday life (Saulnier & Klin, 2007). One of the most extensive and commonly used measures of adaptive functioning in children is the Vineland Adaptive Behavior Scales, Second Edition (Vineland-II; Bishop, Luyster et al., 2008; Sparrow, Cicchetti, & Balla, 2006). The Vineland-II system contains interview and rating forms that can be used with parents and teachers, and it is normed for people from birth through 90 years. The scales of the Vineland-II correspond to broad domains of adaptive functioning: communication, daily living skills, and socialization. Supplemental sections address motor skills and maladaptive behavior.

Considerations for High-Risk Siblings

Practitioners should be particularly vigilant of children who have older siblings diagnosed with ASD. Studies have consistently shown that children with older siblings on the spectrum are at an increased risk for the disorder, due to its strong genetic basis (Chakrabarti & Fombonne, 2001; Constantino et al., 2013; Ozonoff et al., 2011). Recent findings from Ozonoff et al.'s (2011) prospective study of 664 infants, suggest the recurrence rate is as high as 18.7 %. In light of these findings, considerable attention has been directed toward identifying ASD in high-risk infants.

The Autism Observation Scale for Infants (AOSI) is a 20-min behavioral observation system developed by Bryson et al. (2000) to detect symptoms of ASD in high-risk infants (e.g., 6–18 months) with older siblings on the spectrum. Unlike the ADOS-2, The AOSI was created for research purposes only, specifically, to provide a method for systematically studying symptoms of ASD in early life (Bryson et al., 2000). Although the measure is not yet recommended for clinical and diagnostic use due to low sensitivity, it has been shown to reliably measure the behavioral signs of ASD in very young high-risk sibling populations (Bryson & Zwaigenbaum, 2014).

Novel Approaches to Diagnostic Assessment

More research has recently focused on novel approaches to diagnostic assessment. Diagnostic biomarkers are being studied more intensely, with potential promise for identifying autism before behavioral indicators are reliably present. Separately, computer-aided diagnosis is being used to screen for autism more quickly and reduce the burden of screening and comprehensive diagnostic assessment.

Biomarkers are biological indicators of the presence of ASD. Although candidate biomarkers to date have not been sensitive enough and continue to be quite expensive and/or laborious (Walsh, Elsabbagh, Bolton, & Singh, 2011), researchers continue to study several different possibilities. These include gene expression profiles from blood samples, proteomic profiles from serum samples, metabolomics profiles from urine samples, hormonal markers, immunological markers, morphological markers such as head size, electrophysiological markers, neuroanatomical markers such as brain size and structure, brain function, and neuropsychological markers such as visual scanning (Ruggeri, Sarkans, Schumann, & Persico, 2013; Voineagu & Yoo, 2013; Walsh et al., 2011). Given that the biological underpinnings of ASD appear to be complex, it is likely that a panel of biomarkers will prove to have higher sensitivity than any single biomarker (Anderson, 2015; Ruggeri et al., 2013). Selecting a subgroup of individuals with ASD may have more promise than searching for a biomarker applicable to all individuals (Voineagu & Yoo, 2013). Large biobanks, such as the Simons Simplex Collection and the Autism Genetic Resource Exchange, which contain biological data from individuals diagnosed with ASD using gold-standard instruments, will be helpful in generating these panels (Ruggeri et al., 2013). This research also has implicated for targeted psychopharmacological treatment based on an individual's neurodevelopmental pathology (Ruggeri et al., 2013). The research community has been vocal about the potential for ethical considerations with respect to the use of biomarkers (Anderson, 2015; Voineagu & Yoo, 2013).

Computer-aided diagnosis is another novel approach to diagnostic assessment currently being researched. These efforts are based on the concept of using artificial intelligence to mine available data. The artificial intelligence technology discerns patterns that allow it to make decisions that are reliable with trained experts. One such tool has been used to create a 5-min online questionnaire that caregivers fill out and preliminary results have found very high sensitivity and high specificity (Duda, Kosmicki, & Wall, 2014). Other computer-aided diagnostic tools make a digital real-time map of an individual's movements in space, which have been found to be associated with an ASD diagnosis (Hashemi et al., 2012; Torres et al., 2013). These innovations may eventually make it possible to create efficient screening and diagnostic tools that are can be disseminated to large groups of people.

Future Research

Diagnostic assessment is a well-researched topic in ASD; however, there are several future research directions for this topic. Foundationally, efforts are currently being made to capture more accurate prevalence data. Current sampling methods vary widely across studies and therefore limit comparisons across subgroups and comparisons within subgroups over time. The recent changes to the DSM diagnostic criteria may allow for more standardization that will improve comparability of prevalence research. The question of whether incidence of ASD is actually rising can only be answered with better designed research that controls for the systematic biases in prevalence data.

While several screeners are available for general developmental delay and for ASD, there is limited psychometric data or poor psychometric data available on many widely distributed screeners. Further study is important to refine these tools and understand which screeners are best suited for which populations. It is particularly important, given the consistent finding that some populations are under-identified with ASD, to focus on designing and validating screeners in special populations. The diagnostic instruments for ASD continue to be a relatively high clinical burden, requiring a great deal of training, time, and clinician expertise. Continued research is necessary to design tools that reduce this burden to make comprehensive diagnosis accessible to more families and to exert downward pressure on the age of diagnosis to ensure early intervention is available to all children with ASD. Research on novel approaches, including biomarkers and computer-aided diagnosis, is being conducted with larger and larger datasets and may yield more efficient diagnostic tools.

Although enormous public health efforts have been made to introduce and improve universal screening for ASD, these initiatives have not been carefully evaluated for effectiveness over the long-run. It is important that universal screening initiatives are designed to specifically address the reported barriers to obtaining an accurate, timely diagnosis of ASD. Screening initiatives have primarily focused on pediatricians, and preliminary results suggest that multi-pronged approach, where non-medical professionals are also trained to look for signs of developmental delay, may be more effective. Longer-term studies need to follow not just screening rates, but referral, entrance, and engagement with treatment. It is important to understand whether early screening is translating into children accessing evidence-based treatments. Work in this vein should also study how early diagnosis truly affects treatment trajectories and outcomes in the long run, to help the field understanding how much earlier diagnoses need to occur to have real effects for the child and family.

Implications for Practitioners and/or Families

Accurate, early diagnosis is the key to early intensive evidence-based treatment for children with ASD. Research suggests that, while the prevalence of ASD continues to grow, there are several barriers for families seeking diagnosis. A multi-pronged strategy is important to identify children at risk for ASD.

Aggressive, routine screening is recommended for young children, given that research shows that developmental delay may be present in the absence of either parent or physician concern. Given physician concerns about familiarity, time, and cost of using screeners, public health interventions for physician training continue to be important. Training should focus on identifying level one or level two screeners that are appropriate for community practices and how to accurately use these screeners. In addition, given the evidence the pediatric practices do not routinely screen, and that screening in non-medical settings is also effective in capturing developmental delay, public health efforts should equip schools and other community centers with training. Research shows that even children who screen positive for a developmental delay may not be referred for further evaluation or treatment. Training efforts therefore cannot stop teaching how to screen, but must also teach next steps.

It is particularly important that practitioners and families remain aware that certain sociodemographic markers, including minority status and lower socioeconomic status, are associated with greater delays to screening, diagnosis and treatment. It is unclear whether this is due to different symptom presentation in these groups, different levels of awareness or recognition in the family or clinician, or other potential influences. Regardless, training efforts should focus on the importance of capturing all children with a developmental delay and include strategies for screening and referring children and families in these risk groups.

References

Akshoomoff, N. (2006). Use of the Mullen Scales of Early Learning for the assessment of young children with autism spectrum disorders. *Child Neuropsychology, 12*, 269–277.

American Association on Intellectual and Developmental Disabilities. (2013). *Definition of intellectual disability*. Retrieved from http://www.aaidd.org/content_100.cfm

American Psychiatric Association. (2013). *Diagnostic and statistical manual of mental disorders* (5th ed.). Washington, DC: Author.

Anderson, G. M. (2015). Autism biomarkers: Challenges, pitfalls and possibilities. *Journal of Autism and Developmental Disorders, 54*, 1103–1113.

Baghdadli, A., Picot, M. C., Pascal, C., Pry, R., & Aussilloux, C. (2003). Relationship between age of recognition of first disturbances and severity in young children with autism. *European Child and Adolescent Psychiatry, 12*, 122–127.

Baird, G., Charman, T., Baron-Cohen, S., Cox, A., Swettenham, J., Wheelwright, S., & Drew, A. (2000). A screening instrument for autism at 18 months of age: A 6-year follow-up study. *Journal of the American Academy of Child and Adolescent Psychiatry*, *39*, 694–702.

Barbaresi, W. J., Colligan, R. C., Weaver, A. L., & Katusic, S. K. (2009). The incidence of clinically diagnosed versus research-identified autism in Olmstead County, Minnesota, 1976–1997: Results from a retrospective, population-based study. *Journal of Autism and Developmental Disorders, 39*, 464–470.

Baron-Cohen, S., Allen, J., & Gillberg, C. (1992). Can autism be detected at 18 months? The needle, the haystack, and the CHAT. *The British Journal of Psychiatry, 161*, 839–843.

Baron-Cohen, S., Cox, A., Baird, G., Swettenham, J., Nightingale, N., Morgan, K., Drew, A., & Charman, T. (1996). Psychological markers in the detection of autism in infancy in a large population. *The British Journal of Psychiatry, 168,* 158–163.

Baron-Cohen, S., Scott, F. J., Allison, C., Williams, J., Bolton, P., Matthews, F. E., & Brayne, C. (2009). Prevalence of autism-spectrum conditions: UK school-based population study. *The British Journal of Psychiatry, 194,* 500–509.

Barton, M., Dumont-Mathieu, T., & Fein, D. (2012). Screening young children for autism spectrum disorders in primary practice. *Journal of Autism and Developmental Disabilities, 42,* 1165–1174.

Baxter, A. J., Brugha, T. S., Erskine, H. E., Scheurer, R. W., Vos, T., & Scott, J. G. (2014). The epidemiology and global burden of autism spectrum disorders. *Psychological Medicine, 45,* 601–613.

Bayley, N. (2005). *Bayley scale of infant development*. San Antonio, TX: Harcourt Assessment.
Berument, S. K., Rutter, M., Lord, C., Pickles, A., & Bailey, A. (1999). Autism screening questionnaire: Diagnostic validity. *The British Journal of Psychiatry, 175*, 444–451.
Bishop, S. L., Guthriec, W., Coffing, M., & Lord, C. (2011). Convergent validity of the mullen scales of early learning and the differential ability scales in children with autism spectrum disorders. *American Journal on Intellectual and Developmental Disabilities, 116*, 331–343.
Bishop, S. L., Luyster, R., Richler, J., & Lord, C. (2008). Diagnostic assessment. In K. Chawarska, A. Klin, & F. R. Volkmar (Eds.), *Autism spectrum disorders in infants and toddlers* (pp. 23–49). New York, NY: Guilford Press.
Bishop, D. V., Whitehouse, A. J., Watt, H. J., & Line, E. A. (2008). Autism and diagnostic substitution: Evidence from a study of adults with a history of developmental language disorder. *Developmental Medicine & Child Neurology, 50*, 341–345.
Blumberg, S. J., Bramlett M. D., Kogan M. D., Schieve, L. A., Jones, J. R., & Lu, M. C. (2013). Changes in prevalence of parent-reported autism spectrum disorder in school-aged U.S. children: 2007 to 2011–2012. *National health statistics reports* (no 65). Hyattsville, MD: National Center for Health Statistics.
Bölte, S., Westerwald, E., Holtmann, M., Freitag, C., & Poustka, F. (2011). Autistic traits and autism spectrum disorders: The clinical validity of two measures presuming a continuum of social communication skills. *Journal of Autism and Developmental Disorders, 41*, 66–72.
Bryson, S. E., McDermott, D., Rombough, V., Brian, J., & Zwaigenbaum, L. (2000). *The autism observation scale for infants*. Toronto, ON: Unpublished Scale.
Bryson, S. E., & Zwaigenbaum, L. (2014). The AOSI and its development. In V. B. Patel, V. R. Preedy, & C. R. Martin (Eds.), *Comprehensive guide to autism* (pp. 299–310). New York, NY: Springer Science.
Cavagnaro, A. (2009). Autistic spectrum disorders changes in the California caseload an update: June 1987-June 2007. *California Department of Developmental Services, 19*, 536–551.
Centers for Disease Control. (2012). Prevalence of autism spectrum disorders—Autism and developmental disabilities monitoring network, 14 sites, United States, 2008. *Morbidity and Morality Weekly Report Surveillance Summaries, 61*, 1–19.
Centers for Disease Control. (2014). Prevalence of Autism Spectrum Disorder among children aged 8 years—Autism and Developmental Disabilities Monitoring Network, 11 sites, United States, 2010. *Morbidity and Mortality Weekly Report. Surveillance Summaries, 63*, 1–22.
Chakrabarti, S., & Fombonne, E. (2001). Pervasive developmental disorders in preschool children. *JAMA: Journal of the American Medical Association, 285*, 3093–3099.
Chandler, S., Charman, T., Baird, G., Simonoff, E., Loucas, T., Meldrum, D., … Pickles, A. (2007). Validation of the social communication questionnaire in a population cohort of children with autism spectrum disorders. *Journal of the American Academy of Child and Adolescent Psychiatry, 46*, 1324–1332.
Charman, T., Baird, G., Simonoff, E., Loucas, T., Chandler, S., Meldrum, D., & Pickles, A. (2007). Efficacy of three screening instruments in the identification of autistic-spectrum disorders. *The British Journal of Psychiatry, 191*, 554–559.
Charman, T., & Gotham, K. (2013). Measurement issues: Screening and diagnostic instruments for autism spectrum disorders—Lessons from research and practice. *Child and Adolescent Mental Health, 18*, 52–63.
Chawarska, K., Klin, A., Paul, R., & Volkmar, F. (2007). Autism spectrum disorder in the second year: Stability and change in syndrome expression. *Journal of Child Psychology and Psychiatry, 48*, 128–138.
Chawarska, K., Paul, R., Klin, A., Hannigen, S., Dichtel, L. E., & Volkmar, F. (2007). Parental recognition of developmental problems in toddlers with autism spectrum disorders. *Journal of Autism and Developmental Disorders, 37*, 62–72.
Constantino, J. N., Davis, S. A., Todd, R. D., Schindler, M. K., Gross, M. M., Brophy, S. L., … Reich, W. (2003). Validation of a brief quantitative measure of autistic traits: Comparison of the social responsiveness scale with the autism diagnostic interview-revised. *Journal of Autism and Developmental Disorders, 33*, 427–433.

Constantino, J. N., Gruber, C. P., Davis, S., Hayes, S., Passanante, N., & Przybeck, T. (2004). The factor structure of autistic traits. *Journal of Child Psychology and Psychiatry, 45*, 719–726.

Constantino, J. N., Todorov, A., Hilton, C., Law, P., Zhang, Y., Molloy, E., … Geschwind, D. (2013). Autism recurrence in half siblings: Strong support for genetic mechanisms of transmission in ASD. *Molecular Psychiatry, 18*, 137–138.

Coo, H., Ouellette-Kuntz, H., Lloyd, J. E. V., Kasmara, L., Holden, J. J. A., & Lewis, M. E. S. (2008). Trends in autism prevalence: Diagnostic substitution revisited. *Journal of Autism and Developmental Disorders, 38*, 1036–1046.

Coonrod, E. E., & Stone, W. L. (2005). Screening for autism in young children. In F. R. Volkmar, R. Paul, A. Klin, & D. Cohen (Eds.), *Handbook of autism and pervasive developmental disorders, Vol. 2: Assessment, interventions, and policy* (3rd ed., pp. 707–729). John Wiley & Sons: Hoboken, NJ.

Corsello, C., Hus, V., Pickles, A., Risi, S., Cook, E. J., Leventhal, B. L., & Lord, C. (2007). Between a ROC and a hard place: Decision making and making decisions about using the SCQ. *Journal of Child Psychology and Psychiatry, 48*, 932–940.

Cox, A., Klein, K., Charman, T., Baird, G., Baron-Cohen, S., Swettenham, J., … Wheelwright, S. (1999). Autism spectrum disorders at 20 and 42 months of age: Stability of clinical and ADI-R diagnosis. *Journal of Child Psychology and Psychiatry, 40*, 719–732.

Daniels, A. M., Halladay, A. K., Shih, A., Elder, L. M., & Dawson, G. (2014). Approaches to enhancing the early detection of autism spectrum disorders: A systematic review of the literature. *Journal of the American Academy of Child and Adolescent Psychiatry, 53*, 141–152.

De Bildt, A., Oosterling, I. J., van Lang, N. J., Kuijper, S., Dekker, V., Sytema, S., … de Jonge, M. V. (2013). How to use the ADI-R for classifying autism spectrum disorders? Psychometric properties of criteria from the literature in 1,204 Dutch children. *Journal of Autism and Developmental Disorders, 43*, 2280–2294.

De Bildt, A., Sytema, S., Ketelaars, C., Kraijer, D., Mulder, E., Volkmar, F., & Minderaa, R. (2004). Interrelationship between autism diagnostic observation schedule-generic (ADOS-G), autism diagnostic interview-revised (ADI-R), and the diagnostic and statistical manual of mental disorders (DSM-IV-TR) Classification in children and adolescents with mental retardation. *Journal of Autism and Developmental Disorders, 34*, 129–137.

De Giacomo, A., & Fombonne, E. (1998). Parental recognition of developmental abnormalitiesin autism. *European Child and Adolescent Psychiatry, 7*, 131–136.

Dietz, C., Swinkels, S., van Daalen, E., van Engeland, H., & Buitelaar, J. (2006). Screening for autistic spectrum disorder in children aged 14–15 months: Population screening with the early screening of autistic traits questionnaire (ESAT). *Design and general findings. Journal of Autism and Developmental Disorders, 35*, 713–722.

Dosreis, S., Weiner, C. L., Johnson, L., & Newschaffer, C. J. (2006). Autism spectrum disorder screening and management practices among general pediatric providers. *Journal of Developmental and Behavioral Pediatrics, 27*, S88–S94.

Duda, M., Kosmicki, J. A., & Wall, D. P. (2014). Testing the accuracy of an observation-based classifier for rapid detection of autism risk. *Translational Psychiatry, 4*, e424.

Eaves, L. C., Wingert, H. D., Ho, H. H., & Mickelson, E. R. (2006). Screening for autism spectrum disorders with the social communication questionnaire. *Journal of Developmental and Behavioral Pediatrics, 27*, 95–103.

Elliott, C. D. (1990). *Differential ability scales*. San Antonio, TX: The Psychological Corporation.

Elliott, C. D. (2007). *Differential ability scales* (2nd ed.). San Antonio, TX: The Psychological Corporation.

Elsabbagh, M., Divan, G., Koh, Y. -J., Kim, Y. S., Kauchali, S., Marcín, C., … Fombonne, E. (2012). Global prevalence of autism and other pervasive developmental disorders. *Autism Research, 5*, 160–179.

Filipek, P. A., Accardo, P. J., Ashwal, S., Baranek, G. T., Cook, E. H., Dawson, G., … Volkmar, F. R. (2000). Practice parameter: Screening and diagnosis of autism: Report of the Quality Standards Subcommittee of the American Academy of Neurology and the Child Neurology Society, *Neurology, 55*, 468–479.

Fombonne, E. (2009). Epidemiology of pervasive developmental disorders. *Pediatric Research, 65*, 591–598.

Fountain, C., King, M. D., & Bearman, P. S. (2011). Age of diagnosis for autism: Individual and community factors across 10 birth cohorts. *Journal of Epidemiology and Community Health, 65*, 503–510.

Gilliam, J. E. (1995). *Gilliam autism rating scale*. Austin, TX: Pro-Ed.

Gilliam, J. E. (2006). *Gilliam autism rating scale* (2nd ed.). Austin, TX: Pro-Ed.

Gilliam, J. E. (2014). *Gilliam autism rating scale* (3rd ed.). Austin, TX: Pro-Ed.

Goin-Kochel, R. P., Mackintosh, V. H., & Mysters, B. J. (2006). How many doctors does it take to make an autism spectrum diagnosis? *Autism, 10*, 439–451.

Gotham, K., Risi, S., Dawson, G., Tager-Flusberg, H., Joseph, R., Carter, A., … Lord, C. (2008). A replication of the autism diagnostic observation schedule (ADOS) revised algorithms. *Journal of the American Academy of Child and Adolescent Psychiatry, 47*, 642–651.

Gotham, K., Risi, S., Pickles, A., & Lord, C. (2007). The autism diagnostic observation schedule: Revised algorithms for improved diagnostic validity. *Journal of Autism and Developmental Disorders, 37*, 613–627.

Guevara, J. P., Gerdes, M., Localio, R., Huang, Y. V., Pinto-Martin, J., Mikovitz, C. S., … Pati, S. (2012). Effectiveness of developmental screening in an urban setting. *Pediatrics, 131*, 30–37.

Hashemi, J., Spina, T. V., Tepper, M., Esler, A., Morellas, V., Papanikolopoulos, N., & Sapiro, G. (2012, Nov) A computer vision approach for the assessment of autism-related behavioral markers. *Development and Learning and Epigenetic Robotics (ICDL), 2012 IEEE International Conference, 1*, 7–9.

Hertz-Picciotto, I., & Delwiche, L. (2009). The rise in autism and role of age at diagnosis. *Epidemiology, 20*, 84–90.

Holzer, L., Mihailescu, R., Rodrigues-Degaeff, C., Junier, L., Muller-Nix, C., Halfon, O., & Answermet, F. (2006). Community introduction of practice parameters for autistic spectrum disorders: Advancing early recognition. *Journal of Autism and Developmental Disorders, 36*, 249–262.

Honda, H., Shimizu, Y., Imai, M., & Nitto, Y. (2005). Cumulative incidence of childhood autism: A total population study of better accuracy and precision. *Developmental Medicine & Child Neurology, 47*, 10–18.

Hus, V., & Lord, C. (2014). The autism diagnostic observation schedule, module 4: Revised algorithm and standardized severity scores. *Journal of Autism and Developmental Disorders, 44*, 1996–2012.

International Molecular Genetic Study of Autism Consortium. (2001). A genomewide screen for autism: Strong evidence for linkage to chromosomes 2q, 7q, and 16p. *American Journal of Human Genetics, 69*, 570–581.

Johnson, S., Hollis, C., Kochhar, P., Hennessy, E., Wolke, D., & Marlow, N. (2010). Autism spectrum disorders in extremely preterm children. *Journal of Pediatrics, 156*, 525–531.

Johnson, C. P., Meyers, S. M., & The Council on Children with Disabilities. (2007). identification and evaluation of children with autism spectrum disorders. *Pediatrics, 120*, 1183–1215.

Kalbrenner, A. E., Daniels, J. L., Emch, M., Morrissey, J. L., Poole, C., & Chen, J. (2011). Geographic access to health services and diagnosis with an autism spectrum disorder. *Annals of Epidemiology, 12*, 304–310.

Kamio, Y., Inada, N., Moriwaki, A., Kuroda, M., Koyama, T., Tsujii, H., … Constantino, J. N. (2013). Quantitative autistic traits ascertained in a national survey of 22,529 Japanese school children. *Acta Psychiatrica Scandinavica, 128*, 45–53.

Keyes, K. M., Susser, E., Cheslak-Postava, K., Fountain, C., Liu, K., & Bearman, P. (2012). Cohort effects explain the increase in autism diagnosis among children born from 1992 to 2003 in California. *International Journal of Epidemiology, 41*, 495–503.

Kim, S. H., & Lord, C. (2012a). Combining information from multiple sources for the diagnosis of autism spectrum disorders for toddlers and young preschoolers from 12 to 47 months of age. *Journal of Child Psychology and Psychiatry, 53*, 143–151.

Kim, S. H., & Lord, C. (2012b). New autism diagnostic interview-revised algorithms for toddlers and young preschoolers from 12 to 47 months of age. *Journal of Autism and Developmental Disorders, 42*, 82–93.

Kim, S. H., Thurm, A., Shumway, S., & Lord, C. (2013). Multisite study of new Autism Diagnostic Interview-Revised (ADI-R) algorithms for toddlers and young preschoolers. *Journal of Autism and Developmental Disorders, 43*, 1527–1538.

King, M., & Bearman, P. (2009). Diagnostic change and the increased prevalence of autism. *International Journal of Epidemiology, 38*(5), 1224–1234.

Kleinman, J. M., Ventola, P. E., Pandey, J., Verbalis, A. D., Barton, M., Hodgson, S., … Fein, D. (2008). Diagnostic stability in very young children with autism spectrum disorders. *Journal of Autism and Developmental Disorders, 38*, 606–615.

Klin, A., Lang, J., Cicchetti, D. V., & Volkmar, F. R. (2000). Brief report: Interrater reliability of clinical diagnosis and DSM-IV criteria for autistic disorder: Results of the DSM-IV Autism Field Trial. *Journal of Autism and Developmental Disorders, 30*, 163–167.

Le Couteur, A., Haden, G., Hammal, D., & McConachie, H. (2008). Diagnosing autism spectrum disorders in pre-school children using two standardised assessment instruments: The ADI-R and the ADOS. *Journal of Autism and Developmental Disorders, 38*, 362–372.

Liptak, G., Benzoni, L. B., Mruzek, D. W., Nolan, K. W., Thingvull, M. A., Wade, C. M., & Fyer, G. E. (2008). Disparities in diagnosis and access to health services for children with autism: Data from the national survey of children's health. *Journal of Developmental & Behavioral Pediatrics, 29*(3), 152–160.

Lord, C. (1995). Follow-up of two-year-olds referred for possible autism. *Child Psychology and Psychiatry and Allied Disciplines, 36*, 1365–1382.

Lord, C., & Corsello, C. (2005). Diagnostic instruments in autistic spectrum disorders. In F. Volkmar, R. Paul, A. Klin, & D. Cohen (Eds.), *Handbook of autism and pervasive developmental disorders: Vol 2. Assessment, interventions, and policy* (pp. 730–771). Hoboken, NJ: Wiley.

Lord, C., Luyster, R. J., Gotham, K., & Guthrie, W. (2012). *Autism diagnostic observation schedule, second edition (ADOS-2) manual (part II): Toddler module*. Torrance, CA: Western Psychological Services.

Lord, C., Petkova, E., Hus, V., Gan, W., Lu, F., Martin, D. M., … Risi, S. (2012). A multisite study of the clinical diagnosis of different autism spectrum disorders. *Archives of General Psychiatry, 69*, 306–313.

Lord, C., Rutter, M., DiLavore, P. C., Risi, S., Gotham, K., & Bishop, S. L. (2012). *Autism diagnostic observation schedule, second edition (ADOS-2) manual (part I): Modules 1-4*. Torrance, CA: Western Psychological Services.

Lord, C., Rutter, M., DiLavore, P. C., & Risi, S. (1999). *Autism diagnostic observation schedule*. Los Angeles, CA: Western Psychological Services.

Lord, C., Rutter, M., & Le Couteur, A. (1994). Autism diagnostic interview-revised: A revised version of a diagnostic interview for caregivers of individuals with possible pervasive developmental disorders. *Journal of Autism and Developmental Disorders, 24*, 659–685.

Lovaas, O. I. (1987). Behavioral treatment and normal educational and intellectual functioning in young autistic children. *Journal of Consulting and Clinical Psychology, 55*, 3–9.

Mandell, D. S., Ittenbach, R. F., Levy, S. E., & Pinto-Martin, J. A. (2007). Disparities in diagnoses received to a diagnosis of autism spectrum disorder. *Journal of Autism and Developmental Disorders, 37*, 1795–1802.

Mandell, D. S., Listerud, J., Levy, S. E., & Pinto-Martin, J. (2002). Race differences in the age at diagnosis among Medicaid-eligible children with autism. *Journal of the American Academy of Child and Adolescent Psychiatry, 41*, 1447–1453.

Mandell, D. S., Novak, M. M., & Zubritsky, C. D. (2005). Factors associated with age of diagnosis among children with autism spectrum disorders. *Pediatrics, 116*, 1480–1486.

Matson, J. L., & Kozlowski, A. M. (2011). The increasing prevalence of autism spectrum disorders. *Research in Autism Spectrum Disorders, 5*, 418–425.

Miller, J. S., Gabrielsen, T., Villalobos, M., Alleman, R., Wahmhoff, N., Carbone, P. S., & Segura, B. (2011). The each child study: Systematic screening of Autism Spectrum Disorders in a pediatric setting. *Pediatrics, 127*(5), 866–871.

Morelli, D. L., Pati, S., Butler, A., Blum, N. J., Gerdes, M., Pinto-Martin, J., & Guevara, J. P. (2014). Challenges to implementation of developmental screening in urban primary care: A mixed methods study. *BMC Pediatrics, 14*, 16.

Mullen, E. (1995). *The Mullen Scales of Early Learning*. Circle Pines, MN: American Guidance Service.

National Research Council. (2001). *Educating children with autism*. Washington, DC: National Academy Press.

Newschaffer, C., Falb, M., & Gurney, J. (2005). National autism prevalence trends from United States special education data. *Pediatrics, 115*, 277–282.

Norris, M., & Lecavalier, L. (2010). Screening accuracy of level 2 autism spectrum disorder rating scales: A review of selected instruments. *Autism, 14*, 263–284.

Nygren, G., Cederlund, M., Sandberg, E., Gillstedt, F., Arvidsson, T., Gillberg, I.C., … Gillberg, C. (2012.) The prevalence of Autism Spectrum Disorders in toddlers: A population study of 2-year-old Swedish children. *Journal of Autism and Developmental Disorders, 42*, 1491–1497.

Nygren, G., Hagberg, B., Billstedt, E., Skoglund, Å., Gillberg, C., & Johansson, M. (2009). The Swedish version of the diagnostic interview for social and communication disorders (DISCO-10). *Psychometric properties. Journal of Autism and Developmental Disorders, 39*, 730–741.

Oberleitner, R., Reischel, U., Lacy, T., Goodwin, M., & Spitalnick, J. S. (2011). Emerging use of behavior imaging for autism and beyond. *Communicity Medical Care Compunetics, 1*, 93–104.

Ozonoff, S. (2012). Editorial perspective: Autism Spectrum Disorders in DSM-5—An historical perspective and the need for change. *Journal of Child Psychology and Psychiatry, 53*, 1092–1094.

Ozonoff, S., Goodlin-Jones, B., & Solomon, M. (2005). Evidence-based assessment of autism spectrum disorders in children and adolescents. *Journal of Clinical Child and Adolescent Psychology, 34*, 523–540.

Ozonoff, S., Gregory, Y. S., Carter A., Messinger, D., Yirmiya, N., Zwaigenbaum, L., … Stone, W. L. (2011). Recurrence risk for autism spectrum disorders: A baby sibling research consortium study. *Pediatrics, 128*, 488–495.

Pandolfi, V., Magyar, C. I., & Dill, C. A. (2010). Constructs assessed by the GARS-2: Factor analysis of data from the standardization sample. *Journal of Autism and Developmental Disorders, 40*, 1118–1130.

Parner, E. T., Thorsen, P., Dixon, G., de Klerk, N., Leonard, H., Nassar, N., … Glasson, E. M. (2011). A comparison of autism prevalence trends in Denmark and Western Australia. *Journal of Autism and Developmental Disorders, 41*, 1601–1608.

Pierce, K., Carter, C., Weinfeld, M., Desmond, J., Hazin, R., Bjork, R., & Hallager, N. (2011). Detecting, studying and treating autism early: The one year well-baby check-up approach. *Journal of Pediatrics*, 159, 458–465.

Rice, C. E., Rosanoff, M., Dawson, G., Durkin, M. S., Croen, L. A., Singer, A., & Yeargin-Allsop, M. (2013). Evaluating changes in the prevalence of Autism Spectrum Disorders. *Public Health Reviews, 34*(2), 1–22.

Risi, S., Lord, C., Gotham, K., Corsello, C., Chrysler, C., Szatmari, P., … Pickles, A. (2006). Combining information from multiple sources in the diagnosis of autism spectrum disorders. *Journal of the American Academy of Child and Adolescent Psychiatry, 45*, 1094–1103.

Robins, D. L., Fein, D., Barton, M. L., & Green, J. A. (2001). The modified checklist for autism in toddlers: An initial study investigating the early detection of autism and pervasive developmental disorders. *Journal of Autism and Developmental Disorders, 31*, 131–144.

Rogers, S. J., & Vismara, L. A. (2008). Evidence-based comprehensive treatments for early autism. *Journal of Clinical Child and Adolescent Psychology, 37*, 8–38.

Rosenberg, R. E., Landa, R., Law, J. K., Stuart, E. A., & Law, P. A. (2011). Factors affecting age an initial autism spectrum disorder diagnosis in a national survey. *Autism Research and Treatment, 11*, 1–11.

Roux, A. M., Herrera, P., Wold, C. M., Dunkle, M. C., Glascoe, F. P., & Shattuck, P. T. (2012). Developmental and autism screening through 2-1-1: Reaching underserved families. *American Journal of Preventative Medicine, 43*, 457–463.

Ruggeri, B., Sarkans, U., Schumann, G., & Persico, A. (2013). Biomarkers in autism spectrum disorder: The old and the new. *Psychopharmacology, 231*, 1201–1206.

Rutter, M., Bailey, A., & Lord, C. (2003). *The social communication questionnaire manual*. Los Angeles, CA: Western Psychological Services.

Rutter, M., Le Couteur, A., & Lord, C. (2003). *The autism diagnostic interview-revised manual*. Los Angeles, CA: Western Psychological Services.

Santosh, P. J., Mandy, W. L., Puura, K., Kaartinen, M., Warrington, R., & Skuse, D. H. (2009). The construction and validation of a short form of the developmental, diagnostic and dimensional interview. *European Child and Adolescent Psychiatry, 18*, 52–524.

Sattler, J. M. (2008). *Assessment of children: Cognitive applications* (5th ed.). San Diego, CA: Author.

Saulnier, C. A., & Klin, A. (2007). Brief report: Social and communication abilities and disabilities in higher functioning individuals with autism and Asperger syndrome. *Journal of Autism and Developmental Disorders, 37*, 788–793.

Scambler, D., Rogers, S., Wehner, E. (2001) Can the checklist for autism in toddlers differentiate young children with autism from those with developmental delays? *Journal of the American Academy of Child & Adolescent Psychiatry, 40*, 1457–63.

Schopler, E., Van Bourgondien, M. E., Wellman, G. J., & Love, S. R. (2010). *Childhood autism rating scale* (2nd ed.). Los Angeles, CA: Pearson.

Shah, K. (2001). Research in Brief: What do medical students know about autism? *Autism, 15*, 127–133.

Shattuck, P. T. (2006). The contribution of diagnostic substitution to the growing administrative prevalence of autism in US special education. *Pediatrics, 117*, 1028–1037.

Shattuck, P. T., Durkin, M., Maenner, M., Newschaffer, C., Mandell, D. S., Wiggins, L., … Cuniff, C. (2009). Timing of identification among children with an autism spectrum disorder: Findings from a population-based surveillance study. *Journal of the American Academy of Child & Adolescent Psychiatry, 48*, 474–483.

Shattuck, P. T., & Grosse, S. D. (2007). Issues related to the diagnosis and treatment of autism spectrum disorders. *Mental Retardation and Developmental Disabilities Research Reviews, 13*, 129–135.

Siegel, B. (2004). *Pervasive developmental disorders screening test–II (PDDST–II)*. San Antonio, TX: Harcourt Assessment.

Sikora, D. M., Hall, T. A., Hartley, S. L., Gerrard-Morris, A. E., & Cagle, S. (2008). Does parent report of behavior differ across ADOS-G classifications: Analysis of scores from the CBCL and GARS. *Journal of Autism and Developmental Disorders, 38*, 440–448.

Skuse, D. H. (2012). DSM-5's conceptualization of autistic disorders. *Journal of the American Academy of Child and Adolescent Psychiatry, 51*, 344–346.

Skuse, D., Warrington, R., Bishop, D., Chowdhury, U., Lau, J., Mandy, W., & Place, M. (2004). The developmental, dimensional, and diagnostic interview (3di): A novel computerized assessment for autism spectrum disorders. *Journal of the American Academy of Child and Adolescent Psychiatry, 43*, 548–558.

Smith, B., Chung, M. C., & Vostanis, P. (1994). The path to care in autism: Is it better now? *Journal of Autism and Developmental Disorders, 24*, 551–563.

Sparrow, S. S., Cicchetti, D. V., & Balla, D. A. (2006). *Vineland adaptive behavior scale* (2nd ed.). Livonia, MN: Pearson.

Stone, W. L., Coonrod, E. E., & Ousley, O. Y. (2000). Screening tool for autism in two-year-olds (STAT): Development and preliminary data. *Journal of Autism and Developmental Disorders, 30*, 607–612.

Stone, W. L., Lee, E. B., Ashford, L., Brissie, J., Hepburn, S. L., Coonrod, E. E., & Weiss, B. H. (1999). Can autism be diagnosed accurately in children under 3 years? *Journal of Child Psychology and Psychiatry, 40*, 219–226.

Sun, X., & Allison, C. (2009). A review of the prevalence of Autism Spectrum Disorder in Asia. *Research in Autism Spectrum Disorders, 4*, 1561–1567.

Sung, Y., Dawson, G., Munson, J., Estes, A., Schellenberg, G. D., & Wijsman, E. M. (2005). Genetic investigation of quantitative traits related to autism: Use of multivariate polygenic models with ascertainment adjustment. *American Journal of Human Genetics, 76*, 68–81.

Swanson, A. R., Warren, Z. E., Stone, W. L., Vehorn, A. C., Dohrman, E., & Humberd, Q. (2014). The diagnosis of autism in community pediatric settings: Does advanced training facilitate practice change? *Autism, 18*, 555–561.

Swinkels, S. N., Dietz, C., van Daalen, E., Kerkhof, I. M., van Engeland, H., & Buitelaar, J. K. (2006). Screening for autistic spectrum in children aged 14 to 15 months: The development of the early screening of autistic traits questionnaire (ESAT). *Journal of Autism and Developmental Disorders, 36*, 723–732.

Taylor, B., Jick, H., & McLaughlin, D. (2013). Prevalence and incidence rates of autism in the UK: Time trend from 2004–2010 in children aged 8 years. *BMJ Open, 3*, 1–6.

Thoas, K. C., Parish, S. L., Rose, R. A., & Klany, M. (2011). Access to care for children with autism in the context of state Medicaid reimbursement. *Maternal and Child Health Journal, 16*(8), 1636–1644.

Thomas, K. C., Ellis, A. R., McLaurin, C., Daniels, J., & Morrissey, J. (2007). Access to care for autism-related services. *Journal of Autism and Developmental Disorders, 37*(10), 1902–1912.

Thomas, P., Zohorodny, W., Peng, B., Kim, S., Jani, N., Halperin, W., & Brimacombe, M., (2012). The association of autism diagnosis with socioeconomic status. *Autism, 16*, 201–213.

Tolbert, L., Brown, R., Fowler, P., & Parsons, D. (2001). Brief report: Lack of correlation between age of symptom onset and contemporaneous presentation. *Journal of Autism and Developmental Disorders, 31*, 241–245.

Torres, E. B., Brincker, M., Isenhower, R. W., Yanovich, P., Stigler, K. A., Nurnberger, J. I., … Jose, J. V. (2013). Autism: The micro-movement perspective. *Frontiers in Integrative Neuroscience,* 7, 1–32.

Travers, J. C., Tincani, M., & Krezmien, M. P. (2011). A multiyear national profile of racial disparity in autism identification. *Journal of Special Education, 47*, 41–49.

Ventola, P. E., Kleinman, J., Pandey, J., Barton, M., Allen, S., Green, J., … Fein, D. (2006). Agreement among four diagnostic instruments for autism spectrum disorders in toddlers. *Journal of Autism and Developmental Disorders, 36*, 839–847.

Voineagu, I., & Yoo, H. J. (2013). Current progress and challenges in the search for autism biomarkers. *Disease Markers, 35*, 55–65.

Walsh, P., Elsabbagh, M., Bolton, P., & Singh, I. (2011). In search of biomarkers for autism: Scientific, social and ethical challenges. *Nature Reviews Neuroscience, 12*, 603–612.

Wazana, A., Bresnahan, M., & Kline, J. (2007). The autism epidemic: Fact or artifact? *Journal of the American Academy of Child and Adolescent Psychiatry, 46*, 721–730.

Wechsler, D. (2002). *Wechsler preschool and primary scale of intelligence* (3rd ed.). San Antonio, TX: Psychological Corporation.

Wechsler, D. (2003). *Wechsler intelligence scale for children* (4th ed.). San Antonio, TX: Psychological Corporation.

Wetherby, A. M., & Prizant, B. M. (2002). *Communication and symbolic behavior scales developmental profile*. Baltimore, MD: Brookes.

Wetherby, A. M., & Woods, J. (2002). *Systematic evaluation of red flags for autism spectrum disorders in young children*. Tallahassee, FL: Florida State University. Unpublished manual.

Wiggins, L. D., Baio, J., & Rice, C. E. (2006). Examination of the time between first evaluation and first autism spectrum diagnosis in a population-based sample. *Journal of Developmental & Behavioral Pediatrics, 27*, 79–87.

Wiggins, L. D., & Robins, D. L. (2008). Brief report: Excluding the ADI-R behavioral domain improves diagnostic agreement in toddlers. *Journal of Autism and Developmental Disorders, 38*, 972–976.

Williams, J. G., Higgins, J. P. T., & Brayne, C. E. G. (2006). Systematic review of prevalence studies in autism spectrum disorders. *Archives of Disease in Childhood, 91*, 8–15.

Windham, G. C., Smith, K. S., Rosen, N., Anderson, M. C., Gerther, J. K., Coolman, R. B., & Harris. S. (2014). Autism and developmental screening in a public, primary care setting primarily serving Hispanics: Challenges and results. *Journal of Autism and Developmental Disorders,* 44, 1621–1632.

Wing, L., Leekam, S. R., Libby, S. J., Gould, J., & Larcombe, M. (2002). The diagnostic interview for social and communication disorders: Background, inter-rater reliability and clinical use. *Journal of Child Psychology and Psychiatry, 43*, 307–325.

Wing, L., & Potter, D. (2002). The epidemiology of autistic spectrum disorders: Is the prevalence rising? *Mental Retardation and Developmental Disabilities Research Reviews, 8*, 151–161.

Wong, V. C., & Hui, S. L. (2008). Epidemiological study of autism spectrum disorder in China. *Journal of Child Neurology, 23*, 67–72.

Zachary, W., Stone, W., & Humberd, Q. (2009). A training model for the diagnosis of autism in community pediatric practice. *Journal of Developmental and Behavioral Pediatrics, 30*, 442–446.

Chapter 3
Discrete Trial Training

Dorothea C. Lerman, Amber L. Valentino, and Linda A. LeBlanc

Introduction

More than 40 years of research and practice supports the efficacy of Discrete Trial Training (DTT) for remediating the myriad of social, communication, academic, and self-help difficulties that are associated with a diagnosis of autism spectrum disorder (ASD). The term *discrete trial training* originates from the early work of Lovaas (1987) at the University of California—Los Angeles. DTT is a teaching procedure grounded in applied behavior analysis (ABA), but the term also commonly refers to the structured model and curriculum for early intensive behavioral intervention developed by Lovaas, called the UCLA programming model. It is important to note that the terms DTT and the Lovaas or UCLA model are not synonymous. As a teaching procedure, DTT consists of structured learning opportunities that include an antecedent, the learner's response, and a consequence. Taking this framework into account, DTT is often embedded within other approaches to early intervention, such as natural environment teaching and teaching based on verbal behavior taxonomy (i.e., applied verbal behavior; Sundberg & Partington, 1998). Furthermore, early intervention programs that are based on Lovaas' model typically supplement DTT with other ABA-based teaching procedures, such as chaining and incidental teaching (e.g., Fenske, Krantz, & McClannahan, 2001). DTT models focus on establishing early learning repertoires, such as attending and imitation, to facilitate greater fluency in acquisition of all skill sets.

D.C. Lerman (✉)
University of Houston-Clear Lake,
2700 Bay Area Blvd., Campus Box 245, Houston, TX 77058, USA
e-mail: lerman@uhcl.edu

A.L. Valentino • L.A. LeBlanc
Trumpet Behavioral Health, 390 Union Blvd, Suite 300, Lakewood, CO 80228, USA

R. Lang et al. (eds.), *Early Intervention for Young Children with Autism Spectrum Disorder*, Evidence-Based Practices in Behavioral Health,
DOI 10.1007/978-3-319-30925-5_3

Multiple strategies are employed to ensure that the desired behaviors occur under the appropriate stimulus conditions. The goal of this type of programming is to systematically teach the child to respond to language and social stimuli in meaningful ways (e.g., talking, playing).

In this chapter, we focus on DTT as both a teaching procedure and as a model of programming for early intervention. We begin by providing a description of DTT and the characteristic features of DTT programming models. We then describe current research and practice in teaching others to implement DTT, research outcomes for the model, and suggestions for future research.

DTT: Teaching Procedures and Variations

The discrete trial refers to a carefully designed interaction with several critical components: A discriminative stimulus (S^D), a structured prompt sequence as needed, the target behavior, a reinforcer, and an intentionally short interval before the next trial is initiated. The repeated presentation of the S^D with reinforcement for a specific response establishes stimulus control. Thus, in the future, the child will readily respond to that stimulus under naturally occurring conditions. For example, an instructor might present an apple with a prompt "apple" and deliver praise when the child repeats the word apple. Initially, the child will not respond to the presence of the apple by naming it. As a result of the many repeated discrete trials with different apples and with apples in different contexts, the apple begins to exert stimulus control over the child's responses so that he says "apple" when he sees it on a tree, or in a book, or in his kitchen.

Guidelines for implementing DTT procedures published in numerous texts and curriculum manuals over the past 20 years (e.g., Leaf & McEachin, 1999; Lockshin, Gillis, & Romanczyk, 2004; Webber & Scheuermann, 2008) have been drawn largely from the seminal work of Lovaas (1981, 1987). Nonetheless, they also have incorporated some procedural variations based on research findings and clinical experience. In the following sections, we describe commonly recommended components of DTT (e.g., prompt fading, reinforcement, measurement), along with procedural variations and their existing supporting evidence.

Prompt Fading and Error Correction

Prompts are antecedent stimuli that increase the probability of a correct response in the presence of the S^D. Prompts may be combined with the S^D at the start of the discrete trial to ensure that the learner responds without error. In such cases, the prompt must be gradually faded to transfer control from the prompt to the S^D. Prompts also may be delivered as part of an error correction procedure when the learner responds incorrectly or fails to respond to the S^D. The contingent delivery of prompts is intended to evoke the correct response within the same instructional trial and/or to increase the likelihood that the learner will emit the correct response on the next trial. A relatively large number of studies have examined variations of prompt fading and error correction methods.

Research has demonstrated the effectiveness of the most commonly used approaches to fading prompts, including most-to-least prompting (MTL), least-to-most prompting (LTM), graduated guidance, and prompt delay (see MacDuff, Krantz, & McClannahan, 2001, for a review). In general, results of studies comparing these common approaches have resulted in recommendations to use methods that minimize errors. For example, with MTL prompting, the instructor combines the initial S^D with the most intrusive prompt needed to evoke the correct response (e.g., a model prompt). Contingent on correct responding across a certain number of trials, the instructor transitions to less intrusive prompts (e.g., a gesture prompt) until the learner responds correctly in the absence of prompts.

Nonetheless, some recent research suggests that errorless approaches to teaching might lead to overreliance on prompts (Leaf et al., 2014; Libby, Weiss, Bancroft, & Ahearn, 2008). For example, in an interesting variation of MTL, Libby et al. (2008) inserted a 2-s delay between the S^D and prompt to give the subjects an opportunity to respond independently on each trial. Results indicated that this method was just as effective as LTM but was associated with fewer errors.

In addition to these methods, other ways to fade prompts have been described in some texts and curriculum guides. These methods, which include "no-no prompt (NNP)," "flexible prompting," and "simultaneous prompting," have been examined more recently in the literature (e.g., Fentress & Lerman, 2012; Leaf et al., 2013; Leaf, Leaf, Taubman, McEachin, & Delmolino, 2014; Leaf, Sheldon, & Sherman, 2010). With flexible prompting, the therapist does not employ a structured, invariant prompting procedure but instead relies on his or her own judgment about whether to use a prompt on a given trial and, if so, what type of prompt to deliver. The therapist is told to use the least amount of assistance needed while aiming for a high level of success and to provide prompts if the learner has a recent history of making errors with the task (Leaf, Leaf, et al., 2014). Results of several studies indicated that flexible prompting was just as effective in teaching new skills as other more commonly used methods (Leaf, Leaf, et al., 2014; Soluaga, Leaf, Taubman, McEachin, & Leaf, 2008).

With simultaneous prompting, a controlling prompt is always delivered at the same time as the S^D and is not systematically faded across teaching trials. Instead, the learner is periodically given opportunities to exhibit the response independently during "probes" (see Waugh, Alberto, & Fredrick, 2011, for a review). Advantages of this approach are that it does not require the therapist to fade prompts or collect data on performance during instruction (performance is only measured during probes). Although research findings have demonstrated the effectiveness of this approach, results of some comparison studies suggest that other methods may be more successful (e.g., Leaf et al., 2010). NNP is a method of fading in which a prompt is only delivered following two consecutive trials without correct responses. One advantage of this method is that it may reduce the likelihood of prompt dependence. Two studies comparing the effectiveness of this prompt fading method to other methods (simultaneous prompting and MTL prompting) found that learners acquired targeted skills more quickly under the NNP method (Fentress & Lerman, 2012; Leaf et al., 2010). However, Fentress and Lerman further found that skills taught via MTL showed better maintenance than those taught via the NNP procedure.

Instructors also may use a variety of different consequences for errors. These consequences include delivering vocal statements (e.g., saying "no"), withdrawing attention, demonstrating the correct response, and requiring the learner to practice the correct response one or more times (Leaf, Alcalay, et al., 2014; McGhan & Lerman, 2013; Rodgers & Iwata, 1991; Smith, Mruzek, Wheat, & Hughes, 2006; Worsdell et al., 2005). In general, research suggests that all methods can be effective when teaching new skills. Comparisons of different error correction methods have produced inconsistent results but generally have found that strategies that include a response requirement (e.g., learner must practice the correct response one or more times) are more effective than approaches that do not (e.g., providing vocal feedback or demonstrating the correct response).

Reinforcement

Correct responses are followed by brief praise or access to a preferred item. Research has demonstrated the importance of using highly preferred reinforcers during DTT, which are typically identified via systematic preference assessments (e.g., Lang et al., 2014). A procedural variation that may further enhance the effectiveness of DTT is to give the learner opportunities to choose the reinforcer at the moment that it is earned. Reinforcement choice may improve performance by ensuring that the learner receives the most preferred consequence (Sellers et al., 2013) or by reducing the effects of satiation via varied reinforcement (North & Iwata, 2005). Some research findings indicate that choice itself may function as a reinforcer (e.g., Tiger, Hanley, & Hernandez, 2006); in such cases, providing opportunities to choose contingent on responding may enhance the quality or value of the reinforcement contingency (Elliott & Dillenburger, 2014).

A commonly used procedural variation related to the delivery of contingent praise is to refer specifically to the targeted behavior in the praise statement (e.g., "Nice job pointing to the cup!" rather than "Nice job!"). Despite the ubiquity of this recommended variation, few studies have directly examined the benefits of using descriptive (or behavior-specific) versus general praise statements. Furthermore, research findings thus far have not revealed consistent, sustainable, or notable differences in acquisition with these two forms of praise (Polick, Carr, & Hanney, 2012; Stevens, Sidner, Reeve, & Sidener, 2011). As discussed by Polick et al., specific praise may be beneficial for certain individuals (e.g., those with good intraverbal repertoires), suggesting that further research is warranted.

A useful strategy for reducing prompt dependency is to provide differential consequences following prompted versus unprompted responses. Although the use of differential reinforcement is commonly recommended in texts and curriculum guides on DTT, only a handful of studies have examined procedural variations of this approach. Research findings indicate that providing a denser reinforcement schedule (Hausman, Ingvarsson, & Kahng, 2014; Olendick & Pear, 1980; Touchette & Howard, 1984) or higher quality reinforcers (Cividini-Motta & Ahearn, 2013; Karsten & Carr, 2009) for unprompted responses relative to that for prompted responses will enhance acquisition. Furthermore, it appears that acquisition may occur more rapidly for some learners if reinforcement is completely withheld following prompted responses.

Task Interspersal

A common practice is to alternate among two or more instructional targets during teaching sessions with a learner. A number of studies have examined different ways to arrange instructional trials within teaching sessions (Chiara, Schuster, Bell, & Wolery, 1995; Dunlap, 1984; Majdalany, Wilder, Greif, Mathisen, & Saini, 2014; Volkert, Lerman, Trosclair, Addison, & Kodak, 2008). Research findings suggest that learners may acquire skills more quickly when the therapist presents S^Ds for several different targets (e.g., "stand up," "Point to green," "What animal goes 'moo'?") rather than for the same target (e.g., "Point to green.") across consecutive instructional trials (e.g., Chiara et al.; Dunlap). Authors have speculated that task interspersal procedures improve performance by functioning as a motivational operation (MO). However, studies in which unknown targets were alternated with known targets have produced inconsistent findings (see Benavides & Poulson, 2009; Charlop, Kurtz, & Milstein, 1992; Dunlap, 1984; Majdalany et al., 2014; Volkert et al., 2008). As such, the conditions under which task interspersal procedures are beneficial have not yet been delineated and warrant further study. A somewhat different approach to task interspersal is to alter the instructional context by incorporating game-related stimuli (and reinforcers) into DTT. In Geiger et al. (2012), for example, the therapist taught one subject receptive object labels within the context of a train activity. The subject had access to the train activity materials for 30 s. The therapist removed the materials, presented a learning trial with stimuli (attached to pieces of the train track), and provided access to (the additional piece of train track) for 30 s contingent on a correct response. (Another child learned receptive discriminations by jumping to the correct stimulus in a 3-item array that were pasted into a Twister® mat.) Results of a subsequent preference assessment indicated that the (each child preferred their game-based) learning arrangement to a more traditional DTT format conducted at the table in a traditional format.

Intertrial Interval (ITI)

A pause between instructional trials provides a clear demarcation point between the end of a trial and the beginning of the next trial. The length of this ITI may impact performance. For this reason, it is commonly recommended to deliver instructional trials at a rapid pace during DTT. Research findings have shown that acquisition is enhanced with short (e.g., 2-s to 3-s) versus long (e.g., 10-s to 20-s) it is (e.g., Koegel, Dunlap, & Dyer, 1980; Majdalany et al., 2014). Some research, however, also suggests advantages to presenting additional instructional stimuli during ITIs (e.g., Loughrey, Betz, Majdalany, & Nicholson, 2014; Reichow & Wolery, 2011; Vladescu & Kodak, 2013). With this approach, the therapist inserts supplementary information immediately prior to or following instructional trials, with no response required of the learner. The additional stimuli (sometimes called secondary targets) may be related or unrelated to the primary targets (e.g., stating, "Dog have tails," after asking the learner to point to the picture of a dog versus asking the learner to point to the letter "A"). This approach appears to enhance acquisition of the secondary targets without compromising progress on the primary targets. Studies have shown that some learners with autism will acquire the secondary targets either prior to or simultaneously with the primary targets (Reichow & Wolery, 2011; Vladescu & Kodak, 2013). The conditions under which learners will acquire supplementary information in the absence of direct training are unclear, but Vladescu and Kodak noted that their subjects tended to echo (i.e., vocally imitate) the secondary stimuli presented by the therapist. Further research is needed to determine if a strong echoic repertoire is a necessary pre-requisite for learning in this instructional context.

Individual Versus Group Format

DTT is typically conducted within the context of individualized (i.e., one-on-one) instruction. Nonetheless, a number of studies have demonstrated successful learning outcomes when DTT was embedded within a group instruction format (e.g., Leaf et al., 2013; Taubman et al., 2001). In Taubman et al., for example, a teacher delivered the S^D to multiple children who were expected to respond simultaneously. During other lessons, the teacher delivered the instructional trials sequentially across children. Results showed successful acquisition of targets via the group instructional approach. Leaf et al. (2013) directly compared individual versus group instruction formats for six children with autism. The instructor delivered instructional trials sequentially across three children during the group instruction format. Results not only showed that the group format was as effective as individual instruction for teaching new skills, but the children learned some of the targets that had been delivered to other children in the group.

Conditional Discriminations

A large portion of instruction during DTT is devoted to teaching conditional discriminations, in which the correct response in the presence of the S^D depends on the stimulus context. These discriminations are typically taught within the context of match-to-sample tasks. For example, suppose the therapist is teaching a child to discriminate among red, blue, and green. The therapist might present stimuli of each color to the child and state, "Point to blue." In the presence of the blue stimulus, pointing to the blue stimulus is correct only if the therapist has stated, "Point to blue." Curriculum manuals and guides recommend two approaches for teaching this type of auditory-visual discrimination. In one approach (called the "simple-conditional method"), the therapist first targets simple discriminations, in which the learner is taught to respond one stimulus only (e.g., point to blue). The other discriminations (e.g., red and green) are successively introduced, and the learner is then required to respond to each of the stimuli based on the auditory stimulus presented by the therapist. In the other approach (called the "conditional-only method"), the learner is taught all relations simultaneously from the outset of instruction. Results of several recent studies suggest that the conditional-only method is more effective and efficient than the simple-conditional approach (e.g., Grow, Carr, Kodak, Jostad, & Kisamore, 2011; Grow, Kodak, & Carr, 2014). A more detailed overview of instructional strategies for teaching simple and conditional discriminations can be found in Grow and LeBlanc (2013).

Generalization

Ensuring that newly taught skills generalize across relevant responses and contexts (e.g., in different settings and with different people, instructions, and materials) is a critical component of DTT. One of the most common approaches for promoting generalization is to include multiple exemplars in training. The instructor might (a) arrange for different people to deliver the SD (e.g., different instructors, caregivers), (b) present the S^D in multiple locations (e.g., classroom, lunchroom), (c) vary the wording of the S^D (e.g., "Touch green." "Show me green."), and (d) present different stimulus materials (e.g., different sized letters, different colored objects). Research on the multiple exemplar strategy indicates two primary approaches: (a) introducing each new exemplar in a sequential fashion, waiting until the learner demonstrates mastery with an exemplar before introducing the next (often called "serial training"), or (b) teaching multiple new exemplars at a time to the learner (often called "concurrent training"). Both approaches continue until the learner demonstrates generalization across untrained exemplars. Although research findings suggest that both procedural variations lead to the acquisition and generalization of skills, results of several studies indicate that the concurrent training approach may promote generalization more efficiently and effectively for some learners (Schroeder, Schuster, & Hemmeter, 1998; Wunderlich, Vollmer, Donaldson, & Phillips, 2014).

Other approaches for promoting the likelihood of generalization include (a) incorporating materials, situations, and other stimuli from the child's natural environment into training, (b) teaching responses that are likely to contact reinforcement in non-training settings, (c) thinning the schedule of reinforcement in the training setting, and (d) recruiting caregivers and others to prompt and reinforce targeted responses in non-training settings (Stokes & Baer, 1977).

Measurement

Monitoring a learner's progress through trial-based recording of performance is a hallmark of DTT. The authors of many curriculum manuals and guides recommend that therapists record the outcome of every learning trial, summarize performance across blocks of learning trials, and examine the data frequently to make decisions about learner progress and potential program changes. An alternative to this labor-intensive approach to measurement, called continuous recording, is to record learner performance on just a subset of trials or instructional sessions. When using discontinuous recording, the therapist might record the outcome of the first trial, the first three trials, or the first five trials of instructional sessions that consist of nine to ten trials. Despite the potential ease of sampling in this manner, obtaining less data may alter the accuracy or sensitivity of measurement. Results of several studies comparing continuous and discontinuous recording during DTT suggest that the possible benefits of discontinuous recording (in terms of ease and efficiency) may not outweigh the costs (Carey & Bourret, 2014; Cummings & Carr, 2009; Lerman, Dittlinger, Fentress, & Lanagan, 2011; Najdowski et al., 2009; Taubman, Leaf, McEachin, Papovich, & Leaf, 2013). For example, data collected on just a subset of trials may lead therapists to conclude prematurely that a learner has mastered a skill and may be less sensitive to changes in performance (Carey & Bourret, 2014; Lerman et al., 2011). Furthermore, Taubman et al. (2013) found that continuous and discontinuous recording methods required nearly the same amount of therapists' time.

The DTT Programming Model

Many behavioral programs involve similar trial components (i.e., specific antecedent, behavior, and consequence) because the three-term contingency (A-B-C) represents the critical behavioral learning unit. However, DTT programming is typically more structured in the presentations of the trials and the specifics of the prompting sequence, more rapidly paced, and more contrived in the initial learning environment which typically has been stripped of most distracting stimuli. Three critical features of DTT programming likely account for the dramatic and potentially developmental trajectory altering effects for children with autism. First, DTT is initially conducted in a distraction-free environment to promote attending. Second, DTT programs focus heavily on "learning to learn" repertoires that accelerate acquisition in subsequent programming. Third, the DTT programming model emphasizes intensive intervention with teaching occurring across a great number of hours (e.g., 25–40 per week) and with a great density of learning units in each of those hours.

Distraction Free Environment

DTT is typically presented in a distraction free environment to increase the likelihood that the child with autism attends to the teacher and S^D. The distraction free environment is most important for young children who have not yet learned to attend to people or items in a sustained fashion, which is a critical pre-requisite skill for learning. Initial sessions often occur at a small table or with the adult and child sitting face-to-face in chairs. Items such as pictures, posters, toys, television, computers, or other distracting and preferred stimuli are removed from the instructional area. As the child develops attending skills and basic compliance and direction-following skills, teaching begins to occur across settings in more natural contexts to facilitate generalization of newly learned skills.

Structured Curriculum

Typically, a structured curriculum is used as a basis for building the instructional objectives for a DTT program. Commonly used published curricula include those by Leaf and McEachin (1999), Lovaas (2002), Maurice, Green, and Luce (1996), and Sundberg and Partington (1998). These curricula describe the basics of the intervention approach, the specific components of programming, and the progression of skills targeted throughout multi-year intervention efforts (i.e., the curriculum). Initial teaching efforts focus on establishing critical learning repertoires that will facilitate acquisition of later skills and accelerate developmental progress. Children learn to attend, to imitate sounds and movements, to match objects and pictures, and to comply with basic directions. The discriminations become progressively more complex (e.g., two-step directions, three-step directions) and expand to encompass an array of spoken language (e.g., requests, labeling, asking and answering questions), social and play skills (e.g., functional play, parallel play, interactive play, sharing, initiating) and adaptive targets (e.g., toileting skills, self-feeding, dressing) appropriate for children aged 2–6 years. The curriculum is hierarchical in that early skills must be mastered before moving up the hierarchy to later, more difficult skills.

Trials and Intensity of Intervention

The pace of instruction in DTT is typically brisk, particularly for early learners who may have difficulty attending for extended periods of time. An individual trial may last for approximately 5–30 s depending on the targeted skill and the level of prompting required to produce the response. The goal is to have many trials of a specific type of program (i.e., receptive identification) within just a few minutes so that the learner experiences potentially 1000 s of trials across all program types throughout the day almost every day. This volume of learning opportunities actually approximates the number that a typically developing toddler or preschooler might experience in a given day with a difference that the typically developing toddler is often initiating those learning opportunities and readily learning from events happening in their environment without the need for such explicit instruction. Intervention typically occurs at this level of intensity for 1–2 years with an additional year of programming that may occur at lower intensity (e.g., few hours per week, no longer 1–1 ratio) and in natural environments such as preschool or center-based settings.

The critical features described above are common in DTT programs. However, the specific instructional programs and procedures may vary as they are individualized to the learner. A team of professionals typically work together to coordinate and implement programming. For example, the child may work directly with several different instructors for multiple hours per week. This allows for generalization programming so that new skills are more likely to occur in interactions with a wide variety of people. These direct intervention services are overseen by a professional with a higher level of education and credentialing (i.e., Board Certified Behavior Analyst) who creates the programming, assess progress, and develops intervention plans for problematic behavior. This approach to intervention with children with ASD has a substantial evidence base to support the consistent positive effects that are produced when implemented at an early age and at a high level of intensity and duration (see Outcomes Research section below). The following section provides general information to guide a new practitioner through the critical steps for implementing a DTT program effectively.

Guidelines for Implementing the DTT Programming Model

Most curricula and resource manuals for DTT provide information about establishing and monitoring the progress in programs (Leaf & McEachin, 1999; Lovaas, 2002; Maurice, 1994; Maurice et al., 1996). The fact that entire books are devoted to this task is a clear indication that the brief description provided here is only a starting point for those who actually intend to implement this type of programming. Although not detailed enough for a stand-alone resource, this section is designed to provide the process and major milestones for program implementation along with direction to more complete resources for each step.

Starting the DTT Program and Services

Establishing DTT services requires several critical preparatory and preliminary steps. First, families should be oriented to basic information about DTT programming and the evidence regarding effectiveness (i.e., the information provided in sections above and below). This orientation is a critical part of rapport building and should occur in a supportive manner given the stressful and painful context of a newly delivered diagnosis of an ASD for the family. The orientation to services might include a live discussion, provision of reading materials, or a visit to a center-based program to see ongoing services for other children. Consider written materials such as *Right From the Start: Behavioral Intervention for Young Children with Autism* (*2nd Edition*) (Harris & Weiss, 2007) and *Making a Difference: Behavioral Intervention for Autism* (Maurice, Green, & Foxx, 2001), as these materials are family friendly. The orientation should cover the basic expectations about DTT programs (e.g., intensity, location and frequency of sessions, parental involvement in selection of targets and implementation of programming, structure and responsibilities of the treatment team). It may also be useful to provide general information about autism and adjusting to having a child with special needs such as *A Practical Guide to Autism: What Every Family Member, Teacher and Professional Needs to Know* (Volkmar & Wiesner, 2009) or *Children with Autism: A Parent's Guide* (*2nd Edition*) (Powers, 2001).

Second, the instructors and supervising behavior analysts should establish rapport with the child and establish themselves and a wide range of leisure items as highly preferred. This process is often referred to as "pairing" and typically involves conducting preference assessments, engaging in highly preferred play activities with the child, and minimizing instructional demands for the first sessions. Once the treatment team has been paired sufficiently with positive experiences, the child will likely readily approach instructors and willingly interact with them. Instructional demands are gradually introduced and interspersed with ongoing pairing activities to ensure a rich and positive interaction schedule. Many of the first demands that are presented are designed to assess the child's existing skills and deficits with respect to a previously chosen curriculum of programming. The results of these assessment activities are used to select a reasonable array of programs. It is important to distinguish between the term "program" when used to refer to the comprehensive program, which includes all of the tasks, goals and objectives included in an entire DTT program, versus a specific program, which includes a specific goal within the overall comprehensive program. For the purpose of this chapter, the term "program" will be used to refer to the comprehensive program, whereas "specific program" will be used to refer to the specific goals and objectives included in the comprehensive program (e.g., receptive body parts). Many early specific programs and incidental teaching interactions are designed to establish a readiness repertoire (e.g., sitting for a brief period, looking at an adult or items, following simple directions) for more structured programming. The family may be involved in services from the very beginning by participating in pairing sessions and providing information about preferred items and activities.

The next critical step in a successful program is establishing a partnership between the family and the provider team. Participation and input from the family is recruited to establish goals for programming and important behavioral needs (e.g., problem behavior, food selectivity, sleep problems, safety issues). An initial parent interview can be helpful in learning information about environmental determinants of problem behavior, the family's short- and long-term goals for the child, and the behaviors that the family sees as most important and relevant. For example, the behavior analyst might assess skills and determine that a child has receptive language deficits and minimal direction following skills. The behavior analysis would then create a specific program to teach the child to learn the names of common objects (i.e., receptive identification of objects, listener responding) and follow simple directions. The family plays a important role in determining the specific items to target based on information that the family eats a variety of fruit and that they would like their child to be able to "go get a banana" for his snack when asked to do so. Thus, the family provides suggestions and priorities that inform the comprehensive program and enhance its relevance for their lives. The next section will focus on the components and structure of an effective DTT program.

Programs and Targets

The comprehensive program is developed based on the specific curricular assessment conducted, clinical judgment, the current level of the child's functioning, and parental input. Once a specific program is established, individual items, often called "treatment targets," are selected that will serve as the primary focus of intervention. For example, an overall specific program may be "receptive identification of body parts" whereas the treatment targets might be "nose," "head" and "ears." Treatment targets often change as the child masters them until a pre-determined overall goal is met (e.g., the child can receptively identify at least 12 body parts on self, others and in pictures).

The number of specific programs and number of targets in a comprehensive DTT program might vary significantly based on the language level of the learner, number of intervention hours per week, and family goals and priorities. For example, a very early learner may have only three specific programs (e.g., requesting, eye contact, and receptive instructions) with two to three targets in place for each of the programs (e.g., request ball and juice, respond to "sit down," and "clap"). In contrast, a more advanced learner may have 15 or more specific programs across language, social, play, and adaptive skill domains with many targets in each specific program. Generally, the age of the child, number of intervention hours, and type of program (i.e., comprehensive vs. focused) will be important factors guiding decisions about the number of programs and targets within those programs.

Components of the Specific Instructional Program

Each specific instructional program may vary across learner, but a quality DTT program contains the following components: A clear purpose and rationale, a list of needed materials, and a precise procedural description, including specific S^D, description of the target response and acceptable variations, a description of prompts and criteria for fading prompts, reinforcers, and error correction procedures. A quality specific program also includes instructions on target interspersal and target rotation, data collection, and mastery and generalization criteria. For a sample specific program for receptive body parts, see appendix A.

Analysis of Progress and Program Modification

Once specific programs and targets are selected and implementation has begun, the focus shifts to analyzing the learner's progress and making modifications as necessary to ensure optimal efficiency of learning. Data on the learner's behavior must be graphed and analyzed regularly to accomplish this. These data are used to evaluate the effectiveness of a specific program. Consideration may be given to the following points of measurement: At least 80 % of active programs should have multiple targets mastered, the consumer should master a reasonable number of targets every 2–4 weeks ("reasonable" should be based on a consumer's age, number of service hours, and type of service/programming), and the number of trials or probes to criterion for consecutive targets in a program should follow a low stable or decreasing trend. Additionally, mastered targets should maintain over time, or are reintroduced to active status with a maintenance programming component.

As the data are analyzed, complete programs will become mastered and replaced with new ones. The overarching goal is to teach children a variety of language, motor, and adaptive skills to ensure they exhibit skills consistent with those exhibited by same-age peers. A strong focus on generalization of skills in naturally occurring situations is imperative.

Facilitating and Evaluating Progress Towards Socially Meaningful Outcomes

As a child acquires skills in DTT, generalization becomes an important focus of programming. It is important to continuously program for and evaluate both stimulus and response generalization in DTT. This can be an important indicator of both the effectiveness of and necessity for ongoing intervention. Various strategies for promoting generalization, as described above, are embedded into DTT, and a consumer's entire comprehensive program may focus completely on generalization activities.

As stimulus and response generalization occurs, it is important to both assess and facilitate the readiness of the natural environment to sustain treatment gains. For example, a child may have acquired the skill of greeting his peers and due to DTT; he has generalized that skill to use it in the school environment, home environment, at the park and with a variety of peers. An important element of ensuring this skill is sustainable over time is that the individuals in his natural environment will provide appropriate and natural consequences that will maintain this skill over time. That is, just because a child can greet his peers in these situations, does not necessarily mean that when he does so; the natural contingencies of greeting one's peers will maintain responding. It may be important to examine the child's environment and determine any refinement of that skill to ensure the natural contingencies ultimately maintain responding.

As critical repertoires develop, another important consideration is transition into the next environment. This next environment will differ greatly depending on the age and overall functioning of the learner. For example, a small child may need to focus on kindergarten readiness skills, whereas an older child may need to focus on self help and adaptive skills to transition into an independent living situation. An important part of DTT is identifying and specifically planning for the repertoires that will be necessary for success, no matter what the next environment will be. In order to adequately plan for the transition, asking the following questions may prove helpful: first, what do other individuals in this environment do? That is, what are the repertoires that make others successful in the environment? For example, a child in kindergarten may be expected to recite the alphabet, socialize on the playground and sit in a group setting for a period of time. In this case, ensuring the individual with a disability can engage in these behaviors in a similar manner is crucial for success in that new environment. Second, what are the critical behaviors the environment requires for participation? For example, a group home might require independence with dressing or a classroom may require self-initiation of toileting. These behaviors should be specifically incorporated into DTT prior to transition into the new environment to ensure ultimate success.

Teaching Others to Implement DTT

Research findings indicate that therapists with diverse backgrounds and levels of expertise can learn to implement DTT, generalize those skills across learners and targets, and maintain these skills over time. Learner performance, in terms of both acquisition of skills and levels of disruptive behavior, are directly related to the integrity of DTT procedures (e.g., Dib & Sturmey, 2007; Reed, Reed, Baez, & Maguire, 2011). DTT should not be implemented exclusively by specialized behavioral therapists but also by parents, teachers, and any other care providers who are responsible for the social, educational, and behavioral development of the child. The majority of studies showing good outcomes with DTT have included a caregiver training component (see next section below), and results of some studies suggest that DTT outcomes may be similar regardless of whether parents or trained professionals serve as the children's primary therapist (e.g., Sallows & Graupner, 2005). In the following sections, we describe the components of effective staff and caregiver training, along with research findings on alternative modalities for improving the efficiency, accessibility, and cost of training (see also Thomson, Martin, Arnal, Fazzio, & Yu, 2009, for a review).

Behavioral Skills Training

Behavioral skills training (BST), the most commonly used evidence-based approach to training DTT skills, is an explicit, active-response training procedure that involves four critical components—instructions, modeling, rehearsal and feedback (Miltenberger, 2003). Trainers use performance-based criteria to determine when the trainee has mastered the skills. For example, training may continue until the trainee performs the DTT procedures with at least 90 % accuracy across three consecutive practice sessions. Results of numerous studies have shown that BST is highly effective for teaching DTT to teachers, parents, and other staff (e.g., Dib & Sturmey, 2007; Lafasakis & Sturmey, 2007; Lerman, Tetreault, Hovanetz, Strobel, & Garro, 2008; Sarokoff & Sturmey, 2004). Training typically begins with spoken and written instructions that delineate the components of DTT. The next step of BST, modeling, is implemented live or through video and might include examples of both correct and incorrect applications of the procedures and demonstrations of DTT with multiple learner targets. Modeling also might be provided immediately after the trainee has had an opportunity to rehearse (practice), and the trainer demonstrates DTT components that were performed incorrectly by the trainee (e.g., Lafasakis & Sturmey, 2007; Sarokoff & Sturmey, 2004). The rehearsal (practice) with feedback phase may be accomplished through role play with the trainer, through actual teaching sessions with the learner, or both. Practice should include multiple targets and materials to promote generalization of the DTT skills (Ducharme & Feldman, 1992). Feedback typically consists of vocal statements describing DTT components implemented correctly and incorrectly, along with suggestions for correcting implementation errors. Practice with feedback continues until the trainees implement DTT with a high degree of accuracy. However, trainees must continue to receive specific feedback about their performance (McKenney & Bristol, 2015), combined with praise that is contingent upon aspects of DTT implementation, to improve and maintain performance over time (Alvero, Bucklin, & Austin, 2001; Komaki, Desselles, & Bowman, 1989).

A few supplemental procedures have been evaluated for enhancing the effectiveness of BST when teaching DTT skills to others. In May, Austin, and Dymond (2011), for example, therapists engaged in higher levels of accurate responding when BST was combined with stimulus prompts. The prompts consisted of cards listing the learner's targets along with a laminated board showing the differential responses of the therapist for all possible learner responses on each trial. The therapists were taught to place each card in the corresponding section on the laminated board based on the learner's response to the S^D. Thomas (2013) found that DTT implementation of paraprofessionals improved after they were taught to observe and score the accuracy of their peers' teaching sessions.

Alternative Modalities

BST is often considered the gold standard for training others to implement behavioral interventions. However, this approach can be fairly expensive and time-consuming, and it requires the availability of experts to provide the training. Training efficiency is particularly important in settings with high therapist turn-over or when large groups of individuals need to be trained. In some rural or remote areas, experts are not readily available to provide training on DTT. As such, some investigators have developed alternative training modalities to enhance the efficiency, cost, or availability of BST. These approaches vary in terms of the extent to which they incorporate the components of BST.

Training modalities that might eliminate the need for live trainers, including written manuals, videos, and computer-based instruction, have been evaluated in a number of studies on DTT. For example, Thiessen et al. (2009) developed a 37-page manual that provided comprehensive written instructions on (a) the basic principles of applied behavior analysis, (b) preparation for an instructional sessions, (c) antecedents and consequences for correct responses, (d) antecedents and consequences for incorrect responses, and (e) prompt fading. The trainees, undergraduate students, were required to complete a knowledge test after reading each unit in the manual and answer all of the questions correctly before proceeding to the next unit. The manual also instructed trainees to imagine conducting DTT with a child using the components covered in the unit and to evaluate their self-practice via a rating form. After completing the training manual, the trainees demonstrated high levels of procedural integrity when conducting DTT in role play with an experimenter, although integrity decreased somewhat when the trainee implemented DTT with a child with autism. Trainees required 2–5 h to master the manual.

In a subsequent study, Thomson et al. (2012) evaluated the outcomes of the same instructional manual with newly hired tutors providing in-home DTT programs for children with autism. After completing the manual, tutors who did not implement DTT with 80 % accuracy (the mastery criterion) during role play with the experimenter watched a 17-min video that reviewed the information contained in the manual and showed an expert implementing DTT with a child. Five of the eight tutors required the video component following the self-instructional manual and met the mastery criterion after watching the video. Less promising outcomes were obtained when the instructional manual and video were used with parents (Young, Boris, Thomson, Martin, & Yu, 2012). All but one of the five parents required the video component, and two of the parents did not meet the mastery criterion after completing the self-instructional manual and watching the video. In a second experiment, Young et al. replaced the self-practice component of the manual with role play plus feedback. This substitution improved the overall outcomes for the parents, but it required the availability of a trainer. Together, these results suggest that written instructions alone may not be a viable substitute for live BST. However, for some individuals, the addition of video models may be a useful supplement to written instructional manuals.

Results of several studies suggest video instruction alone may eliminate the need for live trainers. In these studies, video modeling with voiceovers that described the critical components of DTT was effective for teaching direct service staff to implement DTT with a high degree of integrity during role play with the experimenter (Catania, Almeida, Liu-Constant, & Digennaro, 2009) and during teaching sessions with children (Vladescu, Carroll, Paden, & Kodak, 2012).

Similar to written manuals, computer-based instruction is designed to eliminate the need for individualized trainers. However, use of the computer permits the inclusion of the modeling component of BST via videos. Nosik, Williams, Garrido, and Lee (2013) compared the outcomes of live BST to computer-based training for direct care staff in a day program for adults. The computer-based instruction included written text, videos, and quizzes with feedback. Results showed that the subjects who received BST implemented DTT with a higher degree of procedural integrity immediately following training and at a 6-week follow up than those who received computer-based instruction. Using a similar computer-based instruction program Pollard, Higbee, Akers, and Brodhead (2014) obtained promising results with four college students who had no prior DTT experience. Three of the four participants met the mastery criterion immediately after completing the training modules and then generalized their teaching skills to a young child with autism. The third participant showed an immediate improvement in performance after receiving a single performance feedback session.

Lack of rehearsal (i.e., hands-on practice with feedback) that is a typical component of BST may compromise the effectiveness of computer-based instruction. If so, one way to improve the outcomes of computer-based instruction would be to incorporate a performance-based component via interactive simulation software. A tested version of this software, called DTkid, permits the trainee to simulate teaching sessions with a child while receiving real-time feedback on performance or an evaluative summary on procedural integrity at the conclusion of the teaching session (Eldevik et al., 2013; Randall, Hall, Bizo, & Remington, 2007). Preliminary research on DTkid suggests that this may be a promising self-instructional approach, but further research is needed.

Another potential approach for increasing the accessibility of staff and caregiver training is to provide BST through videoconferencing. Although this modality does not eliminate the need for live trainers, it may be helpful for reaching individuals who reside far from qualified trainers. Videoconferencing requires access to the internet, a computer, web camera, and conferencing software (e.g., Skype, MoviTM-client). Research suggests videoconferencing is a promising approach for teaching staff and caregivers to implement behavioral assessments and interventions (e.g., Vismara, Young, Stahmer, Griffith, & Rogers, 2009; Wacker et al., 2013a, 2013b).

In one of the few studies to evaluate this modality for teaching DTT, Hay-Hansson and Eldevik (2013) found no differences in the performance of school staff who were taught via live BST versus videoconferencing.

DTT Intervention Research: Large-Scale Outcomes

The landmark study that investigated the effectiveness of DTT with children with autism was conducted by Lovaas (1987). Results of this study are often cited and recognized as the first demonstration that EIBI focused on DTT is highly effective in producing positive outcomes for this population. Specifically, 47 % of the children in the Lovaas study were placed in general education, obtained an average increase in IQ score of 37 points, and had substantial decreases in symptoms of autism. In significant contrast, only 2 % of the control-group children achieved normal educational and intellectual functioning (the remaining were placed in language delayed classes or special classrooms for autism and/or mental retardation).

Since 2000, many researchers have compared the effects obtained with DTT (typically at least 25 h per week of intervention) with those obtained by other non-behavioral (i.e., "eclectic" or "treatment as usual") interventions, with lesser intense DTT models (typically less than 15 h per week), and with no treatment at all. This literature can be categorized into two main areas. First, studies have compared DTT to some other approach, often termed a control group, that either consists of an eclectic approach, no treatment at all, or treatment as usual. The second area includes meta-analyses or systematic reviews in which researchers reviewed and summarized multiple studies to examine the overall effects of DTT.

For the purpose of this chapter, only studies that clearly focused on DTT were included. Although much of the literature on early intensive behavioral intervention (EIBI) includes DTT in some regard, studies were excluded in this review if other approaches were utilized (e.g., Early Start Denver Model, pivotal response training, natural environment teaching, incidental teaching, etc.) either in addition to or in place of DTT. We did not exclude comparisons to these models but excluded any studies that appeared to use these approaches in place of DTT. It should be noted that the terms "early intensive behavioral intervention," "discrete trial teaching," "ABA," the Lovaas method," and "the UCLA model" are often used interchangeably in the literature. However, only studies that focused on structured DTT, as described in this chapter, are included in this review. Studies that did not include a control or comparison group and those that focused on children with disabilities other than autism also were excluded. Although many studies have examined the overall effectiveness of DTT without the use of control groups, these are best reviewed separately (see LeBlanc, Parks, & Hanney, 2014, for a complete review of these studies published between 2000 and 2012).

Two tables are provided to summarize this extensive body of literature (Table 3.1: comparison outcome studies; Table 3.2: meta-analyses and systematic reviews).

Table 3.1 Comparison outcome studies

Authors	Title	Year	Type of article	Purpose	Participant groups	Dependent variables	Summary of findings
Eikeseth, Klintwall, Jahr, Karlsson	Outcome for children with autism receiving early and intensive behavioral intervention in mainstream preschool and kindergarten settings	2012	Comparison outcomes study	To compare DTT group with TAU on adaptive functioning and autism symptoms	35 DTT (23 h/week)	Adaptive	DTT achieved higher scores in adaptive functioning and reduced autism symptoms
					24 TAU	Autism symptoms	No significant difference on adaptive skills or symptoms in TAU group
Eldevik, Hastings, Jahr, and Hughes	Outcomes of behavioral interventions for children with autism in mainstream pre-school settings	2012	Comparison outcomes study	To compare scores on intellectual and adaptive functioning between DTT group and TAU group	31 DTT (13.6 h/week)	Intellect	DTT significantly greater outcomes on intellect and adaptive skills
					12 TAU (eclectic; 5 h/week)	Adaptive	No significant change in IQ or symptoms for control group
Flanagan, Perry and Freeman	Effectiveness of large-scale community-based intensive behavioral intervention: a waitlist comparison study exploring outcomes and predictors	2012	Retrospective outcome comparison study	To compare DTT to treatment waitlist on intellectual functioning, adaptive skills, and symptoms	61 DTT (25.8 h/week)	Intellect	DTT group achieved significantly higher intellectual and adaptive functioning, showed less autism symptoms
					61 no treatment control	Adaptive Autism symptoms	No significant change in IQ, adaptive skills or symptoms for control group

(continued)

Table 3.1 (continued)

Authors	Title	Year	Type of article	Purpose	Participant groups	Dependent variables	Summary of findings
Strauss, Vicari, Valeri, D'Elia, Arima and Fava	Parent inclusion in early intensive behavioral intervention: the influence of parental stress, parent treatment fidelity and parent mediated generalization of behavior targets on child outcomes	2012	Comparison Outcomes study	To compare DTT with eclectic approach on IQ, language, autism severity	24 DTT (35 h/week)	Intellect	DTT achieved higher IQ scores, language and less symptom severity
					20 eclectic (12 h/week)	Language	Both groups made significant gains in adaptive behavior and receptive language
						Autism severity	
						Adaptive	Parents in the eclectic group had significant stress reduction; DTT group parents had not change in stress reduction
						Parental stress	
Fava, Strauss, Valeri, D'Elia, Arima and Vicari	The effectiveness of a cross-setting complementary staff and parent mediated early intensive behavioral intervention for young children with ASD	2011	Comparison outcomes study	To evaluate the effects of DTT and eclectic approach intellectual functioning, autism symptoms and problem behavior	12 DTT (14 h/week)	Intellect	DTT significant increases in intellectual functioning and significant decreases in autism symptoms and problem behavior
					10 eclectic (12 h/week)	Autism symptoms	Eclectic group no significant change in behavior, symptoms and IQ scores
						Problem behavior	

Downs, Downs, Fossum and Rau	Effectiveness of discrete trial teaching with preschool students with developmental disabilities	2008	Longitudinal Comparison Outcome study	Evaluate effects of two levels of DTT on	3 (1 year of three 10–15 min DTT sessions/day)	Communication	Participants acquired more skills and learned more quickly when DTT was provided in one longer session
					3 (1 year of three 30–45 min DTT sessions/day)	Motor skills	
						Language	
						Social	
						Adaptive	
						Cognitive	
Ben-Itzchak, Lahat, Burgin, and Zavhor	Cognitive, behavior and intervention outcome in young children with autism	2008	Comparison Outcome study	Evaluate effects of DTT on IQ and to determine effects of initial cognitive level on outcomes	44 DTT (45 h/week)	Intellect	Greater IQ gains in DTT group after 1 year of treatment; pre-cognitive levels did not predict changes in symptoms
					37 TAU		TAU did not show significant changes in IQ scores
Eikeseth, Smith, Jahr and Eldevik	Outcome for children with autism who began intensive behavioral treatment between ages 4 and 7: a comparison controlled study	2007	Comparison Outcome study	To compare DTT vs. eclectic intervention on IQ, adaptive functioning and social and behavioral problems	13 DTT (28 h/week)	IQ	Significantly greater improvements in IQ and adaptive skills in DTT group
						Adaptive	Less social and behavior problems in DTT group
					12 eclectic (29.1 h/week)	Social	No significant improvements in any area for eclectic group
						Behavior	

(continued)

Table 3.1 (continued)

Authors	Title	Year	Type of article	Purpose	Participant groups	Dependent variables	Summary of findings
Magiati, Charman and Howlin	A 2-year prospective follow-up study of community based early intervention and specialist nursery provision for children with autism spectrum disorders	2007	Prospective comparison outcome study	To compare DTT with autism-specific nursery services on intellect, adaptive, language, play and symptoms	28 DTT (32.4 h/week)	Intellect	Similar outcomes for both groups on all measures, except DTT scored higher on daily living skills
						Adaptive skills	
						Language	
					16 autism specific nursery (25.6 h/week)	Play	
						Symptoms	
Reed, Osborne and Corness	The real-world effectiveness of early teaching interventions for children with autism spectrum disorder	2007	Comparison Outcome study	Compare effects of DTT, eclectic and portage intervention on educational functioning	12 DTT (30.4 h/week)	Educational functioning	DTT higher intellectual functioning than other two groups
					20 eclectic (12.7 h/week)		DTT and eclectic group scored significantly higher on measures of intellectual functioning than portage group
					16 portage (8.5 h/week)		
Reed, Osborne and Corness	Brief report: relative effectiveness of different home-based behavioral approaches to early teach intervention	2007	Comparison Outcome study	Compare effects of high intensity vs. low intensity ABA on intellectual and educational functioning	14 DTT high intensity (30.4 h/week)	Intellect	High intensity group made greater gains in intellect and educational functioning
					13 low intensity (12.6 h/week)	Educational functioning	Low intensity did not show any gains in educational functioning

Remington, Hastings, Kovshoff, Espinosa, Jahr, Brown and Ward	Early intensive behavioral intervention: outcomes for children with autism and their parents after 2 years	2007	Comparison Outcome study	To evaluate the effects of DTT on mental age, intellect, language, adaptive and social interactions	23 DTT (25.6 h/week)	Intellect	DTT achieved significant improvements in mental age, intellectual functioning, language, adaptive, positive social interactions
						Language	
						Adaptive	
					21 control group (15.3 h/week)	Nonverbal communication	No significant difference in any area for control group
						Social interactions	
Cohen, Amerine-Dickens, and Smith	Early intensive behavioral treatment: replication of the UCLA model in a community setting	2006	Replication outcome study	Compare DTT with eclectic intervention on IQ, adaptive skills, receptive language and academic placement	21 DTT (35–40 h/week)	Intellect	DTT achieved higher scores on measures of IQ, adaptive functioning and receptive language. 17/21 DTT children transitioned to mainstream
						Language	
					21 control (eclectic: 35–40 h/week)	Adaptive	No significant difference for control group in any area. One child went to mainstream classroom
						Academic placement	

(continued)

Table 3.1 (continued)

Authors	Title	Year	Type of article	Purpose	Participant groups	Dependent variables	Summary of findings
Eldevik, Eikeseth, Jahr and Smith	Effects of low intensity behavioral treatment for children with autism and mental retardation	2006	Retrospective comparison outcome study	Compare DTT vs. eclectic intervention on IQ, language and communication	13 DTT (12.5 h/week)	Intellect	DTT achieved higher scores in IQ, language functioning and communication and showed less symptoms
					15 eclectic (12 h/week)	Language	No significant difference in IQ, adaptive or language skills in Eclectic group
						Adaptive	
Sallows and Graupner	Intensive behavioral treatment for children with autism: 4 year outcome and predictors	2005	Comparison outcome study	To compare the effects of clinic directed DTT and parent directed DTT	13: clinic directed (37.6 h/week)	Intellect	Both groups made similar gains on all outcome measures
					10: parent directed (31.6 h/week)	Language	
						Adaptive	
						Social	
						Academic	
Howard, Sparkman, Cohen, green and Stanislaw	A comparison of intensive behavior analytic and eclectic treatment for young children with autism	2005	Comparison outcome study	Compare effects of DTT and low intensity eclectic intervention on intellectual functioning, visual spatial skills, language and adaptive functioning	29 DTT (25–40 h/week)	Intellect	DTT significantly higher scores on all domains
					16 intensive eclectic (25–30 h/week)	Visual special skills	
					16 low-intensity eclectic (15 h/week)	Language	The two eclectic groups did not differ in outcomes
						Adaptive	

Eikeseth, Smith, Jahr and Eldevik	Intensive behavioral treatment at school for 4–7 year old children with autism: a 1-year comparison controlled study	2002	Comparison outcome study	To compare the outcomes of DTT and eclectic treatments on adaptive functioning, intellect, visual-spatial skills, and language	13 DTT (28 h/week)	Intellect	DTT group achieved better scores on measures of intellectual functioning, visual-spatial skills and language
					12 eclectic (29.1 h/week)	Visual-spatial skills	Eclectic group showed significantly better increases in adaptive functioning
						Language functioning	
						Adaptive skills	
Smith, Groen, and Wynn	Randomized trial of intensive early intervention for children with pervasive developmental disorder	2000	Randomized clinical control trial	To evaluate outcomes of DTT and parent delivered behavioral intervention on intellectual functioning, visual spatial-skills, language, academic functioning	15 DTT (24.5 h/week)		DTT group scored higher on measures of intellect, visual spatial skills, language and academics
					13 (15–20 h/week)		No difference between the two groups on adaptive skills or problem behavior
Sheinkopf and Siegel	Home-based behavioral treatment of young children with autism	1998	Comparison Outcome study	To evaluate effects of DTT on IQ and severity of symptoms	11 DTT (27 h/week, delivered by parents)	Intellect	DTT achieved significantly higher IQ scores and significantly lower scores on a measure of symptom severity
					11 TAU (11.1 h in school setting)	Symptom severity	TAU groups showed no significant change in IQ scores or symptom severity

(continued)

Table 3.1 (continued)

Authors	Title	Year	Type of article	Purpose	Participant groups	Dependent variables	Summary of findings
Smith, Eikeseth, Klevstrand, and Lovaas	Intensive behavioral treatment for preschoolers with severe mental retardation and pervasive developmental disorder	1997	Comparison Outcome study	To evaluate effects of high intensity DTT on IQ and expressive language skills	11 DTT (30 h/week)	Intellect	DTT greater increases in IQ and expressive language
					10 control (low intensity ABA; 10 h/week)	Expressive language	Average of 8 point IQ increase in DTT group, decrease of 3 IQ points in control group
Birnbauer and Leach	The Murdoch early intervention program after 2 years	1992	Comparison Outcome study	Evaluate effects of DTT on language and intellectual functioning	9 DTT (18.7 h/week)	Intellect	Significantly higher language and nonverbal IQ scores for children in DTT. 4 of the 9 DTT IQ scores within normal range
					5 NTC	Adaptive skills	None of the children in the NTC group scored in the normal range for IQ
						Language	

Codes: *EIBI* Early Intensive Behavioral Intervention, *TAU* treatment as usual, *NTC* no treatment control; unless otherwise specified, intervention was delivered by trained clinicians; hours per week are average, unless otherwise indicated

Table 3.2 Meta analyses and systematic reviews

Authors	Title	Year	Type of article	Number and type of studies	Summary of conclusions
Reichow	Overview of meta analyses on early intensive behavioral intervention for young children with autism spectrum disorders	2011	Overview of meta analyses	5 meta analyses	Four of five analyses concluded DTT was effective intervention for children with autism
Peters-Scheffer, Didden, Korzillius, and Sturmey	A meta analytic study on the effectiveness of comprehensive ABA-based early intervention programs for children with Autism Spectrum Disorders	2011	Meta-analysis	11 total	Experimental groups who received DTT outperformed the control groups on IQ, nonverbal IQ, language (expressive and receptive) and adaptive behavior
Makrygianni and Reed	A meta-analytic review of the effectiveness of behavioural early intervention programs for children with autistic spectrum disorders	2010	Meta-analysis	14 total	Behavioral programs are effective in improving intellectual functioning, language, communication and social skills of children with autism. A moderate to high effect was found for improving adaptive functioning.
Virues-Ortega	Applied behavior analytic intervention for autism in early childhood: Meta analysis, meta-regression and dose-response meta analysis of multiple outcomes	2010	Meta-analysis	22 total	Long term comprehensive ABA intervention leads to positive outcomes (with medium to large effects). Positive outcomes include increases in intellectual functioning, language development, acquisition of daily living skills and social functioning
Howlin and Magiati	Systematic review of early intensive behavioral interventions for children with autism	2009	Systematic review	11 total	DTT results in improved outcomes compared to control/other treatment groups

(continued)

Table 3.2 (continued)

Authors	Title	Year	Type of article	Number and type of studies	Summary of conclusions
Eldevik, Hastings, Hughes, Jahr, Eikeseth and Cross	Meta-analysis of early intensive behavioral intervention for children with autism	2009	Meta-analysis	34 total	DTT produces large to moderate effect sizes for changes in IQ and the Vineland adaptive behavior composite scores for children with ASD compared to no intervention controls and eclectic treatment models
				9 controlled designs with comparison or control group	
Eikeseth	Outcome of comprehensive psych-educational interventions for young children with autism	2009	Systematic review	25 total	DTT is considered well established
				20 (behavioral treatment)	ABA is demonstrated effective in enhancing global functioning in children with ASD and PDD-NOS
				3 (TEACHH)	
				2 (Colorado Health Sciences Project/The Denver Model)	TEACHH and the Denver Model are considered neither well established nor probably efficacious
Reichow and Wolery	Comprehensive synthesis of early intensive behavioral interventions for young children with autism based on the UCLA young autism project model	2009	Comprehensive synthesis (effect size analysis, descriptive analysis, meta-analysis)	14 total	DTT is an effective treatment for children with autism
					May not be effective for all children

Summary of the DTT Outcome Study Literature

Outcome studies allow a comparison of those who experience a particular intervention to those who do not (i.e., no intervention, an alternative intervention, less of the same intervention) on important measures of the effects of the interventions. In the outcome research on DTT, these measures typically involve intellectual functioning, adaptive skills, and other socially significant outcomes that are meaningful for children with autism and their families. DTT is often compared to a community available control (i.e., treatment as usual), eclectic approaches, or a less intensive amount of DTT.

Twenty-two total studies were reviewed here. Thirteen studies between 2000 and 2012 directly compared DTT to eclectic models or treatment as usual (Ben-Itzchak, Lahat, Burgin, & Zachor, 2008; Cohen, Amerine-Dickens, & Smith, 2006; Eikeseth, Klintwall, Jahr, & Karlsson, 2012; Eikeseth, Smith, Jahr, & Eldevik, 2002, 2007; Eldevik, Eikeseth, Jahr, & Smith, 2006; Eldevik, Hastings, Jahr, & Hughes, 2012; Fava et al., 2011; Howard, Sparkman, Cohen, Green, & Stanislaw, 2005; Magiati, Charman, & Howlin, 2007; Remington et al., 2007; Sheinkopf & Siegel, 1998; Strauss et al., 2012), four studies compared higher intensity DTT (i.e., greater number of hours) to lower intensity DTT (i.e., lesser hours) (Downs, Conley-Downs, Fossum, & Rau, 2008; Reed, Osborne, & Corness, 2007a, 2007b; Smith, Eikeseth, Klevstrand, & Lovaas, 1997; Smith, Groen, & Wynn, 2000), two studies compared DTT to no treatment at all (Birnbrauer & Leach, 1993; Flanagan, Perry, & Freeman, 2012), one study compared clinic-directed versus parent-directed DTT (Sallows & Graupner, 2005) and two studies compared high intensity DTT, low intensity DTT, and a no-treatment control (Lovaas, 1987; Reed et al., 2007a, 2007b).

The combined results of these studies consistently show that children participating in high intensity DTT programs achieve significantly greater gains in intellectual functioning, adaptive skills, expressive and receptive language, visual spatial skills, social skills, nonverbal communication, and play skills. Additionally, these studies have shown that DTT results in greater reductions in symptom severity and behavioral problems and results in better academic placement. Some studies (e.g., Eikeseth et al., 2002; Smith et al., 2000; Strauss et al., 2012) have failed to show significant differences between DTT and other approaches/control groups on some variables (behavior problems, adaptive functioning, and parental stress). However, each of the aforementioned studies demonstrated that DTT is most efficacious on the majority of variables investigated. In a rare exception, Magiati et al. (2007) found similar outcomes for autism-specific nursery services and DTT on all measures examined (intellectual functioning, adaptive skills, language, play and symptoms of autism), with the exception that children receiving DTT scored higher on daily living skills. Taken together, this body of literature illustrates superior effects of DTT but also indicates that DTT should include a specific focus on adaptive behavior (e.g., self-care) in addition to the core curriculum that targets intellectual functioning and cognitive skills.

Summary of Meta-analyses/Systematic Reviews

Meta-analyses combine the results from different studies to identify commonalities in findings. The goal of a meta-analysis is to collect and synthesize research results and to allow a more extensive and standard statistical examination of the degree of effect of treatment across multiple independent research investigations. Results of studies are compared by creating a standard "effect size" metric (e.g., degree of change produced) that can be compared and synthesized across multiple evaluations. Systematic reviews are thorough research reviews on a particular topic, aimed at summarizing, synthesizing and identifying gaps in literature.

The systematic reviews and meta-analyses on DTT reviewed in this chapter had varied inclusion criteria. However, taken together, they represent a large analysis of the literature on DTT thus far. The overall results suggest that DTT can produce significant *increases* in intellectual skills (IQ, standardized test scores), cognitive development, language, adaptive and social skills and significant *decreases* in symptoms of autism, problem behavior, and amount of school support needed. It is reasonable to conclude that DTT is an effective intervention for all children with autism. This body of research indicates younger children achieve better outcomes. Older children with more impairment still make substantial gains, but they may not achieve typical IQ and adaptive skills. However, DTT provided to older and more impaired children ensures that they maintain their current level of functioning or achieve better functioning because functioning decreases over time without DTT. Moderately impaired children who receive DTT are highly likely to maintain their level of impairment or to improve to slightly impaired. In contrast, moderately impaired children who receive no intervention at all are likely to become significantly impaired as they age and the gap between their development and that of their same age peers enlarges. Finally, it should be noted that the specific characteristics of intervention delivery (e.g., level of procedural integrity, clinical oversight, training etc.) varied greatly across studies, suggesting we need to define more clearly what constitutes an ideal DTT programming model and identify what ultimately leads to successful outcomes.

Suggestions for Future Research

The existing evidence base suggests that the DTT model and common variations of DTT teaching procedures are highly effective for improving the outcomes of children with ASD. However, additional research is needed to further our understanding of factors that will ensure the best possible outcomes for all children. Despite the positive outcomes of large-scale studies, some children do not appear to benefit as much as others from structured, intensive DTT models. Variables that are likely to impact outcomes include the child's diagnosis and severity of autism; number of treatment hours; duration of treatment; qualifications of the therapists and supervisors; methods of staff training; frequency of progress review; procedural variations of prompting and reinforcement; breadth or range of targets included in programs; strategies to promote generalization; and parental participation in therapy. These factors varied across the large-scale studies, often in unsystematic or unknown ways. Thus, further large-scale research is needed to explicitly explore the relationship between these potentially important variables and therapy outcomes. Results of studies that compare DTT to other comprehensive early intervention approaches, or that evaluate combinations of approaches, also would help parents and practitioners make decisions when selecting treatments.

A number of procedural refinements to DTT procedures (e.g., prompt fading methods, reinforcement schedules; task interspersal arrangements) have not been adequately examined or compared to alternative variations. In particular, systematic evaluation and comparison of strategies to promote generalization have been given surprising little attention in the DTT literature. The number of exemplars needed to promote generalization and the most effective way to select and combine existing generalization strategies should be evaluated in further research. Given that instruction is typically delivered by adults, particular consideration should be given to methods for promoting generalization from adults to same-age peers.

Further development and evaluation of alternatives to traditional BST for teaching staff and caregivers to implement DTT are needed to expand the accessibility of this therapy to those living in rural or remote areas. Self-instructional manuals, computer-based training, and remote coaching may reduce the costs associated with this therapeutic model and the need for expert trainers. Computer-based instruction that incorporates or simulates the components of traditional BST, particularly modeling combined with rehearsal plus feedback, have the greatest potential to be effective across individuals with diverse backgrounds and levels of experience.

Finally, structured DTT programming may be less successful than other instructional models for teaching certain skills. For example, limited information is available about the potential effectiveness of the DTT approach for teaching complex social and emotional responses, particularly those that may impact the likelihood of successful relationships at home, in the community, and on the job. Further research that explores the range of skills that may be successfully taught via this model (e.g., daily living skills; complex social skills), along with modifications to DTT programming or procedures that would increase the breadth of its outcomes, should be considered. As noted previously, DTT instruction is typically combined with a variety of ABA-based interventions, including less structured, more naturalistic instructional approaches (e.g., incidental teaching). Research on the most effective way to supplement DTT instruction with these other approaches could lead to further improvements in the long-term outcomes of early intervention for children with autism.

References

Alvero, A. M., Bucklin, B. R., & Austin, J. (2001). An objective review of the effectiveness and essential characteristics of performance feedback in organizational settings. *Journal of Organizational Behavior Management, 21*, 3–29.

Benavides, C. A., & Poulson, C. L. (2009). Task interspersal and performance of matching tasks by preschoolers with autism. *Research in Autism Spectrum Disorders, 3*, 619–929.

Ben-Itzchak, E., Lahat, E., Burgin, R., & Zachor, A. D. (2008). Cognitive, behavior and intervention outcome in young children with autism. *Research in Developmental Disabilities, 29*, 447–458.

Birnbrauer, J., & Leach, D. J. (1993). The Murdoch early intervention program after 2 years. *Behaviour Change, 10*, 63–74.

Carey, M. K., & Bourret, J. C. (2014). Effects of data sampling on graphical depictions of learning. *Journal of Applied Behavior Analysis, 47*, 1–16.

Catania, C. N., Almeida, D., Liu-Constant, B., & Digennaro, F. D. (2009). Video modeling to train staff to implement discrete-trial instruction. *Journal of Applied Behavior Analysis, 42*, 387–392.

Charlop, M. H., Kurtz, P. F., & Milstein, J. P. (1992). Too much reinforcement, too little behavior: Assessing task interspersal procedures in conjunction with different reinforcement schedules with autistic children. *Journal of Applied Behavior Analysis, 25*, 795–808.

Chiara, L., Schuster, J. W., Bell, J. K., & Wolery, M. (1995). Small-group massed-trial and individually-distributed-trail instruction with preschoolers. *Journal of Early Intervention, 19*, 203–217.

Cividini-Motta, C., & Ahearn, W. H. (2013). Effects of two variations of differential reinforcement on prompt dependency. *Journal of Applied Behavior Analysis, 46*, 640–650.

Cohen, H., Amerine-Dickens, M., & Smith, T. (2006). Early intensive behavioral treatment: Replication of the UCLA model in a community setting. *Developmental and Behavioral Pediatrics, 27*, 145–155.

Cummings, A. R., & Carr, J. E. (2009). Evaluating progress in behavioral programs for children with Autism spectrum disorders via continuous and discontinuous measurement. *Journal of Applied Behavior Analysis, 42*, 57–71.

Dib, N., & Sturmey, P. (2007). Reducing student stereotypy by improving teachers' implementation of discrete-trial teaching. *Journal of Applied Behavior Analysis, 40*, 339–343.

Downs, A., Conley-Downs, R., Fossum, M., & Rau, K. (2008). Effectiveness of discrete trial teaching with preschool students with developmental disabilities. *Education and Training in Developmental Disabilities, 43*, 443–453.

Ducharme, J. M., & Feldman, M. A. (1992). Comparison of staff training strategies to promote generalized teaching skills. *Journal of Applied Behavior Analysis, 25*, 165–179.

Dunlap, G. (1984). The influence of task variation and maintenance tasks on the learning and affect of autistic children. *Renal of Experimental Child Psychology, 37*, 41–64.

Eikeseth, S. (2009). Outcome of comprehensive psycho-educational interventions for young children with autism. *Research in Developmental Disabilities, 30*, 158–178.

Eikeseth, S., Hayward, D., Gale, C., Gitlesen, J., & Eldevik, S. (2009). Intensity of supervision and outcome for preschool aged children receiving early and intensive behavioral interventions: A preliminary study. *Research in Autism Spectrum Disorders, 3*, 67–73.

Eikeseth, S., Klintwall, L., Jahr, E., & Karlsson, P. (2012). Outcome for children with autism receiving early and intensive behavioral intervention in mainstream preschool and kindergarten settings. *Research in Autism Spectrum Disorders, 6*, 829–835.

Eikeseth, S., Smith, T., Jahr, E., & Eldevik, S. (2002). Intensive behavioral at school for 4-to-7 year-old children with autism treatment. *Behavior Modification, 26*, 49–68.

Eikeseth, S., Smith, T., Jahr, E., & Eldevik, S. (2007). Outcome for children with autism who began intensive behavioral treatment between ages 4 and 7: A comparison controlled study. *Behavior Modification, 31*, 264–278.

Eldevik, S., Eikeseth, S., Jahr, E., & Smith, T. (2006). Effects of low-intensity behavioral treatment for children with autism and mental retardation. *Journal of Autism and Developmental Disorders, 36*, 211–224.

Eldevik, S., Hastings, R. P., Hughes, J. C., Jahr, E., Eikeseth, S., & Cross, S. (2009). Meta- analysis of early intensive behavioral intervention for children with autism. *Journal of Clinical Child and Adolescent Psychology, 38*, 439–450.

Eldevik, S., Hastings, R. P., Jahr, E., & Hughes, J. C. (2012). Outcomes of behavioral intervention for children with autism in mainstream preschool settings. *Journal of Autism and Developmental Disorders, 42*, 210–220.

Eldevik, S., Ondire, I., Hughes, J. C., Grindle, C. F., Randell, T., & Remington, B. (2013). Effects of computer simulation training on in vivo discrete trial teaching. *Journal of Autism and Developmental Disabilities, 43*, 569–578.

Elliott, C., & Dillenburger, K. (2014). The effect of choice on motivation for young children on the autism spectrum during discrete trial teaching. *Journal of Research in Special Educational Needs*. doi:10.1111/1471-3802.12073.

Fava, L., Strauss, K., Valeri, G., D'Elia, L., Arima, S., & Vicari, S. (2011). The effectiveness of a cross-setting complementary staff-and parent mediated early intensive behavioral intervention for young children with ASD. *Research in Autism Spectrum Disorders, 5*, 1479–1492.

Fenske, E. C., Krantz, P. J., & McClannahan, L. E. (2001). Incidental teaching: A not-discrete-trial teaching procedure. In C. Maurice & G. Green (Eds.), *Making a difference: Behavioral intervention for autism* (pp. 75–82). Austin, TX: PRO-ED.

Fentress, G. M., & Lerman, D. C. (2012). A comparison of two prompting procedures for teaching basic skills to children with autism. *Research in Autism Spectrum Disorders, 6*, 1083–1090.

Flanagan, H. E., Perry, A., & Freeman, N. L. (2012). Effectiveness of large-scale community-based intensive behavioral intervention: A waitlist comparison study exploring outcomes and predictors. *Research in Autism Spectrum Disorders, 6*, 673–682.

Geiger, K. B., Carr, J. E., LeBlanc, L. A., Hanney, N. M., Polick, A. S., & Heinike, M. R. (2012). Teaching receptive discriminations to children with autism: A comparison of traditional and embedded discrete trial teaching. *Behavior Analysis in Practice, 5*, 49–59.

Grow, L. L., Carr, J. E., Kodak, T. M., Jostad, C. M., & Kisamore, A. N. (2011). A comparison of methods for teaching receptive labeling to children with autism spectrum disorders. *Journal of Applied Behavior Analysis, 44*, 475–498.

Grow, L., Kodak, T. M., & Carr, J. E. (2014). A comparison of methods for teaching receptive labeling to children with autism spectrum disorders: A systematic replication. *Journal of Applied Behavior Analysis, 47*, 600–605.

Grow, L., & LeBlanc, L. (2013). Teaching receptive language skills: Recommendations for instructors. *Behavior Analysis in Practice, 6*(1), 56–75.

Harris, S. L., & Weiss, M. J. (2007). *Right from the start: Behavioral intervention for young children with autism* (2nd ed.). Bethesda, MD: Woodbine House.

Hausman, N. L., Ingvarsson, E. T., & Kahng, S. (2014). A comparison of reinforcement schedules to increase independent responding in individuals with intellectual disabilities. *Journal of Applied Behavior Analysis, 47*, 155–159.

Hay-Hansson, A. W., & Eldevik, S. (2013). Training discrete trials teaching skills using videoconference. *Research in Autism Spectrum Disorders, 7*, 1300–1309.

Howard, J. S., Sparkman, C. R., Cohen, H. G., Green, G., & Stanislaw, H. (2005). A comparison of intensive behavior analytic and eclectic treatments for young children with autism. *Research in Developmental Disabilities, 26*, 359–383.

Howlin, P., Magiati, I., & Charman, T. (2009). Systematic review of early intensive behavioral interventions for children with autism. *American Association on Intellectual and Developmental Disabilities, 114*, 23–41.

Karsten, A. M., & Carr, J. E. (2009). The effects of differential reinforcement of unprompted responding on skill acquisition of children with autism. *Journal of Applied Behavior Analysis, 42*, 327–334.

Koegel, R. L., Dunlap, G., & Dyer, K. (1980). Intertrial interval duration and leaning in autistic children. *Journal of Applied Behavior Analysis, 13*, 91–99.

Komaki, J. L., Desselles, M. L., & Bowman, E. D. (1989). Definitely not a breeze: Extending an operant model of effective supervision to teams. *Journal of Applied Psychology, 74*, 522–529.

Lafasakis, M., & Sturmey, P. (2007). Training parent implementation of discrete-trial teaching: Effects on generalization of parent teaching and child correct responding. *Journal of Applied Behavior Analysis, 40*, 685–689.

Lang R., Werff, M., Verbeek, K., Didden, R., Davenport, K., Moore, M., … Lancioni, G. (2014). Comparison of high and low preferred topographies of contingent attention during discrete trial training. *Research in Autism Spectrum Disorders,* 8, 1279–1286.

Leaf, J. B., Alcalay, A., Leaf, J. A., Tsuji, K., Kassardjian, A., Dale, S., … Leaf, R. (2014). Comparison of most-to-least to error correction for teaching receptive labelling for two chil dren diagnosed with autism. *Journal of Research in Special Educational Needs, 44*(3), 475–498. doi:10.1111/1471-3802.12067.

Leaf, J. B., Leaf, R., Taubman, M., McEachin, J., & Delmolino, L. (2014). Comparison of flexible fading to error correction for children with autism spectrum disorder. *Journal of Developmental and Physical Disabilities, 26*, 203–224.

Leaf, R., & McEachin, J. (1999). *A work in progress: Behavior management strategies and a curriculum for intensive behavioral treatment of autism.* New York, NY: DRL Books.

Leaf, J. B., Sheldon, J. B., & Sherman, J. A. (2010). Comparison of simultaneous prompting and no-no prompting in two-choice discrimination learning with children with autism. *Journal of Applied Behavior Analysis,* 43, 215–228.

Leaf, J. B., Tsuji, K. H., Lentell, A. E., Dale, S. E., Kassardjian, A., Taubman, M., … Oppenheim-Leaf, M. L. (2013). A comparison of discrete trial teaching implemented in a one-to-one instructional format. *Behavioral Interventions, 28*, 82–106.

LeBlanc, L. A., Parks, N., & Hanney, N. (2014). Early intensive behavioral intervention (EIBI): Current status and future directions. In J. Luiselli (Ed.), *Children and youth with Autism Spectrum Disorder (ASD): Recent advances and innovations in assessment, education, and intervention* (pp. 63–75). New York, NY: Oxford.

Lerman, D. C., Dittlinger, L. H., Fentress, G., & Lanagan, T. (2011). A comparison of methods for collecting data on performance during discrete trial teaching. *Behavior Analysis in Practice, 4*, 53–62.

Lerman, D. C., Tetreault, A., Hovanetz, A., Strobel, M., & Garro, J. (2008). Further evaluation of a brief, intensive teacher training model. *Journal of Applied Behavior Analysis, 41*, 243–248.

Libby, M. E., Weiss, J. S., Bancroft, S., & Ahearn, W. H. (2008). A comparison of most-to-least and least-to-most prompting on the acquisition of solitary play skills. *Behavior Analysis in Practice, 1*, 37–43.

Lockshin, S. B., Gillis, J. M., & Romanczyk, R. G. (2004). *Defying autism: Keeping your sanity and taking control.* New York, NY: DRL Books.

Loughrey, T. O., Betz, A. M., Majdalany, L. M., & Nicholson. (2014). Using instructive feedback to teach category names to children with autism. *Journal of Applied Behavior Analysis, 47*, 425–430.

Lovaas, O. I. (1981). *Teaching developmentally disabled children: The Me Book.* Baltimore, MD: University Park.

Lovaas, O. I. (1987). Behavioral treatment and normal educational and intellectual functioning in young autistic children. *Journal of Consulting and Clinical Psychology, 55*, 3–9.

Lovaas, O. I. (2002). *Teaching individuals with developmental delays: Early intervention techniques.* Austin, TX: Pro-Ed.

MacDuff, G. S., Krantz, P. J., & McClannahan, L. E. (2001). Prompts and prompt-fading strategies for people with autism. In G. Maurice, G. Green, & R. Foxx (Eds.), *Making a difference: Behavioral intervention for autism* (pp. 37–50). Austin, TX: Pro-Ed.

Magiati, I., Charman, T., & Howlin, P. (2007). A two-year prospective follow-up study of community based early intensive behavioral intervention and specialist nursery provision for

children with autism spectrum disorders. *Journal of Child Psychology and Psychiatry, 48*, 803–812.
Majdalany, L. M., Wilder, D. A., Greif, A., Mathisen, D., & Saini, V. (2014). Comparing massed-trial instruction, and task interspersal to teach tacts to children with autism spectrum disorders. *Journal of Applied Behavior Analysis, 47*, 1–6.
Maurice, C. (1994). *Let me hear your voice: A family's triumph over autism*. New York, NY: Random House.
Maurice, C., Green, G., & Foxx, R. M. (2001). *Making a difference: Behavioral intervention for autism*. Austin, TX: Pro-Ed.
Maurice, C., Green, G., & Luce, S. (1996). *Behavioral intervention for young children with autism*. Austin, TX: PRO-ED.
May, R. J., Austin, J. L., & Dymond, S. (2011). Effects of a stimulus prompt display on therapists' accuracy, rate, and variation of trial type delivery during discrete trial teaching. *Research in Autism Spectrum Disorders, 5*, 305–316.
McGhan, A. C., & Lerman, D. C. (2013). An assessment of error-correction procedures for learners with autism. *Journal of Applied Behavior Analysis, 46*, 626–639.
McKenney, E. L. W., & Bristol, R. M. (2015). Supporting intensive interventions for students with autism spectrum disorder: Performance feedback and discrete trial teaching. *School Psychology Quarterly, 30*(1), 8–22. Advance online publication. http://dx.doi.org/10.1037/spq0000060.
Miltenberger, R. G. (2003). *Behavior modification: Principles and procedures*. Belmont, CA: Wadsworth Publishing.
Najdowski, A. C., Chilingaryan, V., Bergstrom, R., Granpeesheh, D., Balasanyan, S., Aguilar, B., & Tarbox, J. (2009). Comparison of data-collection methods in a behavioral intervention program for children with pervasive developmental disorders: A replication. *Journal of Applied behavior Analysis, 42*, 827–832.
North, S. T., & Iwata, B. A. (2005). Motivational influences on performance maintained by food reinforcement. *Journal of Applied Behavior Analysis, 38*, 317–333.
Nosik, M. R., Williams, W. L., Garrido, N., & Lee, S. (2013). Comparison of computer based instruction to behavior skills training for teaching staff implementation of discrete-trial instruction with an adult with autism. *Research in Developmental Disabilities, 34*, 461–468.
Olendick, D. L., & Pear, J. J. (1980). Differential reinforcement of correct responses to probes and prompts in picture-name training with severely retarded children. *Journal of Applied Behavior Analysis, 13*, 77–89.
Polick, A. S., Carr, J. E., & Hanney, N. M. (2012). A comparison of general and descriptive praise in teaching intraverbal behavior to children with autism. *Journal of Applied Behavior Analysis, 45*, 593–599.
Pollard, J. S., Higbee, T. S., Akers, J. S., & Brodhead, M. T. (2014). An evaluation of interactive computer training to teach instructors to implement discrete trials with children with autism. *Journal of Applied Behavior Analysis, 47*, 1–12.
Powers, M. D. (2001). *Children with autism: A parent's guide*. Bethesda, MD: Woodbine House.
Randall, T., Hall, M., Bizo, L., & Remington, B. (2007). DTkid: Interactive simulation software for training tutors of children with autism. *Journal of Autism and Developmental Disabilities, 37*, 637–647.
Reed, P., Osborne, L. A., & Corness, M. (2007a). Brief report: Relative effectiveness of different home-based behavioral approaches to early intervention. *Journal of Autism and Developmental Disorders, 37*, 1815–1821.
Reed, P., Osborne, L. A., & Corness, M. (2007b). The real-world effectiveness of early teaching interventions for children with autism spectrum disorder. *Exceptional Children, 73*, 417–433.
Reed, F. D. D., Reed, D. D., Baez, C. N., & Maguire, H. (2011). A parametric analysis of errors of commission during discrete-trial training. *Journal of Applied Behavior Analysis, 44*, 611–615.
Reichow, B. (2012). Overview of meta-analyses on early intensive behavioral intervention for young children with autism spectrum disorders. *Journal of Autism and Developmental Disorders, 42*, 512–520.

Reichow, B., & Wolery, M. (2009). Comprehensive synthesis of early intensive behavioral interventions for young children with autism based on the UCLA young autism project model. *Journal of Autism and Developmental Disorders, 39*, 23–41.

Reichow, B., & Wolery, M. (2011). Comparison of progressive prompt delay with and without instructive feedback. *Journal of Applied Behavior Analysis, 44*, 327–340.

Remington, B., Hastings, R. P., Kovshoff, H., Espinosa, F., Jahr, E., Brown, T., & Ward, M. (2007). Early intensive behavioral intervention: Outcomes for children with autism and their parents after two years. *American Journal on Mental Retardation, 112*, 418–438.

Rodgers, T. A., & Iwata, B. A. (1991). An analysis of error-correction procedures during discrimination training. *Journal of Applied Behavioral Analysis, 24*, 775–781.

Sallows, G. O., & Graupner, T. D. (2005). Intensive behavioral treatment for children with autism: Four year outcome and predictors. *American Journal on Mental Retardation, 110*, 417–438.

Sarokoff, R. A., & Sturmey, P. (2004). The effects of behavioral skills training on staff implementation of discrete-trial teaching. *Journal of Applied Behavior Analysis, 37*, 535–538.

Schroeder, C. M., Schuster, J. W., & Hemmeter, M. L. (1998). Efficiency in programming for generalization: Comparison of two methods for teaching expressive labeling to preschoolers with developmental delays. *Journal of Developmental and Physical Disabilities, 10*, 109–131.

Sellers, T. P., Bloom, S. E., Samaha, A. L., Dayton, E., Lambert, J. M., & Keyl-Austin, A. A. (2013). Evaluation of some components of choice making. *Journal of Applied Behavior Analysis, 46*, 455–464.

Sheinkopf, S. J., & Siegel, B. (1998). Home-based behavioral treatment of young children with autism. *Journal of Autism and Development Disorders, 28*, 15–23.

Smith, T., Eikeseth, S., Klevstrand, M., & Lovaas, O. I. (1997). Intensive behavioral treatment for preschoolers with severe mental retardation and pervasive developmental disorder. *American Journal of Mental Retardation, 102*, 238–249.

Smith, T., Groen, A. D., & Wynn, J. W. (2000). Randomized trial of intensive early intervention for children with pervasive developmental disorder. *American Journal of Mental Retardation, 105*, 269–285.

Smith, T., Mruzek, D. W., Wheat, L. A., & Hughes, C. (2006). Error correction in discrimination training for children with autism. *Behavioral Interventions, 21*, 245–263.

Soluaga, D., Leaf, J. B., Taubman, M., McEachin, J., & Leaf, R. (2008). A comparison of flexible prompt fading and constant time delay for five children with autism. *Research in Autism Spectrum Disorders, 2*, 753–765.

Stevens, C., Sidner, T. M., Reeve, S. A., & Sidener, D. W. (2011). Effects of behavior-specific and general praise, on acquisition of tacts in children with pervasive developmental disorders. *Research in Autism Spectrum Disorders, 5*, 666–669.

Stokes, T. F., & Baer, D. M. (1977). An implicit technology of generalization. *Journal of Applied Behavior Analysis, 10*, 349–367.

Strauss, K., Vicari, S., Valeri, G., D'Elia, L., Arima, S., & Fava, L. (2012). Parent inclusion in early intensive behavioral intervention: The influence of parental stress, parent treatment fidelity and parent-mediated generalization of behavior targets on child outcomes. *Research in Developmental Disabilities, 33*, 688–703.

Sundberg, M. L., & Partington, J. W. (1998). *Teaching language to children with autism or other developmental disabilities*. Pleasant Hill, CA: Behavior Analysts.

Taubman, M., Brierley, S., Wishner, J., Baker, D., McEachin, J., & Leaf, R. B. (2001). The effectiveness of a group discrete trial instructional approach for preschoolers with developmental disabilities. *Research in Developmental Disabilities, 22*, 205–219.

Taubman, M. T., Leaf, R. B., McEachin, J. J., Papovich, S., & Leaf, J. B. (2013). A comparison of data collection techniques used with discrete trial teaching. *Research in Autism Spectrum Disorders, 7*, 1026–1034.

Thiessen, C., Fazzio, D., Arnal, L., Martin, G. L., Yu, C. T., & Keilback, L. (2009). Evaluation of a self-instructional manual for conducting discrete-trials teaching with children with autism. *Behavior Modification, 33*, 360–373.

Thomas, B. R. (2013). Effects of conducting peer behavioral observations on the observer's correct use of discrete trial teaching procedures. *Research in Developmental Disabilities, 34*, 2143–2148.

Thomson, K., Martin, G. L., Arnal, L., Fazzio, D., & Yu, C. T. (2009). Instructing individuals to deliver discrete-trials teaching to children with autism spectrum disorders: A review. *Research in Autism Spectrum Disorders, 3*, 590–606.

Thomson, K. M., Martin, G. L., Fazzio, D., Salem, S., Young, K., & Yu, C. T. (2012). Evaluation of a self-instructional package for teaching tutors to conduct discrete-trials teaching with children with autism. *Research in Autism Spectrum Disorders, 6*, 1073–1082.

Tiger, J. H., Hanley, G. P., & Hernandez, E. (2006). An evaluation of the value of choice with preschool children. *Journal of Applied Behavior Analysis, 39*, 1–16.

Touchette, P. E., & Howard, J. S. (1984). Errorless learning: Reinforcement contingencies and stimulus control transfer in delayed prompting. *Journal of Applied Behavior Analysis, 17*, 175–188.

Vismara, L. A., Young, G. S., Stahmer, A. C., Griffith, E. M., & Rogers, S. J. (2009). Dissemination of evidence-based practice: Can we train therapists from a distance? *Journal of Autism and Developmental Disorders, 39*, 1636–1651.

Vladescu, J. C., Carroll, R., Paden, A., & Kodak, T. M. (2012). The effects of video modeling with voiceover instruction on accurate implementation of discrete-trial instruction. *Journal of Applied Behavior Analysis, 45*, 419–423.

Vladescu, J. C., & Kodak, T. M. (2013). Increasing instructional efficiency by presenting additional stimuli in learning trials for children with autism spectrum disorder. *Journal of Applied Behavior Analysis, 46*, 805–816.

Volkert, V. M., Lerman, D. C., Trosclair, N., Addison, L., & Kodak, T. (2008). An exploratory analysis of task-interspersal procedures while teaching object labels to children with autism. *Journal of Applied Behavior Analysis, 41*, 335–350.

Volkmar, F. R., & Wiesner, L. A. (2009). *A practical guide to autism: What every parent, family member, and teacher needs to know*. New York, NY: Wiley.

Wacker, D. P., Lee, J. F., Padilla Dalmau, Y. C., Kopelman, T. G., Lindgren, S. D., Kuhle, J., … Waldron, D. B. (2013a). Conducting functional communication training via telehealth to reduce the problem behavior of young children with autism. *Journal of Developmental and Physical Disabilities, 25*, 35–48.

Wacker, D. P., Lee, J. F., Padilla Dalmau, Y. C., Kopelman, T. G., Lindgren, S. D., Kuhle, J., … Waldron, D. B. (2013b). Conducting functional analyses of problem behavior via telehealth. *Journal of Applied Behavior Analysis, 46*, 1–16.

Waugh, R. E., Alberto, P. A., & Fredrick, L. D. (2011). Simultaneous prompting: An instructional strategy for skill acquisition. *Education and Training in Autism and Developmental Disabilities, 46*, 528–543.

Webber, J., & Scheuermann, B. (2008). *Educating students with autism: A quick start manual*. Austin, TX: Pro-Ed.

Worsdell, A. S., Iwata, B. A., Dozier, C. L., Johnson, A. D., Neidert, P. L., & Thomason, J. L. (2005). Analysis of response repetition as an error correction strategy during sight-word reading. *Journal of Applied Behavioral Analysis, 38*, 511–527.

Wunderlich, K. L., Vollmer, T. R., Donaldson, J. M., & Phillips, C. L. (2014). Effects of serial and concurrent training on acquisition and generalization. *Journal of Applied Behavior Analysis, 47*, 1–15.

Young, K. L., Boris, A. L., Thomson, K. M., Martin, G. L., & Yu, C. T. (2012). Evaluation of a self instructional package on discrete-trials teaching to parents of children with autism. *Research in Autism Spectrum Disorders, 6*, 1321–1330.

Chapter 4
Pivotal Response Treatment

Lynn Kern Koegel, Kristen Ashbaugh, and Robert L. Koegel

Introduction

Research clearly demonstrates that Applied Behavior Analysis (ABA) interventions (e.g., Discrete Trial Training [DTT]) are effective for the treatment of Autism Spectrum Disorder. The earliest ABA-based interventions were based on the underlying sentiment that intervention had to be implemented in a structured environment that was free from distractions, primarily because the children frequently exhibited off-task behaviors. Although the procedures were effective, it sometimes required thousands of trials to be implemented for the child to learn a single target behavior (Lovaas, 1977). While effective, the children did not seem motivated to engage in the intervention activities due to the high demands of the original ABA procedures. Furthermore, research indicated that the generalization of newly acquired behaviors outside of the clinic setting was often a problem. Due to low motivation in intervention and limited generalizability of treatment gains, we sought to develop procedures derived from the science of ABA that would be helpful in improving the general motivation of the child with autism during intervention. Thus, PRT and many more modern ABA interventions have evolved from highly-structured and adult-driven sessions to more naturalistic and child-focused interactions. In addition, the trend toward inclusion of children with autism in regular education classrooms and community activities, as opposed to segregated settings and institutions, has helped ABA researchers develop treatments that can be incorporated into everyday routines.

L.K. Koegel (✉) • K. Ashbaugh • R.L. Koegel
UCSB Koegel Autism Center, Graduate School of Education, University of California, Santa Barbara, Santa Barbara, CA 93106-9490, USA
e-mail: lynnk@education.ucsb.edu

R. Lang et al. (eds.), *Early Intervention for Young Children with Autism Spectrum Disorder*, Evidence-Based Practices in Behavioral Health,
DOI 10.1007/978-3-319-30925-5_4

From a theoretical point of view, we hypothesized that children with autism displaying challenges in many areas may be exhibiting a deficit in a pivotal area of learned helplessness and thus demonstrating an overall lack of motivation to respond. We speculated that this would produce a general lack of interaction with the children's social and learning environments, resulting in widespread behavioral deficits. Our goal was to develop a Pivotal Response Treatment for autism that would target the key deficit in motivation and reduce symptoms of learned helplessness, and have the potential to produce rapid and widespread improvements in the overall condition of autism.

Theoretical Basis in Learned Helplessness

The theory of learned helplessness was proposed by Seligman (1967), and has since been applied to a number of diverse participants, behaviors and disorders (Hiroto, 1974; Klein, Fencil-Morse, & Seligman, 1976; Maier & Seligman, 1976). Learned helplessness theorizes that exposure to events that are uncontrollable leads participants to believe that behaviors and outcomes are independent, which produces an effect on their motivation, cognition, and emotion (Maier & Seligman, 1976; Miller & Seligman, 1975). Although Seligman's initial work was implemented with animals, it shed light on specific patterns of behavior that appeared to be applicable to human behavior.

Overmier and Seligman (1967) first spearheaded the theory of learned helplessness through an observation of helpless behavior in dogs that were exposed to inescapable and unavoidable electric shocks. Following this observation, Seligman and Maier (1967) conducted an experiment to show that the helpless behavior was caused by the uncontrollability of the original shocks. Through a triad experimental design, they studied three groups of dogs in two phases. In phase one, each group of dogs was strapped in a harness. In the first group, the dogs were simply strapped in the harness and then released. In the second group, the dogs were strapped in the same harness and were subjected to electrical shocks, however they could avoid the shocks by using their nose to press a panel. The third group of dogs were placed in the same harness and received the same shocks as the second group, but in this condition they could not control the duration of the shock and the shocks seemed to be random and outside of their control. In phase two of the experiment, all three groups were placed in a shuttle box. In the shuttle box, shock elimination was controllable for all subjects by jumping over a barrier in the middle of the box. Dogs from the first and second group quickly learned that jumping over the barrier eliminated the shock, but the dogs in the third group made no attempts to escape the shock. Theoretically, the dogs in group three appeared to learn that there was not a relationship between their behavior and the outcome, and therefore they did not initiate an attempt to escape the electric shock while in the shuttle box, despite the fact that they were not harnessed and could escape the shock (Seligman & Maier, 1967). This study paved the road for future research on the effects of repeated exposure to uncontrollable stimuli.

Since Seligman and Maier's (1967) study on the effects of uncontrollable shocks on dogs, similar studies have been conducted to demonstrate the theory of learned helplessness in humans. Hiroto (1974) first applied the concept of learned helplessness to humans by conducting a triad experiment on the effects of uncontrollable noise with humans, and found parallel results of the effects of uncontrollable stimuli between animals and humans. Specifically, college students were separated into three groups. In the first phase, one group received no noise, the second group received loud noise that they could terminate by pushing a button, and the third group received uncontrollable noise that stopped independently of the participant's behavior. In the second phase, all groups were tested in a hand shuttle box and noise termination was controllable for all participants. The results were analogous to the animal studies, in that the groups receiving no noise or controllable noise in phase one readily learned to escape the noise in the shuttle, while the participants that received prior uncontrollable noise did not escape the noise and listened passively (Hiroto, 1974). Similar studies have been conducted with college students that were first presented with unsolvable discrimination problems, and then subsequently it was observed that they "gave up" on solvable anagram puzzles because they previously learned that the outcome was uncontrollable by their response effort (Klein et al., 1976).

In addition to replications of Seligman's original experiment to humans, research also supports strong external validity of the theory (Peterson, Maier, & Seligman, 1993). For example, Hiroto and Seligman (1975) conducted an important experiment to demonstrate that learned helplessness may be considered a "trait" as opposed to a state. They examined the generality of learned helplessness across tasks by conducting experiments that involved an instrumental task (i.e. escaping aversive noise) and/or a cognitive task (i.e. solving an anagram puzzle). They conducted four experiments and found that inescapability in a pretreatment instrumental task (i.e. inescapable aversive tone) produced learned helplessness in both subsequent shuttle box escape testing and subsequent anagram solution testing. This finding showed that participants receiving uncontrollable aversive noises performed poorer during a second phase in the experiment in which they were given anagram puzzles, suggesting that learned helplessness was generalized between an instrumental task and cognitive task. Furthermore, the researchers found that pretreatment insoluble discrimination problems produced deficits associated with learned helplessness in subsequent shuttle box escape testing. This demonstrated cross-modal helplessness, and indicates that learned helplessness may be generalized across tasks (Hiroto & Seligman, 1975).

Deficits Resulting from Learned Helplessness

Research suggests that learned helplessness produces deficits relating to an individual's motivation, cognitive learning, and emotional health. In regard to motivation, when an individual learns that his or her responses are independent of reinforcement, he or she will initiate fewer responses to the stimulus because of their expectancy that the response will not be effective (Klein et al., 1976). This decrease in initiation of voluntary responses is referred to as the motivational deficit (Abramson, Seligman, & Teasdale, 1978). For example, if individuals are exposed to a loud noise that they cannot control or avoid, then they learn to believe that any attempts or effort that they make to eliminate the noise are ineffective. If they are subsequently exposed to a loud noise that they can control, then it is unlikely that they will have motivation to make an attempt at escaping the noise due to the false notion that their response will not be reinforced.

In addition to a motivational deficit as a result of learned helplessness, there is also a cognitive component that results from repeated exposure to uncontrollable events (Klein et al., 1976; Miller & Norman, 1979). More than just a decline in motivation to respond to a stimulus, there is a disruption in the learning of response-reinforcement contingencies (Klein et al., 1976; Peterson et al., 1993). Experience with uncontrollability may hinder the ability to learn that responses have succeeded, even when responding is actually successful (Hiroto, 1974; Maier & Seligman, 1976). For example, in a study by Miller and Seligman (1975), college students were first given escapable, inescapable or no noise in a pretreatment condition, then asked to solve anagrams. In addition to the inescapable noise interfering with the students' ability to solve any given anagram, students that received inescapable noise also required more successes on solving anagrams before catching on to the pattern when compared to students who received escapable noise or no noise (Miller & Seligman, 1975). It took about seven consecutive successes for students that had prior inescapable noise to recognize the pattern solution while it only took about three consecutive successes for students who received escapable or no noise (Miller & Seligman, 1975). This is evidence that perceiving independence between a response and reinforcement may interfere with the ability for individuals to later learn that responses produce outcomes. Peterson et al. (1993) suggest that the cognitive deficit associated with learned helplessness may be due to attentional-perceptual deficits (i.e. not attending to the cues correlated with their own responding) or expectational deficits (i.e. accurately registering the events of a trial but holding a biased expectation that the contingency will not hold on future trials).

A variety of experiments also indicate an emotional effect of uncontrollable events (Maier & Seligman, 1976). Studies generally support the notion that there is a significant increase in feelings of depression, anxiety, stress, frustration and hostility following non-contingent reinforcement (Miller & Norman, 1979). In addition, experiments show that participants who receive repeated uncontrollable events experience fear, which can result in physical symptoms such as increases in stomach ulcers and higher blood pressure than yoked controls (Maier & Watkins, 1998; Seligman, 1975). According to Seligman (1975), learned helplessness produces fear for as long as the subject perceives they do not have control of the outcome.

Learned Helplessness and Autism

From a practical point of view, there are parallel behavior patterns in individuals diagnosed with autism and those experiencing learned helplessness (Barnhill & Myles, 2001; Koegel & Egel, 1979; Koegel & Mentis, 1985; Koegel, O'Dell, & Dunlap, 1988). Children and adolescents with ASD have the ability to learn and communicate, but their communication and behavioral skills as well as their acquisition of new skills can vary depending on the situation (Koegel & Mentis, 1985). This suggests that they may be more capable than some of their behavior suggests, and that part of the difficulty in engaging in appropriate behavior and increasing skill acquisition may be due to learned helplessness.

Historically, researchers were uncertain whether individuals with ASD were unable to learn or if certain variables could be adjusted to increase their learning ability (Koegel & Mentis, 1985). Many felt that children with autism did not have the ability to communicate and engage with others, respond to environmental stimuli, or learn new skills or behaviors (Koegel & Egel, 1979). It was also originally believed that children with ASD were uneducable, and it was common to place them in mental institutions without providing any type of systematic education (Koegel & Koegel, 2006). However, research revealed that children with ASD had the potential to perform appropriate behaviors and learn new skills, but many had developed behaviors that interfered with their performance and learning abilities. For example, if a child with autism is learning how to get dressed, he or she may take a long time and make several mistakes. Consequently, their parents may assist and end up dressing the child themselves. Similarly, children with ASD may try to interact with peers, but communication and socialization deficits may cause their peers to not respond in a positive manner. In these examples, the child made an attempt at a skill but was not reinforced. Other times, they may be reinforced despite not having made an appropriate attempt. Through these types of experiences, children with ASD struggle to learn relevant response-reinforcement contingencies. The individual with ASD may begin to believe that his or her actions cannot control reinforcement, and consequently develop learned helplessness that reduces the likelihood they will initiate in future situations (Koegel & Mentis, 1985). Conceptually, one can imagine that if a child is born with autism and does not engage in the many social-communicative behaviors seen in typically developing children, well-meaning caregivers and teachers may have a tendency to help their child when they exhibit challenges. However, too much assistance may lead to a lack of effort and/or motivation on the child's part and a generalized state of learned helplessness.

Increasing Motivation to Overcome Learned Helplessness

One critical factor in overcoming learned helplessness is increasing the individual's level of motivation by making the response-reinforcement connection more salient (Koegel & Egel, 1979). Research shows that this approach can diminish behaviors associated with learned helplessness and increase the acquisition, generalization and maintenance of treatment gains (Koegel & Egel, 1979; Koegel & Mentis, 1985). Koegel and Egel (1979) first demonstrated that motivation is a critical variable in the behavior of individuals with ASD. Specifically, the researchers found that when children worked on tasks at which they were consistently incorrect, then they had low levels of motivation as measured by their infrequent and decreasing attempts at the task, as well as low levels of enthusiasm when attempting the task (Koegel & Egel, 1979). However, when the children were prompted to keep responding until they correctly completed the task, then the child's motivation increased and they continued working on the tasks with increased enthusiasm (Koegel & Egel, 1979). This suggests that forced exposure to the response-reinforcement contingency can correct the maladaptive behaviors associated with learned helplessness and increase the child's motivation to complete tasks. This appears especially important for individuals with ASD, because their disability may make it more challenging to correctly complete tasks that typically developing individuals may be able to complete more easily. However, assisting the child or adult with ASD to respond to a task before they receive reinforcement is critical in developing a sense of the response-reinforcement contingency, which is important in determining how the individual will behave in future situations (Koegel & Egel, 1979; Koegel & Koegel, 2006).

Instructions for Implementing PRT Procedures

Because of the importance of the pivotal area of learned helplessness proposed by Koegel and Egel (1979), many researchers have worked to develop effective treatment techniques to improve the motivation of individuals with ASD. Pivotal Response Treatment (PRT) was developed based on the theory of learned helplessness, and procedures were specifically designed to increase motivation (Koegel & Koegel, 2006, 2012). Increasing motivation has been shown to produce broad improvements in other areas of sociability, communication, behavior and academic skill building for individuals with ASD (Koegel & Koegel, 2006). It is important to note that the effective interventions prior to a focus on the pivotal area of motivation targeted single behaviors individually, making the intervention time-consuming and laborious. Our goal in creating an iteration of the previous effective ABA techniques was to develop an intervention that resulted in more widespread generalized gains, or to find "pivotal areas" that, when targeted, would result in improvements in a variety of untargeted areas.

Beginning in the early 1980s, our research efforts concentrated on developing procedures to increase motivation, and were directed towards developing techniques that would improve the overall responsiveness, engagement, and affect for children on the autism spectrum. Several techniques were studied individually, including child choice, reinforcing attempts, using natural reinforcers, and interspersing maintenance and acquisition tasks (Simpson, 2005). Research indicated that these treatment strategies were individually effective in producing positive behavioral and affective changes for children with ASD. We also found that combining these techniques as a package intervention had a large positive effect on learning and responding in children with autism. Specifically, the combined approach reduced behaviors related to learned helplessness due to an increase in the child's overall level of motivation (Koegel & Koegel, 2006; Koegel, O'Dell, & Koegel, 1987). In the remainder of this chapter, we will discuss each of these experimentally validated treatment components and provide illustrations for implementing the specific procedures.

Child Choice

Incorporating child choice involves using child-preferred materials, activities, topics and toys, and can help increase the child's responsiveness during interactions (Koegel, Dyer, & Bell, 1987). This can be accomplished by asking the child what he or she would like to play with, or by observing the child to see what items he or she gravitates toward. These items can then be incorporated into treatment sessions and used to stimulate and prompt responding. Children that tend to become overwhelmed when presented with many options can be offered a choice between a few preferred options. For example, the adult can ask the child, "Would you like to play with the trains or the cars?" In PRT, adults are instructed not to attempt to redirect the child to a specific item, but to be vigilant and attentive to items that the children find enjoyable as evidenced by their seeking out the item. Allowing the child to have some choice in the treatment creates higher levels of responding and improved positive affect (Dyer, Dunlap, & Winterling, 1990). A child's preference can vary over time and sometimes within a single intervention session, so it is important for the clinician to adjust when necessary and constantly reassess preference to assure that the most desired and sought after items and activities are being used to buttress and maintain motivation. Simply incorporating child choice into the treatment can improve a variety of areas, including social play, pragmatic behaviors, and language development. Furthermore, research shows that incorporating child choice into the intervention sessions can lead to improved generalization outside of the teaching setting (Carter, 2001).

Reinforcing Attempts

Reinforcing attempts is another component of PRT that has been shown to effectively increase motivation for individuals with ASD. Some children escape or avoid situations because previous failures have led them to believe that they cannot be successful (Hedley & Young, 2006; Koegel et al., 1987). However, when their attempts to complete tasks are reinforced, they tend to continue to make further attempts (Koegel & Koegel, 2006). For children with autism, these attempts frequently lead to some remarkable successes. Koegel et al. (1988) confirmed that reinforcing attempts is effective in increasing motivation and correct responding by comparing two different treatment conditions for nonverbal children with autism. One condition reinforced successive approximations of speech sounds through operant shaping, and the second "motivational" condition reinforced any attempts to produce speech sounds even if they were not correct. Results demonstrated that the experimental motivational condition was far more effective than reinforcing increasingly correct speech sounds via a strict shaping paradigm. Specifically, the motivational condition was superior with respect to improvements in the children's speech production and the children's interest, enthusiasm and general behavior (Koegel et al., 1988). Not only did the target speech sounds improve more quickly, but numerous important collateral gains were also observed. In contrast to the previous interventions, wherein it was believed that the children needed clear feedback for specific speech sounds and were regularly provided with clear consequences (e.g. "good job" or treats for correct responses or "no" for incorrect responses), we found that reinforcing all attempts produced more correct responding and improved affect. For example, if a child was learning first words and the target word was "ball", then reinforcing attempts would mean rewarding both a clear production of the word as well as a reasonable attempt, such as "ba." As long as the child was trying, then he or she was reinforced. However, it is important to remember that if the child made a perfect production but was not making an attempt (e.g. looking away uninterested or engaging in repetitive ritualistic behavior, etc.), then the child was not reinforced. This is critical, because we are focusing on the basic pivotal construct of improving motivation, not simply reinforcing the child for correct responses. Thus, reinforcing attempts at tasks and behaviors can provide response-reinforcement contingencies that will increase motivation and decrease symptoms of learned helplessness.

Direct and Natural Reinforcers

The purpose of using natural reinforcers directly related to the target response is to strengthen the child's understanding of the contingency between their response and the natural reinforcer, better than might be possible using an arbitrary reinforcer unrelated to the target behavior. In a simple example, when targeting verbal expressive communication, reinforcing a child's verbal request to play with a ball by giving him the ball can be considered natural because it resembles the contingencies likely to be experienced in the criterion environment (natural environment outside of treatment sessions). Whereas, reinforcing the child's social labeling of a flash card of a ball with a piece of candy would not resemble the likely consequence in the real world and would therefore be considered arbitrary. Response-reinforcement contingencies are strengthened through the use of direct and natural reinforcers for individuals with ASD, meaning the reinforcers directly relate to the task or behavior that is being taught (Koegel & Williams, 1980). It is still common to observe treatment providers using flash cards and other artificial stimulus materials, and then providing a favorite treat or other desired reinforcer. This will strengthen responding to the flash cards, but it may not teach the relationship between responding and reinforcement, a key point in remediating learned helplessness. Alternatively, a more effective teaching strategy is when the child is provided with a desired item or activity contingent upon a correct response that is inherently and naturally connected to the behavior (e.g. given an actual ball to play with after making a valid attempt at saying "ball"). Research shows that using direct and natural reinforcers improves the motivation level of the child, and enhances the strength of the response-reinforcement contingency (Koegel & Williams, 1980).

Interspersing Maintenance and Acquisition Tasks

Another component of PRT involves interspersing maintenance and acquisition tasks to increase motivation and decrease learned helplessness (Dunlap & Koegel, 1980). Incorporating and interspersing reinforcement for mastered tasks creates more frequent exposure to a favorable and well-established response-reinforcer contingency (Dunlap & Koegel, 1980). For example, data suggest that when a child with autism is learning mathematics, incorporating some math problems that the child can easily complete into the assignment in addition to the more difficult problems resulted in improved motivation, increased confidence, and more exposure to successful response-reinforcer contingencies. It is sometimes tempting to keep presenting difficult problems when a child is responding well, but incorporating a mix that includes some easier (mastered) tasks will result in increased attempts and improved engagement in more difficult tasks through the operant mechanism of behavioral momentum (Matson et al., 1996).

Task Variation

PRT also uses task variation to help improve motivation and responsiveness. Dunlap and Koegel (1980) first showed the differential effectiveness of using a constant task condition versus a varied task condition when teaching children with autism discrimination tasks. In the constant task condition, a single task was presented repeatedly throughout the session. During the varied task condition, the target task was interspersed with a variety of other tasks from the child's curricula. Results demonstrated that the children's correct responding declined during the constant task condition. In contrast, there was improved and more stable responding during the varied task condition. Affect was also measured using a Likert scale wherein naive observers scored tapes of the children and provided an overall subjective opinion of the children's affect during the sessions. The observers judged the children to be more enthusiastic, interested, and happier during the varied task sessions. This study led us to understand the importance of varying the task to improve responsiveness. Although there is a paucity of data and this area warrants further research to determine how to best accomplish task variation, it is likely that task variation can be accomplished using different stimuli and activities throughout the sessions. For example, if a clinician is working on helping the child discriminate between big versus little and having the child select his or her favorite toys based on size, the clinician may want to only present a few size trials and then move on to another target behavior (e.g., identifying color). Although it is tempting to present the same activity repeatedly with the intention of giving the child more consolidated and focused practice, research has shown that, in the end, this may actually result in slower rates of learning and an increase in behavior problems (Dunlap, 1984).

The Motivational Package of PRT

Pivotal Response Treatment consists of combining the aforementioned motivational components as a package. Prior to this development, studies that focused on verbal communication found that only about 50 % of children with autism became verbal (Prizant, 1983). However, when motivational components were incorporated into a treatment package, upwards of 90 % of children who began intervention during preschool years learned to use verbal expressive language as their primary mode of communication (Koegel, 2000). Researchers have also shown that PRT is equally effective at producing verbal communication when compared to alternative and augmentative communication (AAC) systems. This is helpful to understand, as parents prefer their young children be taught verbal communication over AAC (Schreibman & Stahmer, 2014). This is not to suggest that AAC systems are unimportant. For a small percentage of children who are unable to learn to use expressive verbal communication, AAC systems are highly recommended and the motivational procedures described above can be used to encourage communication via picture cards, speech generating devices, and manual signs or gestures in older children. However, given parental preference and the fact that at this point in time only about 20 % of nonverbal children over 5 years old are able to learn verbal communication as a primary mode of communication suggests that AAC should be considered after age 5 when a verbal-only approach using motivational procedures has been ineffective (Koegel, 2000; Koegel & Koegel, 2012).

Pivotal Areas

As previously mentioned, Pivotal Response Treatment is focused on targeting specific "pivotal" areas that when modified, produce very rapid and widespread gains in other areas relating to social, communication and behavioral skills. In addition to the pivotal area of motivation, our research indicates additional critical skill areas that when taught also result in broad improvements. Specifically, these pivotal areas include initiations, self-management, and response to multiple cues. Further, emerging data from preliminary studies suggest that empathy may also be a pivotal behavior that can be taught.

Initiations

Despite the increased level of responsiveness when children are motivated during Pivotal Response Treatment, we continue to perceive some disparities between the development of typical children's communication and the communication of children with autism. Additionally, there are also differential outcomes for children with autism (i.e. some children improved much more than others). Having the advantage of years of videotaped samples allowed us to go back to early videos of the children before they had received any intervention and assess for any differences that might have predicted differential treatment outcomes. This eventually allowed us to understand why some children had more positive outcomes than others, even though they all received what we believed to be very similar and intensive state-of-the-art programs with parent participation and inclusive educational settings whenever possible. In this retrospective videotape study, we examined archival data of adolescents and adults who had very poor outcomes and compared them with individuals who had very good outcomes (Koegel, Koegel, Shoshan, & McNerney, 1999). We first selected two groups of children, all of whom had seemingly good prognostic indicators (i.e. verbal communication skills and verbal intelligence quotients above 50 in the preschool years) with the intention of studying why some children with these apparently similar early signs would have very different outcomes. Interestingly, when we analyzed archival videotapes of the children, we found that the individuals who eventually had the most favorable long-term treatment outcomes had a higher number of verbal and nonverbal initiations during the toddler years. Specifically, in a simulated waiting room setting, the children with the best outcomes had engaged in more verbal and nonverbal initiations with their mothers, such as bringing them toys or labeling items during their preschool years. From this analysis, it appeared that initiations were an important prognostic indicator for positive long-term outcomes for children with ASD.

Based on this first phase of the study, we became interested in whether we could teach initiations to children with autism who did not initiate to others and, if so, would those children then have more favorable treatment outcomes. Through our research, we found that children with autism who did not engage in initiations during baseline could be taught to initiate to others. Furthermore, they did indeed have improved outcomes that were similar to children in the first study after receiving the intervention focused on teaching initiations (Koegel et al., 1999). That is, those children who learned to initiate were more likely to have success in school, go to college, develop friendships, and so on.

We first started teaching initiations by examining whether we could teach children with autism a common verbal initiation, such as asking the first questions that are generally acquired during a toddler's development. Specifically, we first assessed if we could teach the children to ask, "What's that?" (frequently shortened to "Dat?" while pointing to an item) which is typically within a toddler's first lexicon. A few question-asking studies had been published that taught individuals with autism but, researchers had reported difficulty with generalization to other peers and settings (Hung, 1977) or the need for nonverbal prompting to evoke a question (Raulston et al., 2013; Taylor & Harris, 1995). After difficulties with several intervention iterations while trying to teach question-asking, we incorporated motivational components into the intervention to assess whether this would increase spontaneous and generalized use of question-asking (Koegel, Camarata, Valdez-Menchaca, & Koegel, 1998). We placed a variety of child preferred items in an opaque bag and prompted the children to ask, "What's that?" about items in the bag. Furthermore, before giving the desired items to the child, we had them repeat the label. Conceptually, our goal was to provide a context wherein both child choice and natural reinforcers could be used when the child initiated a question. This procedure was highly effective in increasing question-asking for children with ASD. After question-asking was occurring at a high rate, we began fading out the child-preferred items and gradually (beginning with every fourth item) replacing the preferred items with neutral items that the child was not able to label. Eventually, we also faded the opaque bag, so that we could use items naturally placed around the room. As a result of this intervention, vocabulary tests showed that the children began learning the targeted words as a result of increases in question asking, and generalization measures indicated that the children used their newly learned questions and their new vocabularies in the home and school. One might argue that the question originally functioned as a request for obtaining the item, because the children were very likely anticipating that one of their favorite items was in the bag. That is, one might suspect that the children were merely asking for an item in the bag, rather than asking an information-seeking question about the label of the item in the bag. However, that did not appear to be the case, as the generalization probes showed that the children also asked questions in other appropriate contexts for the more social purpose of seeking information regarding the labels of items, and not as requests to obtain them.

After successfully teaching "What's that?" we began developing procedures to teach a variety of other questions. The second question we taught was "Where is it?" which usually comes next in the developmental sequence (Bellugi, 1965; Rowland, Pine, Lieven, & Theakston, 2003). To teach this initiation, we hid the child's favorite items in various locations, and then prompted the child to ask where the item was. After the child initiated the question "Where is it?" the adult informed the child of the location so that the child could seek out the desired item. Following the successful teaching of "Where is it?" we have also taught additional questions, such as "Whose is it?" to result in the acquisition of possessive pronouns (e.g. "mine" and "yours") and the possessive "s" (e.g. "Daddy's"). To teach "Whose is it?" we used favorite items in a collection of items that were possessed by the child, and neutral items in a collection of items that were possessed by the clinician. Eventually, we were able to use neutral items in both collections, with the children continuing to ask the question, "Whose is it?" We then went on to teach additional questions such as "What's happening?" and "What happened?" to increase the child's use of verbs and verb endings by using pop-up books centered on themes around the child's interest (e.g., "-ing" and past tense such as "ed."). Specifically, we manipulated the tab of the pop-up in the book and prompted the children to ask "What's happening?" or "What happened?" Following the query, we responded with a conjugated verb. The results showed increases in questions, and consequently verb diversity as well as the targeted verb ending (-ing or past tense) (Koegel, Carter, & Koegel, 2003). Finally, we targeted non-question initiations such as "Help" and "Look" so the children could learn to initiate attention-seeking and assistance-seeking strategies. In order to provide natural reinforcers for "Help" and "Look" we arranged situations such as putting a treat or desired item in a tightly sealed jar, then prompting the child to request "Help" so that a natural reinforcer followed when the adult helped the child open the jar. Similarly, just before a child was provided with a favorite item or activity, we prompted the child to say "Look!" or "Look, Mommy!" then provided that opportunity to demonstrate play with the favorite item or to demonstrate the desired activity.

This second phase of our study showed that children who were taught initiations also had rapid and broad areas of behavioral improvements, resulting in greatly improved long-term outcomes (Koegel et al., 1999). For example, the participants in our studies who initially focused their very limited initiations for functions of requests and protests were not exhibiting communicative competence in a broad range of language functions. In contrast, teaching question-asking and other related initiations in a motivational context resulted in collateral gains in a variety of areas, including naive raters judging the children as appearing more appropriate on normalcy scales (Koegel et al., 1999; Koegel, Koegel, Green-Hopkins, & Barnes, 2010). Thus, due to the widespread positive effect of improving initiations on broad areas of the children's functioning, we came to consider initiations a pivotal area.

Self-Management

In addition to identifying the pivotal areas of motivation and initiations, we have also identified self-management as a pivotal area for individuals with autism. This came about when we realized that individuals with autism spectrum disorder often do not control their behaviors in the absence of an interventionist. It is interesting that this area of study came about relatively late in intervention research for autism. This was largely due to the fact that professionals believed that self-management might not be possible for children with autism. In the 1970s, self-management was considered a viable and desirable treatment for other populations besides individuals with autism and for a variety of target behaviors such as weight reduction (Horan & Johnson, 1971), health issues (Mitchell & White, 1977), marital discord (Goldiamond, 1965), study habits (Fox, 1962) and smoking cessation (Roberts, 1969). For the most part, these studies focused on adults with average intellectual functioning. Few studies focused on children with disabilities, and many believed a child with a severe disability (e.g. autism) would be unable to engage in self-management due to cognitive impairments. Similar to other researchers, our early work focused on using self-management with children who did not have autism, but rather who demonstrated more limited disabilities such as difficulties with speech sound production (Koegel, Koegel, & Ingham, 1986). However, we rapidly began to speculate that the procedures might be effective for individuals with autism, and decided to embark on a line of research to assess whether self-management might indeed be possible for children with autism. In an early study by Koegel and Koegel (1990) we targeted loud and repetitive stereotypic responding that occurred by children with autism in full-inclusion public school classrooms. We found that students with autism could learn self-management skills. For example, the children were able to learn to use alarms to signal them to evaluate a previous time period as to whether or not a disruptive behavior had occurred, and then record on a piece of paper the presence or absence of the disruptive behavior. Later, contingent upon a pre-determined number of appropriately recorded responses, the students could self-reward or turn in their points to obtain a reinforcer. For example, one older elementary child with whom we worked earned points at school for quietly staying on task as opposed to engaging in loud verbal repetitive behaviors and not completing his assignments. Once he earned a predetermined number of points for successful intervals through self-management, he was able to take out his earphones and electronic music device and listen to one his favorite jazz music pieces. Some children require a bit more adult direction, but others can be taught to self-administer their own rewards, such as the example above.

Several steps are required to teach self-management skills. First, we carefully define and measure the behavior. Next, a system for self-monitoring is created and reinforcers are identified with the help of the individual with autism. If the response is measurable by frequency, such as each time the child asked a question or responded to a question, responses were tallied using a counter. If the behavior is measurable by using a time period with appropriate behavior, such as an extended period of time with appropriate classroom behavior (e.g. staying in seat, engaging in assigned work) then an alarming timer (such as an iPhone) or watch (with a repeat chronographic alarm function) that can be set to the predetermined time interval can be used. Next, the individual needs to understand what behavior is to be self-evaluated. Examples of appropriate and inappropriate behaviors are described and demonstrated, and then the individual practices monitoring their own behavior. Generally, we try to use the self-management of a positive behavior (e.g., "Did you stay in your seat?") rather than an undesired behavior ("Did you get out of your seat?"). After it is clear that the individual understands the target behavior, a time period or number of responses is specified in order to receive the predetermined reinforcer. It is important that the initial interval or response requirement be small enough (we based this on pretreatment assessments) so that the individual experiences success and is motivated to continue with the intervention. After the individual is engaging in the desired behavior and accurately monitoring behavior, then the self-management program is ready to be implemented. As the individual continues to self-monitor, the time interval or number of responses required to receive a reinforcer is gradually and systematically increased until it more closely approximates that of a typical individual in the same environment. For example, if typical children in the classroom usually work for a period of 30 min, then we use a 30-min interval for our final target.

Self-management has now been shown to be effective with a variety of behaviors in individuals with autism including on-task behavior in school (Dunlap, Dunlap, Koegel, & Koegel, 1991), responsiveness to questions, decreasing disruptive behavior (Koegel, Koegel, Hurley, & Frea, 1992), and many other areas. For children who have limited or no expressive verbal communication, pictorial self-management can be used (Pierce & Schreibman, 1994). For example, a variety of pictures depicting the desired behavior (e.g., setting the table, brushing teeth, and putting away toys) can be given to the individual to use as guides to manage their behavior. To be sure that the self-management is being used rather than just following a routine, the order of the pictures can be varied. Again, it is important to note that self-management has been shown to be an excellent tool to teach the engagement of a desired response or behavior in the absence of a treatment provider. The ability to become self-aware of a desired or undesired behavior, and to be able to self-control that behavior, has been shown to result in positive improvements in a variety of other untargeted behaviors. For example, when an individual with autism is taught to self manage one pragmatic behavior, such as appropriate body posturing toward the conversational partner, other areas (such as eye contact) can improve without having to be directly targeted (Koegel & Frea, 1993). Thus, self-management appears to be another pivotal area.

Response to Multiple Cues

Research indicates that responding to multiple cues is another pivotal area for individuals with autism. Overselective responding to only a limited part of a complex stimulus (e.g. a father's glasses, rather than the father's face as a whole) has been a particularly problematic for individuals on the autism spectrum. One of the first studies addressing this issue showed that, while typically developing children may take in three relevant cues from a stimulus (e.g., a face), children with autism may only respond to one cue (Lovaas, Schreibman, Koegel, & Rehm, 1971). In a laboratory setting, the study showed that when simultaneously presented with visual, auditory, and tactile cues, the children with autism only responded to one of the cues. This same phenomenon may occur when only two stimuli are presented; the children with autism often just respond to one cue (Koegel & Wilhelm, 1973). Later studies suggested that this may also occur in relation to social stimuli and complex teaching cues where extra stimuli are presented as prompts. In this latter example, children would often become heavily prompt dependent, and fail to learn the actual skill targeted. For example, during classwork many children with ASD would respond to the teacher's eye gaze at the correct stimulus or to a crease in the corner of a flash card rather than learning the targeted skill.

Similarly, social competence requires that an individual respond to a multiplicity of cues, which can change to some extent on a daily basis. For example, initial work in this area demonstrated that children with autism could be taught to recognize a male versus a female doll, but when certain irrelevant characteristics (e.g., the doll's belts) were switched, then the children were unable to respond correctly as to which stimulus was the male versus the female (Schreibman & Lovaas, 1973). Although typically developing young children may also respond on the basis of a limited number of cues, they appear to rapidly learn which cues are most relevant. That is, a typically developing young child generally responds to the head of the doll and not the clothing or other body parts and, when the head is changed (keeping all other stimuli constant), a typical developing child will continue to respond correctly when asked to identify the doll's gender. In contrast, the children with autism responded based on one cue that was usually irrelevant (e.g. the belt), such that when the pants or skirt were removed, the child with ASD was no longer able to discriminate whether the doll was male or female. One can imagine how this may cause numerous difficulties in social settings, particularly when the relevant features of a stimulus that a child responds to may not include the face or head.

Having said that, it should be noted that the original work conducted in the 1970s was during a time when the motivational components had not yet been discovered, the children tended to be excluded from most community settings, and treatment was provided in structured environments that were free from distractions (Lovaas, 1977). These types of unnatural, sterile teaching environments may have compounded the problem of overselective responding. Now that we use motivational components through PRT and provide treatment in natural settings, many children do not need specialized work on multiple cues. It may be that motivating the children results in broadening the children's attention. It has been shown that response to multiple stimuli involved in joint attention can improve without any special intervention if motivation is targeted (Bruinsma, 2004; Vismara & Lyons, 2007).

However, for the small percentage of children that do continue to have difficulties responding to multiple cues, there are intervention procedures to address this deficit (Burke & Cerniglia, 1990). For example, multiple cues can be presented in the context of child choice. If a child enjoys coloring with markers, the adult can offer him a variety of markers and sizes, such as the big blue marker, the little blue marker, the big red marker, and the little red marker. If the child selects the marker based on both size and color, we know that he or she is responding to both cues. It is possible to be creative and incorporate multiple cues into daily routines, such as getting dressed (e.g., "Put on your blue short sleeved shirt and your jean shorts"), cooking (e.g. "Can you hand me the long wooden spoon?"), and so on, as long as other items cues are available for the child to discriminate. Research shows that this type of embedded teaching can improve overall consistency of responding to complex stimuli, as well as decrease the social and academic difficulties caused by not responding to all of the relevant cues. Therefore, responding to multiple cues also appears to be a pivotal area in the sense that it produces widespread improvements across a variety of areas.

Empathy

The final pivotal area that we are beginning to research relates to empathy (Koegel, Ashbaugh, Koegel, Detar, & Regester, 2013). The development of social understanding is complicated and is clearly affected by many variables. The fact that most individuals with ASD report that they prefer to be with other people and want to have friends (Muller, Schuler, & Yates, 2008), as well as the variability in testing patterns, suggests that it is not completely accurate to state that individuals on the autism spectrum simply cannot understand others' feelings. However, some behaviors, particularly social skills, necessitate the ability to "mentalize" or be able to understand others' thoughts (Frith & Happé, 1994). Some have hypothesized that this challenge for individuals with ASD may be caused by some type of cognitive deficit. However, most agree that whether or not an individual has a cognitive deficit, the problem would be greatly exacerbated by a lack of social interaction. Further, we have begun intervention and are finding that areas related to the expression of empathy can improve with intervention. We have used a variety of approaches including self-management, visual cues, and video-feedback to teach adolescents and adults to respond in an empathetic manner. Teaching both the expression of empathetic understanding and empathetic interests (e.g., question-asking related to another person's interests) in response to leading statements has been helpful. Specifically, while we engage in social conversation, we may say, "I had a great weekend." If the individual does not continue the conversation by showing understanding and interest of the other person's situation, then we may prompt them to say "That sounds like fun, did you go out of town?" or "That is good to hear, what did you do?" or "Glad you had a nice weekend, did you see friends?" With repeated practice in response to a variety of leading statements, individuals with ASD learn to express empathetic understanding and interest, and respond in a way that continues the social conversation (Ashbaugh, 2014). Again, while this is a new area of our research, we are finding that these empathetic responses can be learned, and individuals who respond empathetically are judged to be more desirable conversational partners, have improved social conversation, and hypothetically will have an easier time developing and maintaining relationships. Due to the preliminary results that indicate targeting empathy produces widespread gains in areas of social interaction and improving relationships (Ashbaugh, 2014), we believe that it is a potential pivotal area.

Review of Research on PRT Procedures

A large number of published studies support the use of PRT. Some focus on the individual components (i.e. child choice, direct and natural reinforcers, rewarding attempts, interspersing maintenance tasks, and task variation) and additional research has evaluated the components as a package. Studies have been conducted using single case experimental designs as well as group designs. Research has been conducted both within our center and at additional sites. Table 4.1 represents some of the many studies that provide an empirical base for PRT.

Suggestions for Future Research

There are a number of areas related to PRT that would benefit from future research. First, there are likely additional pivotal responses that have yet to be discovered. Second, future research is necessary to examine issues relating to parent stress for families with an individual on the autism spectrum. While our research has found that the implementation of PRT is less stressful for parents to implement than more structured approaches (Koegel, Bimbela, & Schreibman, 1996), there is still a

Table 4.1 A sampling of articles demonstrating the empirical support for pivotal response treatment[a]

Study	Design	Treatment	Dependent variables	Treatment outcome
Support for PRT as a package intervention				
Mohammadzaheri, Koegel, Rezaee, and Rafiee (2014)	Randomized clinical trial	PRT targeting language vs. Structured ABA	Mean Length of Utterance and Pragmatics	PRT approach was significantly more effective in improving targeted and untargeted areas after 3 months of intervention.
Voos et al. (2012)	Single case series	PRT targeting pivotal areas of development, including motivation, social initiation and responsivity in order to improve social and language functioning in both participants.	Total Fixation Duration and percent of looking time at adult faces	PRT resulted in increased activation in regions recruited by typically developing children during social perception.
			Neural mechanisms supporting social perception	
			Skills in communication, daily living and socialization	
			Pragmatic skills	
			Number of on topic comments, questions, total narrative details, and conversations	
Baker-Ericzen, Stahmer, and Burns (2007)	Clinical replication	Large-scale community-based 12-week parent education	Communication	Following parent education in
			Daily living skills	PRT, all children showed significant improvement in communication, daily living skills, socialization, motor skills, and Adaptive Behavior Composite domains of the *Vineland Adaptive Behavior Scales* regardless of gender, age, and race/ethnicity of the families.
		PRT intervention and examined whether child variables are associated with treatment outcome	Socialization	
			Motor skills	
			Adaptive behaviors	
Schreibman, Kaneko, and Koegel (1991)	Group design with random assignment	Traditional Discrete Trial vs. PRT	Parental affect	Parents in the PRT condition displayed significantly more positive affect than parents trained in Discrete Trial.

(continued)

Support for PRT components				
Child choice				
Koegel, Dyer, et al. (1987)	Three studies: correlational analysis, repeated reversals design with three children, community setting	Manipulation of child-preferred and arbitrary activities	Number of social avoidance behaviors (gaze aversion, closed eyes, etc.)	Child-preferred activities and social avoidance behaviors were significantly negatively correlated in terms of both objectively scored behavior and subjective ratings of social responsiveness in unmanipulated settings.
			Subjective measures of social responsiveness	
Reinforcing attempts				
Koegel et al. (1988)	Within-subject repeated reversals design	Compared two different reinforcement conditions:	Ratings of affect	While each condition produced some improvement in the children's speech, the data indicate that considerably more rapid and consistent progress occurred when the children were reinforced within the framework of a speech attempts contingency rather than when they were reinforced solely on the basis of their correct speech production.
		Successive motor approximates of speech sounds reinforced	Measures of improvement in speech production	
		"Motivation" condition in which attempts to produce speech sounds were reinforced; no motor shaping of speech		
Task variation				
Dunlap and Koegel (1980)	Within subject design, multiple baseline across participants	Varied task condition vs. constant task condition	Number of correct unprompted responses to questions	Declining trends in correct responding during the constant task condition, with substantially improved and stable responding during varied task condition.
			Enthusiasm, happiness and interest	Children more enthusiastic, interested, and better behaved during the varied task sessions.
Natural reinforcers				
Koegel and Williams (1980)	Multiple baseline design across participants	Two different response-reinforcer relationships: (1) target behaviors were a direct part of the response chain required to procure a reinforcer and (2) where target behavior was an indirect part of chain leading to reinforce	Percentage of correct responses	Results showed rapid acquisition only when the target behavior was a direct part of the chain leading to the reinforcer.

(continued)

Table 4.1 (continued)

Study	Design	Treatment	Dependent variables	Treatment outcome
Support for pivotal areas				
A. *Motivation*				
Koegel, Singh, Koegel, Hollingsworth, and Bradshaw (2013)	Multiple baseline design across participants	Modified PRT was used to assess the feasibility of rapidly increasing infant motivation to engage in social interaction	Percentage response to name	Results demonstrated that consistently low or erratic levels of social behavior were evident during baseline period, and these patterns could be improved with PRT. Social engagement immediately increased and social engagement remained at a stable and high level at follow-up.
			Avoidance of eye contact	
			Affect (interest and happiness)	
			Fidelity of implementation	
Koegel, Singh, and Koegel (2010)	Multiple baseline design across participants	Specific motivational variables such as choice, interspersal of maintenance tasks, and natural reinforcers incorporated into academic tasks	Academics (writing and math performance)	For all children, disruptive behavior decreased immediately following implementation of the intervention and remained low throughout the intervention and post intervention phases.
Koegel and Egel (1979)	Multiple baseline design across subjects	Influence of correct versus incorrect task completion on children's motivation to respond to such tasks. Treatment procedures designed to prompt children to keep responding until they completed the tasks correctly.	Proportion of time child attempted to complete tasks without engaging in non-related behavior	Effective treatments were those that increased exposure to a response-reinforcement contingency for completing the tasks.
			Enthusiasm level	
B. *Initiations*				
Koegel, Carter, et al. (2003)	Multiple baseline design across participants	Assessed whether children with autism could be taught a child-initiated query as a pivotal response to facilitate the use of grammatical morphemes.	Language	Both children learned the self-initiated strategy and both acquired and generalized the targeted morpheme. Additionally, generalized use of the self-initiation into other question forms and concomitant increases in mean length of utterance, verb acquisition, and diversity of verb use occurred for both children.
			Use of morphemes	

Koegel, Koegel, Shoshan, and McNerney (1999)	Retrospective analysis of archival data	Examined treatment outcomes for children initiating social communication at high and low rates	Number of initiations	Retrospective analysis of archival data showed that children who exhibited high levels of spontaneous initiations at pre-intervention had more favorable post-intervention outcomes. In addition, children who were taught to initiate social communication (when such initiating was low) showed highly favorable post-intervention outcomes.
			Pragmatic ratings	
			Social/community functioning	
		Assessed an intervention to teach initiations	Adaptive behavior scale scores	
C. *Language*				
Koegel, Koegel, et al. (2010)	Multiple baseline design across participants	Taught children to use the question "Where is it?" using intrinsic reinforcers	Language acquisition	The children could rapidly acquire and generalize the query, and that there were collateral improvements in the children's use of language structures corresponding to the answers to the questions the children asked.
			Number of unprompted "where" questions asked	
			Number of prepositions/ordinal markers correctly produced	
Koegel, O'Dell, et al. (1987)	Multiple baseline design across participants	Traditional Discrete	Imitative child utterances	Children produced more imitative and spontaneous utterances in the PRT condition. Generalization of treatment gains occurred only in the PRT condition.
		Trial vs. PRT (called Analogue Treatment[a] vs. NLP[a])	Spontaneous child utterances	
			Generalization	
D. *Self-management*				
Koegel et al. (1992)	Multiple baseline design across participants	Self-management used to improve responsiveness to verbal initiations from others in multiple settings without the presence of a treatment provider.	Responsiveness to verbal initiations	Collateral reductions in disruptive behavior occurred when the children's responsivity improved.

[a]Historically, various terms have been used synonymously in these empirical articles. For example, PRT was previously called the Natural Language Paradigm (NLP) when intervention focuses on language. PRT has also been referred to as training in the pivotal areas of motivation, self-initiations and self-management

generalized level of stress that accompanies a parent after their child is diagnosed with ASD. Our preliminary work suggests that PRT can be effectively implemented when also incorporating parent-preferred activities, and this may be helpful in lowering parental stress levels (Kim, 2014). It would be beneficial for future research to examine procedures that assist in reducing stress for parents with autism.

Another recent area in which research should be expanded relates to the age of beginning intervention for a child displaying signs of ASD. We are now adapting PRT to be implemented with infants who show early at risk signs of autism (Koegel, Singh, et al., 2013). This early intervention may be especially important in improving outcomes, and discovering procedures that result in improvements in prelinguistic communication. Several recent pilot studies suggest that intervention may be helpful in decreasing concerning behavioral symptoms and improving early social communication for infants at risk for autism (Rogers et al., 2014). Studies are beginning to show that components of PRT can be used to improve gestural communication (e.g. pointing) as early as 12 months (Steiner, Gengoux, Klin, & Chawarska, 2013) and social engagement for infants under 12 months (Koegel, Singh, et al., 2013). PRT components that appear to be effective with infants generally involve using infant preferred items and activities in natural settings. Further, most of the infant interventions programs utilize parent education. Thus, infant intervention can be cost and time efficient (Koegel, Koegel, Ashbaugh, & Bradshaw, 2014). Furthermore, concerned parents can actively begin implementing intervention rather than following a "wait and see" approach, thereby improving child behavior as well as reducing levels of parental stress (Bradshaw, Steiner, Gengoux, & Koegel, 2014).

Lastly, additional research is necessary for developing procedures to improve employment outcomes for individuals on the autism spectrum. Securing and maintaining employment is often challenging for adults with ASD. We have published a promising study suggesting that improvement in social interactions can also improve job acquisition (Koegel, Singh, et al., 2013). This is an important area to address, as the literature indicates that individuals with ASD that participate in the workforce enjoy an improved quality of life and increased cognitive abilities (Garcia-Villamisar, Ross, & Wehman, 2000). Additionally, improving employment outcomes for the population with ASD has economic advantages for both individuals on the autism spectrum and the general public (Cimera & Burgess, 2011; Mawhood & Howlin, 1999).

Implications for Families and Practitioners

While we discussed a variety of issues relating to PRT, we would like to emphasis some underlying considerations for families and practitioners. First, it appears to be important that treatment is implemented in natural environments and individuals with ASD are included with their typical peers whenever possible (Koegel, Matos-Fredeen, Lang, & Koegel, 2012). This means utilizing items and activities found in natural settings, and including children with ASD with their typically developing peers as often as possible. There are a plethora of studies discussing the social and academic benefits of inclusion and treatment in the natural environment for individuals with ASD (Watkins et al., 2015).

Second, it is important to remember that parent education is a critical component of PRT (Koegel, Brookman, & Koegel, 2003; Koegel, Koegel, Kellegrew, & Mullen, 1996; Koegel, Symon, & Koegel, 2002; Santarelli, Koegel, Casas, & Koegel, 2001). It appears that parents should be active participants in the child's treatment program, and should understand how to conduct and incorporate PRT procedures (Lang, Machalicek, Rispoli, & Regester, 2009). It seems to be essential that parents implement the treatment procedures frequently throughout the child's waking hours so that the child is able to receive the maximum amount of treatment, under easy to administer naturalistic conditions. It also seems to us that it may be helpful to provide parents with feedback while they work with their child, in order to create consistency across settings and treatment providers.

Third, Fidelity of Implementation (FoI) is important to consider when conducting treatment. We have identified very specific researched components that individuals must implement at 80% criteria in order to meet Fidelity of Implementation. Treatment providers who do not meet FoI will most likely be ineffective and may even be counterproductive to the child's progress. Staff and family members should be consistently monitored to ensure that they are implementing the correct procedures and that the components are well coordinated across settings.

Closely related to making sure that providers are implementing PRT properly is the importance of regularly collecting data. Data collection helps objectively assess whether the individual is responding favorably to the intervention program, or if the treatment goals and interventions need to be adjusted. It is important that data are collected in a discrete and logical manner. It is common for clinicians to collect data on every response, which can interfere with the naturalness of the interaction and reduce teaching opportunities. Data collected at carefully-planned and logical times through probes can be just as revealing and accurate as response-by-response data, and may be easier for clinicians (Kuriakose, 2012). Of course, if a child is nonverbal and the target response is first words or word attempts that the child emits extremely infrequently, data should be collected on each trial. In contrast, if a child is producing hundreds of words an hour, recording every response may interfere with the interaction. In short, be smart about methods for data collection. Make a logical plan for data collection so that you will be able to assess progress for the individual with ASD.

Next, we would like to emphasize a strength-based approach when working with individuals with ASD (Cosden, Koegel, Koegel, Greenwell, & Klein, 2006). Oftentimes, professionals that work with an individual who has disabilities focus on the deficits and forget that those with autism have many areas of strength upon which we can build. Research shows that focusing on an individual's strengths while developing goals and interventions has a measured positive effect on parents (Steiner, 2011). Furthermore, strengths can be used as a positive tool for targeting areas relating to academics, communication, and social areas (Pituch et al., 2011).

Finally, multi-component programs are necessary for teaching many behaviors (e.g. conversation skills, increasing social activities, etc.). Most social communication goals and disruptive behaviors require several interventions to be implemented simultaneously. Again, data should be collected on a regular basis for multi-component programs to continuously assess if the child is making progress. It is also important to coordinate multi-component programs across settings to ensure that all treatment providers are well-trained. While PRT greatly improves efficiency, and dramatically reduces the number of interventions required, it appears that at this point in time it is still necessary to implement several interventions in an efficient multi-component package.

In summary, PRT is a well-researched intervention for individuals with ASD. Incorporating techniques to increase motivation for individuals with ASD can efficiently decrease symptoms of learned helplessness and increase skill acquisition. Studies show that PRT can be applied to a variety of areas including communication, socialization, and academics. Using PRT has also been shown to produce observable improvements in affect and responsiveness, and decreases in disruptive and off-task behavior. By focusing treatment on pivotal areas, we can produce widespread gains that will efficiently improve core challenges for individuals on the autism spectrum.

References

Abramson, L. Y., Seligman, M. E., & Teasdale, J. D. (1978). Learned helplessness in humans: Critique and reformulation. *Journal of Abnormal Psychology, 87*, 49.

Ashbaugh, K. (2014, September). *Improving success for adults with ASD in higher education and employment settings*. Paper presented at the Seventh Annual Pivotal Response Treatment Conference. University of California, Santa Barbara.

Baker-Ericzen, M. J., Stahmer, A. C., & Burns, A. (2007). Child demographics associated with outcomes in a community-based Pivotal Response Training program. *Journal of Positive Behavioral Interventions, 9*, 52–60.

Barnhill, G. P., & Myles, B. S. (2001). Attributional style and depression in adolescents with Asperger syndrome. *Journal of Positive Behavior Interventions, 3*, 175–182.

Bellugi, U. (1965). The development of interrogative structures in children's speech. In K. Riegel (Ed.), *The development of language functions* (pp. 103–138). Ann Arbor, MI: University of Michigan Language Development Program.

Bradshaw, J., Steiner, A. M., Gengoux, G., & Koegel, L. K. (2014). Feasibility and effectiveness of very early intervention for infants at-risk for Autism Spectrum Disorder: A systematic review. *Journal of Autism and Developmental Disorders, 45*, 778–794.

Bruinsma, Y. (2004). *Increases in the joint attention behavior of eye gaze alternation to share enjoyment as a collateral effect of Pivotal Response Treatment for three children with autism*. Santa Barbara, CA: University of California.

Burke, J. C., & Cerniglia, L. (1990). Stimulus complexity and autistic children's responsivity: Assessing and training a pivotal behavior. *Journal of Autism and Developmental Disorders, 20*, 233–253.

Carter, C. M. (2001). Using choice with game play to increase language skills and interactive behaviors in children with autism. *Journal of Positive Behavior Interventions, 3*, 131–151.

Cimera, R. E., & Burgess, S. (2011). Do adults with autism benefit monetarily from working in their communities? *Journal of Vocational Rehabilitation, 34*, 173–180.

Cosden, M., Koegel, L. K., Koegel, R. L., Greenwell, A., & Klein, E. (2006). Strength-based assessment for children with autism spectrum disorders. *Research and Practice for Persons with Severe Disabilities, 31*, 134–143.

Dunlap, G. (1984). The influence of task variation and maintenance tasks on the learning and affect of autistic children. *Journal of Experimental Child Psychology, 37*, 41–64.

Dunlap, L. K., Dunlap, G., Koegel, L. K., & Koegel, R. L. (1991). Using self-monitoring to increase students' success and independence. *Teaching Exceptional Children, 23*, 17–22.

Dunlap, G., & Koegel, R. L. (1980). Motivating autistic children through stimulus variation. *Journal of Applied Behavior Analysis, 13*, 619–627.

Dyer, K., Dunlap, G., & Winterling, V. (1990). Effects of choice making on the serious problem behaviors of students with severe handicaps. *Journal of Applied Behavior Analysis, 23*, 515–524.

Fox, L. (1962). Effecting the use of efficient study habits. *Journal of Mathematics, 1*, 75–86.

Frith, U., & Happé, F. (1994). Autism: Beyond "theory of mind". *Cognition, 50*, 115–132.

Garcia-Villamisar, D., Ross, D., & Wehman, P. (2000). Clinical differential analysis of persons with autism in a work setting: A follow-up study. *Journal of Vocational Rehabilitation, 14*, 183–185.

Goldiamond, I. (1965). Self-control procedures in personal behavior problems: Monograph supplement 3-V17. *Psychological Reports, 17*, 851–851.

Hedley, D., & Young, R. (2006). Social Comparison Processes in Depressive Symptoms in Children and Adolescents with Asperger Syndrome. *Autism, 10*(2), 139–153.

Hiroto, D. S. (1974). Locus of control and learned helplessness. *Journal of Experimental Psychology, 102*, 187.

Hiroto, D. S., & Seligman, M. E. (1975). Generality of learned helplessness in man. *Journal of Personality and Social Psychology, 31*, 311.

Horan, J. J., & Johnson, R. G. (1971). Coverant conditioning through a self-management application of the Premack principle: Its effect on weight reduction. *Journal of Behavior Therapy and Experimental Psychiatry, 2*, 243–249.

Hung, D. W. (1977). Generalization of "curiosity" questioning behavior in autistic children. *Journal of Behavior Therapy and Experimental Psychiatry, 8*, 237–245.

Kim, S. (2014). *Incorporating parent preferred interests into social interventions*. Paper presented at the Seventh Annual Pivotal Response Treatment Conference. University of California, Santa Barbara.

Klein, D. C., Fencil-Morse, E., & Seligman, M. E. (1976). Learned helplessness, depression, and the attribution of failure. *Journal of Personality and Social Psychology, 33*, 508–516.

Koegel, L. K. (2000). Interventions to facilitate communication in autism. *Journal of Autism and Developmental Disorders, 30*, 383–391.

Koegel, L. K., Ashbaugh, K., Koegel, R. L., Detar, W. J., & Regester, A. (2013). Increasing socialization in adults with Asperger's syndrome. *Psychology in the Schools, 50*, 899–909.

Koegel, R. L., Bimbela, A., & Schreibman, L. (1996). Collateral effects of parent training on family interactions. *Journal of Autism and Developmental Disorders, 26*, 347–359.

Koegel, R. L., Brookman, L., & Koegel, L. K. (2003). Autism: Pivotal response intervention and parent empowerment. *The Economics of Neuroscience, 5*, 61–69.

Koegel, L. K., Camarata, S. M., Valdez-Menchaca, M. C., & Koegel, R. L. (1998). Teaching children with autism to use self-initiated strategy to learn expressive vocabulary. *American Journal of Mental Retardation, 102*, 346–357.

Koegel, L. K., Carter, C. M., & Koegel, R. L. (2003). Teaching children with autism self-initiations as a pivotal response. *Topics in Language Disorders, 23*, 134–145.

Koegel, R. L., Dyer, K., & Bell, L. K. (1987). The influence of child-preferred activities on autistic children's social behavior. *Journal of Applied Behavior Analysis, 20*, 243–252.

Koegel, R. L., & Egel, A. L. (1979). Motivating autistic children. *Journal of Abnormal Psychology, 88*, 418–426.

Koegel, R. L., & Frea, W. D. (1993). Treatment of social behavior in autism through the modification of pivotal social skills. *Journal of Applied Behavior Analysis, 26*, 369–377.

Koegel, R. L., & Koegel, L. K. (1990). Extended reductions in stereotypic behaviors through self-management in multiple community settings. *Journal of Applied Behavior Analysis, 1*, 119–127.

Koegel, R. L., & Koegel, L. K. (2006). *Pivotal response treatments for autism: Communication, social, and academic development*. Baltimore, MD: Brookes.

Koegel, R. L., & Koegel, L. K. (2012). *The PRT pocket guide: Pivotal response treatment for Autism Spectrum Disorders*. Baltimore, MD: Brookes.

Koegel, L. K., Koegel, R. L., Ashbaugh, K., & Bradshaw, J. (2014). The importance of early identification and intervention for children with or at risk for autism spectrum disorders. *International Journal of Speech-Language Pathology, 16*, 50–56.

Koegel, L. K., Koegel, R. L., Green-Hopkins, I., & Barnes, C. C. (2010). Brief report: Question-asking and collateral language acquisition in children with autism. *Journal of Autism and Developmental Disorders, 40*, 509–515.

Koegel, L. K., Koegel, R. L., Hurley, C., & Frea, W. D. (1992). Improving pragmatic skills and disruptive behavior in children with autism through self-management. *Journal of Applied Behavior Analysis, 25*, 341–353.

Koegel, L. K., Koegel, R. L., Kellegrew, D., & Mullen, K. (1996). Parent education for prevention and reduction of severe problem behaviors. In L. K. Koegel, R. L. Koegel, & G. Dunlap (Eds.), *Positive behavioral support* (pp. 3–30). Baltimore, MD: Paul H. Brookes.

Koegel, L. K., Koegel, R. L., Shoshan, Y., & McNerney, E. (1999). Pivotal response intervention II: Preliminary long-term outcome data. *Research and Practice for Persons with Severe Disabilities, 24*, 186–198.

Koegel, L. K., Koegel, R. L., & Ingham, J. C. (1986). Programming rapid generalization of correct articulation through self-monitoring procedures. *Journal of Speech and Hearing Disorders, 51*, 24–32.

Koegel, L. K., Matos-Fredeen, R., Lang, R., & Koegel, R. (2012). Interventions for children with autism spectrum disorders in inclusive school settings. *Cognitive and Behavioral Practice, 19*, 401–412.

Koegel, R. L., & Mentis, M. (1985). Motivation in childhood autism: Can they or won't they? *Journal of Child Psychology and Psychiatry, 26*, 185–191.

Koegel, R. L., O'Dell, M., & Dunlap, G. (1988). Producing speech use in nonverbal autistic children by reinforcing attempts. *Journal of Autism and Developmental Disorders, 18*, 525–538.

Koegel, R. L., O'Dell, M. C., & Koegel, L. K. (1987). A natural language teaching paradigm for nonverbal autistic children. *Journal of Autism and Developmental Disorders, 17*, 187–200.

Koegel, L. K., Singh, A. K., Koegel, R. L., Hollingsworth, J. R., & Bradshaw, J. (2013). Assessing and improving early social engagement in infants. *Journal of Positive Behavior Interventions, 16*, 69–80.

Koegel, L. K., Singh, A. K., & Koegel, R. L. (2010). Improving motivation for academics in children with autism. *Journal of Autism and Developmental Disorders, 40*, 1057–1066.

Koegel, R. L., Symon, J. B., & Koegel, L. K. (2002). Parent education for families of children with autism living in geographically distant areas. *Journal of Positive Behavior Interventions, 4*, 88–103.

Koegel, R. L., & Wilhelm, H. (1973). Selective responding to the components of multiple visual cues by autistic children. *Journal of Experimental Child Psychology, 15*, 442–453.

Koegel, R. L., & Williams, J. A. (1980). Direct versus indirect response-reinforcer relationships in teaching autistic children. *Journal of Abnormal Child Psychology, 8*, 537–547.

Kuriakose, S. (2012). Making data collection easy in PRT. In R. L. Koegel & L. K. Koegel (Eds.), The PRT pocket guide: Pivotal response treatment for Autism Spectrum Disorders. Baltimore, MD: Brookes.

Lang, R., Machalicek, W., Rispoli, M. J., & Regester, A. (2009). Training parents to implement communication interventions for children with autism spectrum disorders: A systematic review of training procedures. *Evidenced Based Communication Assessment and Intervention, 3*, 174–190.

Lovaas, O. I. (1977). *The autistic child: Language development through behavior modification*. Oxford: Irvington.

Lovaas, O. I., Schreibman, L., Koegel, R., & Rehm, R. (1971). Selective responding by autistic children to multiple sensory input. *Journal of Abnormal Psychology, 77*, 211.

Maier, S. F., & Seligman, M. E. (1976). Learned helplessness: Theory and evidence. *Journal of Experimental Psychology: General, 105*, 3.

Maier, S. F., & Watkins, L. R. (1998). Cytokines for psychologists: Implications of bidirectional immune-to-brain communication for understanding behavior, mood, and cognition. *Psychological Review, 105*, 83.

Matson, J. L., Benavidez, D. A., Stabinsky Compton, L., Paclawskyj, T., & Baglio, C. (1996). Behavioral treatment of autistic persons: A review of research from 1980 to the present. *Research in Developmental Disabilities, 17*, 433–465.

Mawhood, L., & Howlin, P. (1999). The outcome of a supported employment scheme for high-functioning adults with autism or Asperger syndrome. *Autism, 3*, 229–254.

Miller, I. W., & Norman, W. H. (1979). Learned helplessness in humans: A review and attribution-theory model. *Psychological Bulletin, 86*, 93–119.

Miller, W. R., & Seligman, M. E. (1975). Depression and learned helplessness in man. *Journal of Abnormal Psychology, 84*, 228–238.

Mitchell, K. R., & White, R. G. (1977). Behavioral self-management: An application to the problem of migraine headaches. *Behavior Therapy, 8*, 213–221.

Müller, E., Schuler, A., & Yates, G. B. (2008). Social challenges and supports from the perspective of individuals with Asperger syndrome and other autism spectrum disabilities. *Autism, 12*(2), 173–190.

Mohammadzaheri, F., Koegel, L. K., Rezaee, M., & Rafiee, S. M. (2014). A randomized clinical trial comparison between Pivotal Response Treatment (PRT) and structured Applied Behavior Analysis (ABA) Intervention for Children with Autism. *Journal of Autism and Developmental Disorders, 44*, 2769–2777.

Overmier, J. B., & Seligman, M. E. (1967). Effects of inescapable shock upon subsequent escape and avoidance responding. *Journal of Comparative and Physiological Psychology, 63*, 28–33.

Peterson, C., Maier, S. F., & Seligman, M. E. P. (1993). *Learned helplessness: A theory for the age of personal control*. New York, NY: Oxford University Press.

Pierce, K. L., & Schreibman, L. (1994). Teaching daily living skills to children with autism in unsupervised settings through pictorial self-management. *Journal of Applied Behavior Analysis, 27*, 471–481.

Pituch, K. A., Green, V. A., Didden, R., Lang, R., O'Reilly, M. F., Lancioni, G. E., & Sigafoos, J. (2011). Parent reported treatment priorities for children with autism spectrum disorders. *Research in Autism Spectrum Disorders, 5*, 135–143.

Prizant, B. M. (1983). Language acquisition and communicative behavior in autism toward an understanding of the whole of it. *Journal of Speech and Hearing Disorders, 48*, 296–307.

Raulston, T. Carnett, A., Lang, R. Tostanoski, A., Lee, A., Machalicek, W., … Didden, R. (2013). Teaching individuals with autism spectrum disorder to ask questions: A systematic review. *Research in Autism Spectrum Disorders, 7*, 866–878.

Roberts, J. W. (1969). Termination factor for RNA synthesis. *Nature, 224*, 1168–1174.

Rogers, S. J., Vismara, L., Wagner, A. L., McCormick, C., Young, G., & Ozonoff, S. (2014). Autism treatment in the first year of life: A pilot study of infant start, a parent-implemented intervention for symptomatic infants. *Journal of Autism and Developmental Disorders, 44*, 2981–2995.

Rowland, C. F., Pine, J. M., Lieven, E. V., & Theakston, A. L. (2003). Determinants of acquisition order in wh-questions: Re-evaluating the role of caregiver speech. *Journal of Child Language, 30*, 609–636.

Santarelli, G., Koegel, R. L., Casas, J. M., & Koegel, L. K. (2001). Culturally diverse families participating in behavior therapy parent education programs for children with developmental disabilities. *Journal of Positive Behavior Interventions, 3*, 120–123.

Schreibman, L., Kaneko, W. M., & Koegel, R. L. (1991). Positive affect of parents of autistic children: A comparison across two teaching techniques. *Behavior Therapy, 22*, 479–490.

Schreibman, L., & Lovaas, O. I. (1973). Overselective response to social stimuli by autistic children. *Journal of Abnormal Child Psychology, 1*, 152–168.

Schreibman, L., & Stahmer, A. C. (2014). A randomized trial comparison of the effects of verbal and pictorial naturalistic communication strategies on spoken language for young children with autism. *Journal of Autism and Developmental Disorders, 44*, 1244–1251.

Seligman, M. E. P. (1967). The disruptive effects of unpredictable shock. Doctoral Dissertation. University of Pennsylvania, Philadelphia, Pennsylvania.

Seligman, M. E., & Maier, S. F. (1967). Failure to escape traumatic shock. *Journal of Experimental Psychology, 74*, 1–9.

Seligman, M. E. P. (1975). *Helplessness: On depression, development, and death*. W H Freeman/ Times Books/ Henry Holt & Co, New York, New York.

Simpson, R. L. (2005). Evidence-based practices and students with autism spectrum disorders. *Focus on Autism and Other Developmental Disabilities, 20*, 140–149

Steiner, A. M. (2011). A strength-based approach to parent education for children with autism. *Journal of Positive Behavior Interventions, 13*, 178–190.

Steiner, A. M., Gengoux, G. W., Klin, A., & Chawarska, K. (2013). Pivotal response treatment for infants at-risk for autism spectrum disorders: A pilot study. *Journal of Autism and Developmental Disorders, 43*, 91–102.

Taylor, B. A., & Harris, S. L. (1995). Teaching children with autism to seek information-acquisition of novel information and generalization of responding. *Journal of Applied Behavior Analysis, 28*, 3–14.

Vismara, L. A., & Lyons, G. L. (2007). Using perseverative interests to elicit joint attention behaviors in young children with autism theoretical and clinical implications for understanding motivation. *Journal of Positive Behavior Interventions, 9*, 214–228.

Voos, A. C., Pelphrey, K. A., Tirrell, J., Bolling, D. Z., Vander Wyk, B., Kaiser, M. D., … Ventola, P. (2012). Neural mechanisms of improvements in social motivation after pivotal response treatment: Two case studies. *Journal Autism Developmental Disorders, 43*, 1–10.

Watkins, L., O'Reilly, M., Kuhn, M., Gevarter, C., Lancioni, G., Sigafoos, J., & Lang, R. (2015). A review of peer-mediated social interaction interventions for students with autism in inclusive settings. *Journal of Autism and Developmental Disorders, 45*, 1070–1083.

Chapter 5
Early Start Denver Model

Meagan R. Talbott, Annette Estes, Cynthia Zierhut, Geraldine Dawson, and Sally J. Rogers

Introduction

The Early Start Denver Model (ESDM) is a comprehensive, developmental, relationship-based behavioral treatment for toddlers with ASD. It is both manualized and empirically-validated. The ESDM fuses developmental principles with empirically based teaching strategies from applied behavior analysis incorporated throughout the routines that fill children's daily lives—during play with both objects and people, caretaking, family meals, bathing, outdoor play, community outings, and so on. The focus on embedding learning opportunities within these varied contexts supports generalization of skills learned when working with an individual therapist and also means that parents are able (and expected) to take an active role in incorporating ESDM strategies into their interactions with their children. The emphasis on learning via positive, socially engaging, and child-led interactions inside everyday routines means that the learning that takes place in ESDM is fun for both children and adults. In fact, fostering these kinds of warm, socially rewarding interactions is one of the main goals of the ESDM approach.

The ESDM is one of small number of treatments, including both behavioral and pharmacological, with empirical support for its effectiveness in improving outcomes for young children with ASD. In the first randomized, controlled trial comparing

M.R. Talbott (✉) • C. Zierhut • S.J. Rogers
UC Davis MIND Institute, 2825 50th Street, Sacramento, CA 95817, USA
e-mail: Meagan.talbott@ucmc.ucdavis.edu

A. Estes
UW Autism Center, University of Washington, Seattle, WA 98195, USA

G. Dawson
Duke Center for Autism and Brain Development, Duke University, Durham, NC 27705, USA

R. Lang et al. (eds.), *Early Intervention for Young Children with Autism Spectrum Disorder*, Evidence-Based Practices in Behavioral Health,
DOI 10.1007/978-3-319-30925-5_5

ESDM to standard community care, toddlers received 15 h/week of 1:1 ESDM delivered by paraprofessionals and supervised by trained professionals. Children receiving ESDM intervention had significantly better outcomes in terms of their cognitive, language, and social skills, adaptive functioning, and autism diagnosis after 2 years of treatment (Dawson et al., 2010, 2012). Results from ongoing follow-up of this sample suggest that these cognitive gains are maintained through age 6 and that core autism symptoms are reduced, despite the cessation of intensive intervention (Estes, Rogers, Greenson, Winter, & Dawson, 2015). Other controlled studies have shown that both parents and professionals trained in ESDM techniques acquire the skills at high fidelity in a relatively short amount of time (weeks), and that use of these techniques is associated with increases in children's rates of spontaneous language use, imitation, and social initiations as well as their scores on standardized developmental measures (Rogers, Estes, et al., 2012; Vismara, Colombi, & Rogers, 2009; Vismara, McCormick, Young, Nadhan, & Monlux, 2013; Vismara & Rogers, 2008; Vismara, Young, & Rogers, 2012; Vismara, Young, Stahmer, Griffith, & Rogers, 2009).

In this chapter, we begin with an overview of the theoretical underpinnings, procedures, and implementation of the ESDM. The information presented here is described in much greater detail in the published ESDM Manual, *Early Start Denver Model for Young Children with Autism: Promoting Language, Learning, and Engagement* (Rogers & Dawson, 2010). Interested readers are encouraged to refer to this manual for more detailed information on all aspects of the ESDM, including both theoretical grounding and practical application of this model. We have also provided an overview of the currently published research involving training, implementation, and child outcomes using the ESDM treatment approach. The results of these studies have been summarized in a table. We conclude this chapter with a discussion of some of considerations for practitioners and families interested in applying the ESDM.

The Early Start Denver Model: Origins and Implementation

Background and Theory

ESDM conceptualizes ASD as a disorder that can impact development across all domains beginning early in life, and thus focuses on improving functioning in all affected domains: fine and gross motor, cognitive, self-care, and play skills as well as the core domains of language and social communication. However, given the core deficits defined by studies of toddlers with ASD, five developmental domains receive particular attention in the ESDM: imitation, nonverbal communication including joint attention, verbal communication, social development, and pretend play. Imitation is considered a core skill for children to master and also a critical teaching strategy for adults to use in each targeted domain. ESDM specifically targets children's ability to imitate people's sounds, words, gestures, actions on objects, and oral-facial movements.

In addition to this comprehensive developmental perspective, ESDM incorporates affective and relational theories of ASD. These features were first specified in the original Denver Model approach developed by Rogers and colleagues in the 1980s (Rogers & DiLalla, 1988; Rogers, Herbison, & Lewis, 1984; Rogers & Lewis, 1989; Rogers, Lewis, & Reis, 1987). In the Denver Model, deficits in emotion sharing and affective synchrony were assumed to underlie the difficulties in intersubjectivity observed in children with ASD—difficulty in joint attention, imitation, perspective taking, and social communication. This perspective arose from Stern's model of interpersonal development, and the Denver Model addressed these particular areas of difficulty for children with ASD by focusing on development within affectively rich (positive) social-communicative exchanges. The ESDM retains these relationship- and play-based approaches. The Denver Model was developed in a preschool setting, and consequently, the ESDM provides a great deal of specificity and insight into how to implement the teaching techniques and program into a group format. There is empirical support for the effectiveness of group delivery of both the Denver Model and ESDM in preschool settings (Eapen, Crnčec, & Walter, 2013; Rogers et al., 1984, 1987, Rogers & DiLalla, 1988; Rogers & Lewis, 1989; Vivanti et al., 2014).

The ESDM also conceptualizes ASD as involving fundamental differences in children's motivation for seeking out social interactions. The social motivation hypothesis proposed by Dawson and colleagues argues that children with autism find social interactions less rewarding and as a result, spend less time seeking out, attending to, and interacting with people and more time interacting with objects (Dawson et al., 2002; Dawson, Webb, & McPartland, 2005). The consequence of this reduction in the reward value of social interaction is an altered developmental course in both brain development and child learning (Dawson, 2008). ESDM targets this social motivational difference through a variety of strategies both developed within the original Denver Model and also some that were developed within Pivotal Response Training (PRT; described in detail in Chap. 4) and adapted into ESDM. Some of the motivational strategies are: (1) increasing both the strength and the frequency of rewards embedded in social interactions, (2) emphasizing social interactions that engender positive affect, (3) following children's interests, goals, and initiations in choosing activities and materials, (4) emphasizing very pleasurable play with people, (5) using least to most prompting strategies, (6) alternating maintenance and acquisition learning targets, (7) providing novel, interesting activities by addressing multiple objectives in an activity and by developing themes and variation in activities, (8) imitating children's actions and interacting reciprocally, (9) sharing control of the interaction, and (10) providing functional communication strategies that immediately help children achieve their goals.

ESDM differs sharply from traditional early intervention approaches such as discrete trial (DTT) procedures, in a variety of ways. The frame of learning inside ESDM is not a discrete trial, but rather a joint activity that allows for multiple objectives to be taught and is built upon the introduction of a theme to an interaction and then providing variations on that theme. Joint activity routines may include object-related play and non-object routines including songs (e.g.

itsy bitsy spider, row-row-row your boat) and social games (e.g. peekaboo, pattycake). In the ESDM, joint activities focused on non-object routines emphasizing social and affective engagement are termed sensory social routines. These activities occur during all kinds of daily living routines including meals, bath, community outings, outdoor play, and chores. Whereas DTT is adult-led with an emphasis on establishing control over the child's behavior, ESDM is child-led and involves shared control of activities and materials; children are active partners who select and shape the content of joint activities and interactions in which learning takes place. This requires therapists to be spontaneous and flexible in their teaching, as the specific learning prompts for a given objective will vary according to how the interaction unfolds. The process of skill-building also differs in ESDM. In DTT, teaching occurs through rote repetition, with each skill broken down into targeted subfeatures, which are later combined to produce the target complex behavior. In ESDM, while individual skills are also built up over time using prompting, shaping, chaining, and other techniques from applied behavior analysis, there is an explicit emphasis on building multisensory complex skills in naturalistic contexts (rather than decontextualized rote learning), using developmentally appropriate sequences. The naturalistic context for learning also includes the use of intrinsic reinforcers (e.g. obtaining the toy a child requests via gesture, continuing a pleasurable song routine a child requests via directed vocalization), rather than extrinsic reinforcers (e.g. receiving food after vocalizing in response to a prompt).

Additional key components of ESDM include the use of positive behavior support strategies (described in O'Neill, Jenson, & Radley, 2014) for managing unwanted behavior and the inclusion of parents and families in all aspects of treatment, including the formation of children's learning objectives, training to mastery in treatment techniques, and incorporation of these techniques into daily household and play routines.

A variety of published studies have now demonstrated that children who begin receiving ESDM treatment, whether in a group setting or in 1:1 instruction from parents and/or paraprofessionals, show significant developmental acceleration compared to baseline and to control groups. These studies include two randomized controlled trials of ESDM vs. community treatment, two controlled studies of group delivered ESDM, and five single subject designs. A full discussion and listing of the existing empirical support for ESDM is found later in this chapter.

Practice and Implementation

The ESDM was designed as a comprehensive treatment for children between 12 and 60 months—the developmental curriculum covers skills typically emerging between 7–9 and 48 months of age. Children chronologically older than 60 months or who have skills beyond the 48 month range would be better served by other treatment methods that are more appropriate to their chronological ages and educational needs, in both style and content. ESDM is interdisciplinary in nature and assumes that a team of professionals from a variety of disciplines is providing oversight and support for the child's treatment. However, it is delivered via a generalist model in that an ESDM trained, certified therapist from any of the licensed professions is able to deliver and supervise parents and paraprofessionals in delivering the comprehensive treatment on a daily or weekly basis. There is no preferred setting for delivering ESDM. It is a flexible intervention designed to be carried out wherever young children spend their days and thus is appropriate for home based interventions, integrated settings involving day care and preschool, and individual therapist delivered hours in a clinical setting. The best outcomes thus far have been reported when children receive an average of 15 h per week of ESDM from trained and supervised paraprofessionals augmented with parent coaching for a 2 year period. While less intensive delivery formats have also demonstrated positive outcomes, it is not yet known whether the best group outcomes that have been reported from ESDM can be achieved within less intensive formats. This is a research question that needs to be answered.

Child Initial Skill Evaluation

The ESDM Curriculum Checklist was designed to assess children's skills across ten developmental domains, and is used to help guide the development of individualized objectives to target during each 12-week quarter of treatment. The curriculum checklist covers the following developmental domains: receptive communication, expressive communication, social interaction, imitation skills, cognitive skills, play skills, fine motor skills, gross motor skills, independence/behavior, and joint attention. Each of these domains are broken into four developmental levels which roughly represent typically developing age ranges of 12–18, 18–24, 24–36, and 36–48 months. These levels have been designed to reflect the pattern of abilities typically observed in children with ASD, such that for any particular level, social and communicative skills are relatively less advanced than the visual motor skills included in the same level. At the outset of treatment, children's abilities are assessed across each of these ten domains. The assessment should be conducted using the same general approach and style used in ESDM treatment—through joint- and play-based activities. Conducting the assessment in this style allows the assessor to evaluate children's skills across multiple domains simultaneously, including social communicative abilities. Skills are scored as mastered (Pass, P), emerging or inconsistent (Pass/Fail, P/F), or not observed or reported (Fail, F). The entire assessment requires observation over several joint activities during a 1- or 1.5-h-long session, with the assessor pausing between activities to record the behaviors they observed and to note the behaviors they should try to elicit and evaluate in subsequent activities. Some behaviors are not easily observed during these sessions and should be evaluated using parent report or other sources of information. The checklist also serves as a measure for monitoring developmental progress over the course of treatment.

Development of Children's Individualized Learning Objectives

From this initial assessment using the curriculum checklist, a set of concrete, developmentally appropriate, short-term objectives are derived. Typically, this includes 2–3 objectives in each domain (approximately 20 in total). Objectives are constructed using data gathered from the curriculum checklist, from parent report, and from other assessment data. Objectives are not specific curriculum items, and they do not represent the child's first failures on the curriculum. Rather, they are constructed from both data on children's current behavioral abilities and from parent goals and represent new skills that are culturally important in that family, important for functioning in everyday life, and are generalized across people, environments, and materials. For example, a 12-week objective might focus on teaching the child to spontaneously and imitatively use conventional play materials (hat, sunglasses, etc.) on himself, a play partner, and a character (i.e. stuffed animal). Accomplishing this objective would result in a "Pass" for checklist items across social skills, imitation, and play domains, but would also satisfy the family's goal of increasing their child's play with peers and siblings.

Objectives are designed to target skill acquisition to be accomplished in a 12 week period. Subgoals for each objective are also written that break down each objective into small steps that can be achieved in roughly a 2-week period. Thus, while the final step of each objective defines a 12-week goal, progress can be monitored in an ongoing fashion via mastery of the smaller steps for each objective, and adjustments made if the initial objective is found to be gauged inappropriately for a 12 week period of time. Objectives encompass items the child currently shows uneven or emerging abilities in (the P/F items), but also include ceiling items on the curriculum—items the child is currently unable to pass (F items), but that they will be likely to accomplish over the next few months. Objectives are written with the therapist's best estimate of what learning can be accomplished in the coming 12 weeks, and thus are tailored for children's individual learning rates and profiles of strengths and weaknesses. Objectives in the ESDM are written in a very specific format that always includes four elements: the specific behavioral antecedent that precedes and will eventually elicit the specific targeted behavior, the targeted behavior itself, the criteria that will define mastery of the skill and finally, the criteria that indicate generalization of the skill to other people, contexts, and materials.

Antecedents

The antecedent may take many forms, but as much as possible, should represent a stimulus that elicits the behavior in typically developing children of the same age. Antecedents may include other people's behavior (peers, adults, parents), environmental cues (e.g. an auditory signal, items specific to a location or activity), internal cues (physiological cues for states like hunger), or behaviors occurring in a chain, where one behavior cues the next behavior in the sequence (e.g. putting on a jacket after putting on rain boots). Care needs to be taken to ensure the specified antecedent is truly a discriminative stimulus for the behavior you are teaching and *not* simply the context or setting in which the behavior typically occurs. For example, the bathroom is a setting, whereas flushing the toilet is a discriminative stimulus for washing one's hands if your target behavior is spontaneously washing hands after toileting.

Specifying the Target Behavior

Targeted behaviors also need to be specified using concrete, observable definitions in order to monitor progress and mastery of that behavior. For example, it is rather difficult to determine whether a child 'has the concept of big vs. small'; it is relatively easy to observe and monitor whether a child 'matches five sets of objects on the basis of size (big vs. small)'. Additionally, the specified behaviors may be complex or require multiple components, particularly as children progress towards developmentally advanced skills. Complex behaviors might involve multiple steps involved in setting a table for snack or sorting items into bins and putting bins on a shelf for cleaning up (with the particular antecedents for these behaviors clearly specified).

Specifying the Mastery Criterion

In addition to selecting a target behavior and the stimulus it should follow, objectives in the ESDM also need to include an observable criterion for determining whether the skill has been successfully learned. This requires consideration of the child's individual learning rate and expected progress. For some children, learning and using eight newly learned expressive verbs in 4/5 consecutive hour-long sessions will be an achievable 12-week objective. For others, learning and using two verbs will be more appropriate, though both children are ultimately working towards the goal of producing ten or more verbs both imitatively and spontaneously to label the actions of both themselves and a partner. Mastery criteria should reflect developmentally appropriate frequencies, latencies, percentages, etc. of occurrence. For example, typically developing children do not combine gaze with gesture 100 % of the time, so this would be an inappropriate criterion for mastery level use of eye contact combined with gesture.

Specifying the Generalization Criterion

The final component of children's objectives in the ESDM is an explicit measure of skill generalization. Generalization is more generally supported by both the naturalistic context and the selection of naturally-occurring and developmentally appropriate antecedents for target behaviors utilized in the ESDM. Including an explicit measure of generalization in children's learning objectives takes this one step further and ensures deep learning of the targeted skills, rather than context-specific performance. In terms of objective writing, the generalization criterion should include a demonstration of the target behavior with multiple people, contexts, and materials.

Taking Data and Monitoring Children's Progress

Once the child's learning objectives for the quarter (12 weeks) have been selected and defined, these objectives are broken down further into the components/learning steps that will be the focus of daily teaching. This is accomplished through a developmental task analysis for each objective—detailing the specific steps that will move the child from their current baseline ability towards successful mastery of the full written objective. The ESDM Manual (Rogers & Dawson, 2010) outlines strategies for writing steps for five different types of behavior objectives. These include the following types of sequences: (1) developmental sequences, in which children with ASD are expected to follow a pattern of skill acquisition observed in typically developing children; (2) behavior chains or 'bundled' behaviors, including behavior chains often observed for self-care skills like dressing, or adding gaze to communicative gestures; (3) increasing the frequency and diversity of existing behaviors, such as increasing the number or frequency of sounds in the child's verbal repertoire; (4) linking existing behaviors to new antecedents, such as vocalizing in response to another person, instead of randomly; (5) the steps involved in building a completely new skill, which will likely focus on prompting, shaping, and fading of the target behavior. There are most often 5–6 steps written for an objective, though the number of steps is will vary and ultimately is chosen based on how the skill will be built up from the child's current performance.

These individual learning objective steps define the specific skills to be taught in a specific session. The initial step of each objective is the child's current baseline performance of the skill at the time the steps are written, and thus represents the current maintenance level of skill. The second step describes the current acquisition step—the specific behavior to be learned immediately. Once the second step is learned,. it becomes a maintenance skill, and the third step is now the acquisition step. This makes it easy for the therapist to vary maintenance and acquisition skills and to track both on a data sheet. Therapists record data related to each objective's current acquisition step as well as the step immediately preceding it—the maintenance step-every 15 min during treatment. At a natural stopping point in the therapy session (or one the therapist has created), the therapist should stop and record performance on the acquisition and maintenance step of each objective that has been taught in the preceding 15 min. Not all objectives will have been targeted during this time frame, and will depend on the specific activities that have occurred. As the session progresses, the therapist monitors which objectives still need to be addressed and provides activities and opportunities to address them. In ESDM practice, one addresses all objectives in each treatment session, and by recording every 15 min the therapist sees what is left to be accomplished in the hour. This use of an interval recording system was developed specifically for ESDM and is supported by strong inter-rater agreement about child performance on the acquisition and maintenance steps. At the conclusion of an hour-long therapy session, the therapist summarizes the data recorded across the 15-min intervals into a Data Summary Sheet. This summary sheet provides an overview, at the session level, of child performance on objectives. When mastery criteria are met for a step, the mastered step becomes the maintenance step and the next step becomes the acquisition target.

Altering Teaching Strategies: Addressing Individual Children's Response to Intervention

The sub-steps for each objective are designed to be mastered in approximately a 2-week period, and if there are 5–6 steps written for an objective, with the first one a maintenance level of skill, then in principle the child should master most objectives in 12 weeks of teaching. That is the expectation. For a step to be mastered in 2 weeks, one should see changes in the daily performance data within the first few days of teaching with failure giving away to occasional success, and then more frequent successes, and then consistent successes. No change in the data over the first week or so of teaching should trigger an immediate review of teaching procedures and amount of practice being given. If the child is receiving ten or more interspersed teaching trials per day on the skill, and if the therapist is using high fidelity ESDM teaching techniques, then the next step is to change the teaching procedure. ESDM has developed a decision tree that lays out the process of changing the teaching strategy *for the particular skill that is not progressing*. Applying the decision tree to individualize a teaching approach is described in detail in the teaching manual and will not be reiterated here. In general however, one begins by assessing reinforcer strength and assuring that the child is highly motivated for the reinforcer. If not, then adaptations begin there to enhance child motivation. If maximizing reinforcer strength does not improve performance over the next few days, one moves to the next level of individualization involving the consistency and salience of the teaching event. The therapist follows a hierarchy that systematically limits variability and masses practice trials to assist learning. If learning performance does not improve following these steps, then a third level of individualization is brought in which involves use of visual supports.

Once adaptations are made to the teaching of a particular skill that result in improved performance, the individualized teaching approach is continued until the objective is mastered. During the next 12-week period of intervention, one begins again with naturalistic behavioral teaching. While readers often assume that these adaptations are used most frequently for children with the slowest learning rates, this has not been our experience. The adaptations are also used for when motivation and initiation problems hinder the performance of children with rapid learning rates. For some children, modifications are temporary and after a few quarters the child can make rapid progress using the naturalistic teaching paradigms defined as the default teaching strategy in ESDM. However, a small number of children in our experience will need modifications involving reinforcer strength, teaching consistency, and/or visual supports, throughout their ESDM treatment in order to progress as rapidly as possible. This reflects individual learning needs and allows one to use the full range of empirically supported teaching techniques, chosen in a systematic fashion, within ESDM. Thus, it is incorrect to describe ESDM as a play-based teaching approach. It is a comprehensive, individualized intervention approach that addresses the needs of all young children with autism by matching teaching strategies with child learning performance. Its default teaching approach is naturalistic; we begin by following children's leads, sharing control, using child preferred materials and activities and embedding learning activities into everyday play and routines in natural contexts, delivered by familiar, sensitive, and highly responsive adults because research has demonstrated that this combination of variables fosters rapid language learning, improved child cooperation and social motivation, decreased levels of problem behaviors, and acceleration of development rate, in typically developing children and in children with developmental delays and because rigorously designed studies have demonstrated very positive outcomes that are at least comparable to the most effective approaches that have been published. This teaching approach is also considered best practice for young children in general (National Association for the Education of Young Children, 2009) and is in practice in high quality preschools and centers for children all over the world, which may support readiness and rapid integration into typical learning environments during the preschool and kindergarten years for many or most young children with autism.

Training and Certification Procedures

The ESDM materials are publically available and there is no restriction in accessing them. The specific training process and requirements for becoming a certified ESDM therapist can be found on the ESDM website maintained through the UC Davis MIND Institute (http://www.ucdmc.ucdavis.edu/mindinstitute/research/esdm/pdf/certification_steps.pdf). Training is offered at several institutions throughout the world. Steps involved in becoming a certified therapist are briefly summarized below. Individuals seeking ESDM certification must work regularly with 12–48 month-old children with ASD, have a terminal educational degree (usually a graduate degree) and professional license or credential for independent practice in their location, work as part of an interdisciplinary team (or have regular contact with and/or access to other specialists outside one's discipline), have the resources to complete the post-training supervisory process, and have thoroughly read through and begun to try out some ESDM practices described in the Manual (Rogers & Dawson, 2010).

Steps for ESDM Certification

1. Attend an Introductory ESDM training workshop.
   (a) The Introductory workshop provides an overview of the ESDM through didactic instruction, videotaped exercises and group discussion.
2. Attend an Advanced ESDM workshop.
   (a) The Advanced workshop provides hands-on experience in evaluating children's skills, developing objectives, and carrying out a treatment plan. Attendees are provided with training and feedback on these skills, including fidelity measures.
3. Begin to practice ESDM, and after 6 months of experience apply for certification supervision
   (a) This initiates the formal process for submitting the follow-up materials required to receive official certification as an ESDM Certified Therapist.
4. Following acceptance, submit post-training materials for evaluation and supervision
   (a) Required materials include curriculum checklists, objectives, teaching steps, videotapes of direct intervention, self- and peer-rated fidelity measures, and child data sheets (from submitted video session) for one practice child and two official submissions (only one is required if the trainee meets fidelity for the practice child submission).
   (b) Continue to work with a supervisor through 2–3 rounds of materials that demonstrate ESDM competencies.

Fidelity of Direct Implementation

Therapists providing treatment must demonstrate high fidelity in ESDM technique use. The ESDM Teaching Fidelity Rating System uses a likert-based rating system, where 1 reflects no competent teaching and 5 reflect extremely competent teaching practices, to assess therapist competence in 13 critical skills. The 13 domains assessed are: a) Management of child attention; b) quality of the A-B-C teaching episode; c) quality of instructional techniques; d) modulation of child affect and arousal; e) management of unwanted behavior; f) dyadic engagement; g) child motivation; h) adult affect; i) adult sensitivity and responsivity; j) communicative opportunities and functions; k) appropriateness of adult's language; l) elaboration of activities; m) transitions between activities.

To achieve treatment fidelity, interventionists must a) demonstrate 85 % of the number of points possible in each play activity, *and* b) consistently score at least a 4 on each skill, *and* c) have no scores lower than a 3. Interventionists are encouraged to use the fidelity rating system to evaluate their own treatment sessions.

Delivering ESDM in a Group Format

The basic principles of ESDM were first developed from the Denver Model preschool approach, which involved mainly small group activities in a 1:2 ratio for approximately 5 h per day. The group model followed developmentally appropriate practices and a typical schedule of activities for toddlers and very young children. As in the current ESDM delivery, each child was evaluated quarterly and individualized objectives were developed in all domains. Each child's objectives were targeted across the day inside the ongoing activities that make up early childhood centers: hello circles, center activities, outdoor play, meal and snack time activities, and toileting and handwashing routines.

The use of ESDM in group programs is described in a chapter of the ESDM manual (Rogers & Dawson, 2010), and two independent research groups in Australia have led the way in setting up model programs and conducting studies to assess efficacy of ESDM delivered in groups. Even though these two settings had a much higher ratio of children to staff than did the original Denver site, their positive findings add to and extend the earlier positive findings from the original Denver Model studies. Additionally, the staff to child ratio in these settings reflects current practice in many childcare and inclusive settings for young children with ASD. Vivanti et al. (2014) have conducted the most rigorous study to date, comparing the effects of 12 months of ESDM group treatment to a reasonably sized group of children contrasted to a carefully matched comparison group of children also receiving specialized autism services. As described later in this chapter, the data demonstrate significantly more acceleration of child learning in ESDM than in the specialty community program. Another group from Australia has reported that problem behavior was greatly improved following group ESDM intervention (Fulton, Eapen, Crnčec, Walter, & Rogers, 2014).

While the basic principles and practices of ESDM are unchanged in group settings, several challenges unique to the group setting require particular attention. Most group settings involve paraprofessionals in the classroom, and the paraprofessional training for classroom staff needs to be similar in rigor to the training provided to supervised paraprofessionals delivering intensive 1:1 ESDM to children at home. The largest challenges in the group setting are: developing activities that will support the learning objectives of several different children at the same time, holding children's attention long enough to deliver high quality learning opportunities while at the same time moving rapidly enough from one child to the next that child attention is maintained across the group, data recording.

While these ESDM papers come from group settings in which all children had autism, other group programs coming from the naturalistic behavioral paradigm have provided models of integrated preschools that also have strong effects on child change for children with autism. As first articulated by Gail McGee from Walden Preschool (McGee, Morrier, & Daly, 1999; McGee, Paradis, & Feldman, 1993) and later refined and examined by Aubyn Stahmer at the Toddler Center (Stahmer & Ingersoll, 2004) group instruction using naturalistic behavioral strategies can result in positive behavior changes. To these earlier models, ESDM contributes a developmental curriculum, a means of describing adult behavior that captures interpersonal and relationship qualities as well as teaching behavior, and a method for taking interval data during the ongoing activities.

It is not yet known whether ESDM delivered in groups can accomplish the same amount of change over time as it does in 1:1 delivery. While the higher ratio of children to adults likely results in fewer planned teaching interactions, the presence of peers, especially typically developing peers or peers with a wide range of language and play skills, provides other potential sources of learning opportunities, and the greater number of hours that are provided in a child day care setting or all day preschool may provide more learning opportunities than can be carried out in 15 h per week of 1:1 intervention in homes. Few other preschool group approaches for ASD have provided controlled outcome data to compare to the Vivanti et al. (2014) effects (Strain & Bovey, 2011; Boyd et al., 2014). Hopefully this area of research need will result in more outcome data in the next few years, since group delivery of services to preschoolers is a typical model of educating young children across a wide range of cultures and socioeconomic groups.

Parent Coaching and Procedures for Involving Parents

Thus far, we have described the process and procedure for implementing ESDM in a 1:1, therapist-delivered model. As described above, parent involvement and parent coaching is an essential component of this comprehensive model, which emphasizes incorporating treatment practices into children's daily lives. As such, highly skilled parents who understand the principles and approaches of ESDM and ABA are optimally positioned to complement treatment delivery by professionals by incorporating ESDM techniques into their own dyadic and familial interactions with their children. The interventionists providing the bulk of treatment hours in the 2010 RCT (Dawson et al., 2010) had a bachelors-level educational background, without advanced training or degrees, aside from the specific training they received in ESDM theory and delivery. They were supervised by trained and certified ESDM professionals. Thus, many parents are equally well-prepared to use the ESDM treatment techniques and theoretically, can learn to apply them with equal efficacy. This is an exciting possibility, because parent-delivered intervention provided as part of a comprehensive, multidisciplinary team can help to bridge timing common gap in service delivery between diagnosis and commencement of community services. Although parent-delivered intervention is not a substitute for evidence-based practices implemented by professionally trained, multidisciplinary teams, there are often gaps in funding to provide community services at the level of intensity and individualization that has been demonstrated to improve developmental outcomes for young children with ASD. Adjunctive parent-delivered intervention can supplement community services and provide high-quality learning opportunities at home during early childhood when learning and developmental change is occurring at a rapid pace. Parent involvement is consistent with best practices in early childhood intervention and Part C services. Parent involvement in setting treatment objectives is critical for delivering culturally sensitive treatment and applying ESDM in diverse communities, individualized to each families unique needs. The skills and approaches parents learn as partners with ESDM providers sets the course for positive parent-child interaction and effective parent advocacy across the lifespan.

The concepts, strategies, and skills used in parent coaching sessions are described in detail in a parent manual designed for parents and professionals wishing for more information on how parent-implemented ESDM (P-ESDM) can be learned and applied by parents at home and in the community (Rogers, Dawson, & Vismara, 2012). The parent manual describes ten intervention themes essential to P-ESDM: (a) social attention and motivation for learning, (b) sensory social routines, (c) dyadic engagement, (d) non-verbal communication, (e) imitation, (f) antecedent-behavior-consequence relationship (ABCs of learning), (g) joint attention, (h) functional play, (i) symbolic play, and (j) speech development. Primary caregivers receive systematic instruction on how to embed each theme in daily play and caretaking routines at home. Over the course of intervention, parents are taught the interactive principles associated with P-ESDM and gain mastery in applying these principles with their children. They are not taught to elicit specific behavioral learning objectives (e.g., "child will vocalize six different consonants in 10 min of play"), though therapists develop these types of objectives and track change using this approach. Daily data on child progress are gathered by the therapists during coaching sessions with parents and child. Typically one parent will self-identify as the primary caretaker and that parent will attend all parent coaching sessions. However, ESDM parent coaching can be used with additional caretakers, including parents, grandparents, and childcare providers.

The first step in parent involvement is a collaborative process in which treatment objectives are set during an initial 1.5 h treatment evaluation session in which the child is evaluated by a therapist to determine the child's level on the ESDM Curriculum. The results of this evaluation are reviewed with the primary caregiver and the caregiver provides the ESDM therapist with his or her own goals for the child. Out of this meeting, 12–15 learning objectives are generated for the child that will guide intervention for the next 12 weeks. Objectives are broken down into 4–6 teaching steps. The therapist uses these objectives and teaching steps to help the parent identify appropriate toys and learning activities for their child, and to track weekly child progress. It is very useful to conduct this session in the home to assess the learning environment and help the parent optimize the home for increasing learning opportunities for the child.

After this initial session, a parent coaching schedule is determined. Depending upon the needs of the family and child, parent coaching may be conducted as part of an intensive, in-home ESDM intervention program. In this situation, parents meet with the lead ESDM supervisor twice per month. Parent coaching can also be carried out prior to initiating an intensive treatment program, to start intervention while on a waiting list, for example. In this case, coaching sessions may be held up to twice per week. And finally, when infants under 12 months of age are identified as showing early signs of ASD, parent coaching sessions implemented 2–3 times per week for 12 weeks is a developmentally appropriate approach to delivering individualized intervention (Rogers et al., 2014).

Parent coaching sessions follow a consistent structure. 1–1.5 h treatment sessions are broken into six 10–15 min periods, each with a different activity. At the start of the session, parents share their progress practicing the previous week's theme at home with discussion of triumphant moments (e.g., "my child looked up at me and smiled when eating his cheerios in his high chair"). In the next 10–15 min block parents and their child engage in a preferred play activity (e.g., toy play, books, bubbles) to demonstrate experiences from the past week Sessions can be analyzed for parent fidelity to the P-ESDM model and parent learning can be measured over time. Parent experiences and observations in that play period are discussed and followed up on later in the session. In the next 10–15 min, the therapist explains the next P-ESDM theme verbally while providing written materials. The therapist then models the techniques with the child while parents observes. In the following 10–15 min, parents practice the new concepts while the therapist coaches them as needed. The next 10–15 min involves another parent practice with coaching using a different type of activity to support parent generalization at home. The final 10–15 min addresses any remaining parent interest or question and ends with an action plan of daily times and activities when parents feel they could embed the targeted topics and facilitate child learning within home routines.

The parent coaching process and practices, and the interactive strategies used by the therapist throughout the session, are based on the work of Hanft, Rush, and Shelden (2004). An important characteristic of coaching is a partnership model, in which the strengths, existing knowledge, values and goals of the parent are acknowledged and directly sought in order to set goals, and shape how the treatment will be delivered. This is in contrast to a traditional parent training model in which the therapist sets the goals and provides information to the parent in the role of expert. A related set of approaches coaching strategies comes from the Motivational Interviewing literature. The ESDM therapist uses information on the parent's readiness for change (DiClemente & Marden Velasquez, 2002; Prochaska, Redding, & Evers, 2002) to individualize intervention goals and help parents move into actively implementing new skills at home with their child.

Review of Existing Literature

As of this writing, there are 15 published research studies involving direct application of the ESDM. They include data on the effectiveness of ESDM in improving children's outcomes, research on dissemination and training procedures for parents and professionals, impacts of ESDM parent coaching on parental stress and competence, children's outcomes from ESDM delivery in a group setting, and finally, initial findings related to a downward extension of ESDM to infants showing risk signs of ASD in the first year of life. These studies are summarized in Table 5.1. Additionally, several additional studies are also currently underway. They are not included in Table 5.1, but are described below.

Table 5.1 Published research studies on the Early Start Denver Model efficacy and training procedures, by publication year

	Participant Characteristics	Study Characteristics					
Study	N and age	Primary setting	Study objectives	Method	Length and intensity	Primary outcomes	Primary Limitations
Vismara and Rogers (2008)	One infant with risk signs identified at 9 months of age	Parent coaching in laboratory, parent delivery in home	Pilot testing a parent-implemented model for ESDM treatment	Case study	Weekly 90-min parent coaching session for 12 weeks. Follow up through 24 months of age.	Parent achieved fidelity in ESDM implementation after 7 weeks.	Single case study.
						Infant increased spontaneous vocalizations, imitation, social initiation and attentiveness	
Vismara, Colombi, et al. (2009)	8 children; 7 with ASD diagnoses at enrollment, one with risk signs at 10 months of age who received a diagnosis at 18 months.	Parent coaching in laboratory; parent delivery in home.	Piloting parent coaching and delivery of P-ESDM	Non-concurrent multiple baseline	One weekly hour-long therapist/parent coaching session for 12 sessions for P-ESDM group; follow up assessment 3 months after end of treatment	The majority (7/8) of parents who completed training reached 85 % fidelity for ESDM implementation.	Clinic-based delivery of parent coaching and monitoring of parent implementation.
	10–36 months					Children increased vocalization frequency and attentiveness during treatment; increases were maintained at follow-up for 6/8 children.	No non-treatment control group.

Vismara, Young, et al. (2009)	10 Adults (5 live, 5 distance)	Laboratory	Evaluating telehealth procedure for training professionals	Quasi-experimental: Training via distance education technology or live; comparison of three training conditions (self-instruction, didactic training seminar, team supervision)	Phase 1 (5 months): direct intervention using ESDM; Phase 2 (5 months): parent coaching of ESDM.	No group differences in fidelity of direct implementation or parent coaching.	Training conditions occurred in the same order for all participants, specific contribution of each training type to learner competence unclear.
						90 % of trainees achieved fidelity of at least 80 % for direct intervention.	Alternative parent-training practices were not included.
						Children made significant gains in verbal utterances, attention, and initiation during direct phase.	
						One therapist met fidelity in parent coaching techniques, but 50 % of parents achieved fidelity of 85 %.	
Dawson et al. (2010)	48 with ASD (24 treatment, 24 community control);	Home	Evaluating the efficacy of ESDM versus community treatment for children younger than 2½.	Randomized controlled trial with a treatment-as-usual control group	20 h/week for 2 years	ESDM group improved 17.6 standard score points on IQ measures (versus 7.0 for comparison group) and maintained their trajectory of adaptive behavior growth while comparison group declined.	Long-term follow up needed (underway).
	18–30 months at treatment; 48–77 months at follow up.					ESDM group more likely to move into a less severe diagnosis (AD to PDD NOS).	Non-manualized control intervention.

(continued)

Table 5.1 (continued)

Study	Participant Characteristics	Study Characteristics					
	N and age	Primary setting	Study objectives	Method	Length and intensity	Primary outcomes	Primary Limitations
Dawson et al. (2012)	48 with ASD (24 treatment, 24 community control);	Laboratory	Determining whether and how early intensive behavioral intervention (ESDM) alters brain development.	EEG measures (ERP and spectral power) collected during passive viewing of faces and objects; data collected at end of 2010 Dawson et al. RCT	Single session following 2-year treatment RCT	ESDM group and typical controls showed a shorter Nc latency and increased cortical activation (decreased α power and increased θ power) when viewing faces versus objects. The ASD comparison group showed the opposite pattern—shorter Nc latency and increased cortical activation for objects than for faces. Children receiving ESDM showed improved social behavior which correlated with improved patterns of brain activity.	EEG data available for 60 % of ASD participants (due to non-tolerance of procedures or movement artefacts).
	18–30 months at treatment; 48–77 months at follow up.						No baseline (pre-treatment) EEG data available.
Rogers, Dawson, et al. (2012)	98 (49 ESDM, 49 Community)	Parent coaching in laboratory; Parent delivery in home.	Evaluating parent coaching and delivery of P-ESDM	Randomized controlled trial with treatment-as-usual control group	One weekly hour-long therapist/ parent coaching session for 12 sessions for P-ESDM group	No group differences in parent-child interaction characteristics or child outcomes. Both increased parent interaction skills and in child developmental progress. P-ESDM group reported significantly stronger therapist alliance.	Community treatment group received nearly twice the number of intervention hours.
	12–24 months					Across groups, younger children and those receiving more hours of treatment had more positive outcomes.	Children unlikely to receive 'full dose' until the end of 12 week training course.
							Parent fidelity monitored in laboratory, not home.
							Non-manualized control intervention.

Vismara et al. (2012)	9 families with a child between 16 and 38 months diagnosed with ASD	Home	Piloting telehealth ESDM parent coaching procedures (video-conferencing therapy sessions and instructional DVD)	Single-subject, multiple baseline	Baseline periods ranged from 4 to 11 probes (collected twice per week). Active treatment included 12 weeks of hour-long coaching sessions conducted via telehealth services. Follow up included 3 h-long sessions every 2 weeks.	P-ESDM implementation fidelity increased significantly during active phase. Average time to fidelity was 6.41 weeks.	Parents reported frustration with some aspects of the telehealth delivery system, including technical issues (internet connection freezing, intermittent problems with video cameras).
						Parent and child engagement ratings significantly increased during active treatment.	Small and homogeneous sample.
						Significant increases in children's spontaneous speech and imitation, and vocabulary production and understanding.	
						Parents rated the telehealth procedure as satisfactory.	

(continued)

Table 5.1 (continued)

Study	Participant Characteristics	Study Characteristics					
	N and age	Primary setting	Study objectives	Method	Length and intensity	Primary outcomes	Primary Limitations
Vismara, Young, and Rogers (2013)	24 Adults	Laboratory	Training workshop development; evaluating ESDM training procedures, and provider fidelity posttraining and at follow up	One-group pre-post test	4 day intensive workshop, follow up evaluation after 4 months	Post-training, all professionals reached fidelity (80 % or higher) for delivery implementation and reached 80 % agreement between self-evaluations and trainer ratings.	Only 11 or 24 (46 %) of trainees submitted follow-up materials. Follow-up materials included only one treatment session (versus multiple children and sessions).
						At 4-month follow-up, fidelity of treatment delivery was maintained, but self-ratings were less accurate than immediately post training.	No data on barriers to community practice was obtained.
						Training methods and participants' knowledge of ESDM practices and techniques were rated as highly satisfactory at posttraining. Responses to open-ended comments revealed an appreciation of hands-on interaction with children, live coaching, and videotape rating exercises as well as requests for more time to practice these skills.	No comparison group receiving alternative training procedure.

Vismara, Young, et al. (2013)	8 families with a child between 18 and 45 months diagnosed with ASD	Home	Evaluating telehealth ESDM parent coaching procedures (video-conferencing therapy sessions and a self-guided website) and associated child outcomes	Single-subject, multiple baseline	Baseline periods ranged from 3 to 8 probes (collected twice per week). Active treatment included 12 weeks of 1.5 h long telehealth intervention sessions. Follow up included 3 1.5 h long monthly sessions.	Parents rated the internet platform and therapist conferencing sessions as highly satisfactory.	Long-term costs and feasibility of implementation unclear.
						Parent fidelity ratings increased significantly during active treatment; 6/8 parents reached 80 % fidelity by the end of treatment.	Small and homogenous sample.
						Ratings of parent engagement increased significantly during active treatment.	Decline in parental website use over time.
						At follow up, children's language was significantly positively correlated with parental engagement ratings and ESDM technique use.	
Vivanti, Dissanayake, Zierhut, and Rogers (2013)	21 children with ASD, 22–58 months	Preschool (Victorian ASELCC)	Evaluating potential predictors of response to group-based ESDM intervention: functional use of objects, goal understanding, social attention, imitation	Quasi-experimental pre- and post-design with a single treatment group; regression analyses predictors of change.	15–25 h/week of group-based ESDM for full calendar year	Significantly higher age equivalent scores for all MSEL subscales at post-test.	Other, untested variables may be significant moderators of response to treatment (for both ESDM and/or other intervention approaches).
						No significant decreases in ADOS severity scores.	Lack of a control group and non-randomized design.
						Use of objects, goal understanding and imitation were related to receptive and non-verbal cognitive gains.	
						Symptom severity explained 40 % of variance in expressive language gains.	
						Social attention unrelated to outcome.	

(continued)

Table 5.1 (continued)

Study	Participant Characteristics	Study Characteristics					
	N and age	Primary setting	Study objectives	Method	Length and intensity	Primary outcomes	Primary Limitations
Eapen et al. (2013)	26 children with ASD, 36–58 months	Preschool (Sydney ASELCC)	Evaluating efficacy of group-based ESDM on children's adaptive behavior, developmental, and ASD outcomes.	Quasi-experimental pre- and post-design with a single treatment group.	15–20 h/week of group-based and 1 h/week of 1:1 ESDM for 12 months	Significant increase in MSEL DQ scores for receptive and expressive language and visual reception subscales.	Lack of a control group and non-randomized design.
						Significant increases in receptive language scale score and motor skills domain on VABS.	
						Significant decrease in SCQ scores.	
Fulton et al. (2014)	38 children with ASD, 38–64 months (including the 26 children from the Eapen et al., 2013 study)	Preschool (Sydney ASELCC)	Evaluating impact of ESDM on children's maladaptive behavior.	Quasi-experimental pre- and post-design with a single treatment group	15–20 h/week of group-based and 1 h/week of 1:1 ESDM for 12 months	Significant reduction in clinician-rated ESDM behavior ratings (presence of maladaptive behaviors).	Lack of a control group and non-randomized design.
						At entry 2 % of children were rated as having compliant or above average behavior; post-treatment, 79 % were rated as such.	Clinician ratings of problem behaviors were not blind.
						No significant changes in VABS Adaptive Behavior Composite, Maladaptive Behavior Index, or in SCQ total scores.	
Vivanti et al. (2014)	57 children with ASD (27 ESDM, 30 community education control); aged 18–60 months	Preschool (Victorian ASELCC)	Evaluating efficacy of group-based ESDM.	Quasi-experimental pre- and post-design with ESDM treatment and community education control group	15–25 h/week of group-based ESDM for full calendar year	Both groups made gains in cognitive skills (MSEL), adaptive functioning, and social communication (VABS total and communication subscales).	Non-randomized design.
						ESDM group made significantly more gains on MSEL DQ for Total Scores (14 vs. 7 DQ points) and Receptive subscales (20 vs. 10).	Non-manualized control intervention.
						The ESDM program was rated as highly satisfactory by parents and staff.	Resource-heavy implementation (increased staff responsibilities), resulting in limited access.

Estes et al. (2014)	98 parents of toddlers (aged 12–24 months) with ASD	Parent coaching in laboratory/clinic.	Evaluating the impact of parent coaching in P-ESDM on parents' stress and sense of competence.	Randomized controlled trial with a treatment-as-usual control group (same subjects as Dawson et al., 2010)	One weekly hour-long therapist/parent coaching session for 12 sessions for P-ESDM group.	Parents in P-ESDM group reported significantly lower parenting stress than parents in community group.	Short intervention period (12 weeks).
						There were no group differences in parental sense of competence.	Non-manualized control intervention.
						Negative life events were associated with increases in parenting stress and decreases in competence for both groups.	
Rogers et al. (2014)	25 infants aged 7–15 months at enrollment.	Parent coaching in laboratory; Parent delivery in home.	Pilot development and evaluation of infant-appropriate, parent-delivered ESDM	Single case design (parent fidelity data); quasi-experimental with a treatment group and 4 control groups matched on autism symptoms and MSEL scores at 9 months.	Hour-long parent coaching sessions in clinic weekly for 12 weeks; hour-long maintenance sessions every other week for 6 weeks; hour-long booster sessions for infants showing poor progress during maintenance; follow up assessments at 15, 18, 24, and 36 months of age.	From 18 to 36 months, infants in treatment group had fewer ASD symptoms than AO and DR infants, but more symptoms than HR and LR.	Limited sample size.
	7 highly symptomatic of ASD.					All 7 parents achieved treatment fidelity (80 %) by the end of treatment; the parent coaching was rated as highly satisfactory.	Non-randomized design.
	Comparison infants: 7 high risk infant siblings later diagnosed (AO), 7 high risk siblings not diagnosed (HR), 7 low risk infant siblings (LR), and 4 infants eligible for intervention who declined to enroll (DR, $n=4$)						Parent fidelity assessed in laboratory.

Evidence for ESDM Efficacy in Promoting Child Change

The ESDM has primarily been used in three main intervention delivery contexts: a) intensive, group-based, preschool delivery, with staff ratio of 1:3–4 children, for 15–25 h per week; b) intensive, in-home, 1:1 delivery by paraprofessionals for at least 15 h per week; c) a low intensity parent coaching and delivery program, generally consisting of 12 h-long weekly sessions of clinician contact for parent coaching and limited direct delivery (P-ESDM). The data from each of these lines of research clearly show that children receiving ESDM make significant developmental progress in language and social communication, cognition, and adaptive functioning (Dawson et al., 2010, 2012; Eapen et al., 2013; Fulton et al., 2014; Rogers, Estes, et al., 2012; Vismara, Colombi, et al., 2009; Vivanti et al., 2013, 2014).

Initial support for the ESDM approach came from studies of the Denver Model, which had been implemented in a preschool setting (Rogers et al., 1984, 1987, Rogers & DiLalla, 1988; Rogers & Lewis, 1989). These Denver Model studies focused primarily on evaluating the developmental growth and outcomes of young children with both autism and other non-spectrum developmental disorders (i.e. ADHD, Reactive Attachment Disorder) who attended a specialized preschool for at least 10 h per week. The preschool-implemented Denver Model focused primarily on fostering play, symbolic cognition, social reciprocity, interpersonal relationships, and communication, through the use of positive affect, developmentally sensitive adult responses to children's emerging communication, scaffolding of symbolic and interactive play routines with peers, and physical space carefully designed to support children's attentional focus and learning. Over the course of several years of monitoring, children in this treatment program made significant gains across several developmental domains—cognitive, communication, social/emotional, motor, and symbolic play (Rogers et al., 1984; Rogers & DiLalla, 1988; Rogers & Lewis, 1989). Children with ASD made as many gains in communication and cognition as children with non-spectrum emotional/behavioral disorders, despite more significant initial impairments in these areas (Rogers & DiLalla, 1988). After 6 months in treatment, children showed significantly higher scores than expected based on their initial developmental rate, indicating that not only did they make progress, they made gains beyond those attributable simply to maturation (Rogers et al., 1984; Rogers & DiLalla, 1988; Rogers & Lewis, 1989). In children with longer-term outcomes available, the accelerated developmental rate observed over the first 6 months of treatment was maintained for the next 9–12 months (Rogers & DiLalla, 1988; Rogers & Lewis, 1989). These studies demonstrate that the core features of the Denver Model that have been incorporated into the ESDM—the interactive style, developmental orientation, focus on social relationships, positive affect, and play—are all associated with significant developmental change.

More recently, several investigations have evaluated the efficacy of ESDM implemented in community preschools offering autism-specific services in Sydney and Melbourne, Australia (Eapen et al., 2013; Fulton et al., 2014; Vivanti et al.,

2013, 2014). At both sites, children attended community-based day care centers for 15–25 h per week for nearly a year. Classrooms were limited to ten children and had a staff to child ratio of 1:3 or 1:4. Children also received 1 h per week of 1:1 treatment, delivered either separately (Sydney site) or within the classroom (Melbourne). Both sites provided parent coaching sessions, but parent use at home was not monitored. Thus, the bulk of high quality treatment hours came from this center- and group-based format. Outcome measures common to both sites included the Mullen Scales of Early Learning (MSEL, Mullen, 1995), a developmental assessment, and the Vineland Adaptive Behavior Scale, a parent-report measure of adaptive functioning (VABS-II, Sparrow, Balla, & Cicchetti, 2005). Children receiving ESDM in this group format showed significant increases in MSEL Overall Developmental Quotient (DQ) scores, MSEL receptive language, expressive language, visual reception subscale scores, as well as VABS-II communication subscale scores (Eapen et al., 2013; Vivanti et al., 2014). Children at both sites also demonstrated decreases in autism symptoms on both parent-report and observational measures. This included significantly lower total scores on the Social Communication Questionnaire (SCQ; Rutter, Bailey, & Lord, 2003), and the Social Affect scale of the gold-standard observational measure, the Autism Diagnostic Observation Scale (ADOS; Lord et al., 2000) (Eapen et al., 2013; Vivanti et al., 2014). The Sydney site also assessed changes in children's maladaptive behaviors using behavior ratings from ESDM Data Sheets (described in earlier sections of this chapter) recorded during children's 1:1 sessions. At the outset of treatment, only one child (of 38) was rated as compliant or above average, indicating that nearly all of the children were rated as displaying maladaptive behaviors. After 12 weeks, the number of children rated as compliant or above average increased to 26 children (68 %), and 30 children (79 %) were rated as such by the end of the program (Fulton et al., 2014).

In addition to evaluating developmental growth amongst children in this ESDM group program, Vivanti et al. (2014) compared their outcomes to those enrolled in non-ESDM, but ASD-specific community education programs. The treatment offered in the community comparison group also included an individualized treatment plan, but consisted of an eclectic approach—incorporating features of multiple evidence-based treatment approaches, rather than a single, manualized program. While both groups demonstrated significant increases in both MSEL Overall DQ and VABS-II scores and decreases in ADOS Social Affect scale scores, children in the ESDM group made significantly more MSEL DQ gains than children in the comparison group (15 vs. 7 points) (Vivanti et al., 2014).

In sum, the implementation of ESDM in group-based settings is associated with significant developmental progress in cognitive, social, and adaptive skills. This is particularly evident for children's cognitive abilities, as children enrolled in ESDM-based group programs showed significantly larger increases in MSEL Developmental Quotients than children enrolled in non-ESDM comparison programs. It is important to note that the programs implemented in these initial studies were of very high quality, delivered by teachers who had undergone the ESDM certification process, with ongoing monitoring and evaluation of treatment fidelity. More details on research analyzing the process and feasibility of implementing

ESDM in these community settings are described in later sections of this chapter. While future investigations using a fully randomized design and well-matched comparison groups to further evaluate the efficacy and feasibility of community- and group-based ESDM models is warranted, the existing studies indicate that intensive, high-quality group ESDM programs are associated with significant and clinically meaningful changes in children's development.

A second mechanism for intensive delivery involves individual, rather than group-based, delivery, accompanied by parent coaching. Dawson et al. (2010) published the results of a randomized controlled trial comparing ESDM to a community treatment control group in 48 toddlers with ASD. They found that after 2 years, children receiving 15 h per week of ESDM delivered in the home 1:1 by paraprofessionals and parents who had received coaching and reported using ESDM techniques themselves, made significantly more developmental progress than children receiving community treatment. Children in the ESDM group gained an average of 17.6 standard score points on the MSEL, while the community group gained an average of 7.0 points. The ESDM group also had better receptive and expressive language and adaptive functioning outcomes. While the community group declined in adaptive skills, the ESDM group maintained their standard scores, indicating that although still delayed overall, they gained adaptive skills at the same rate as the normative sample. Dawson et al. (2012) analyzed children's social behavior outcomes, based on the Pervasive Developmental Disorder—Behavior Inventory (PDD-BI; (Cohen & Sudhalter, 1999), as well as their neurophysiological responses (event-related brain potentials and EEG spectral power) in response to face and non-face stimuli at the conclusion of treatment in the same cohort. Children who had received community treatment demonstrated an electrophysiological pattern of responses indicating greater attentional and cognitive processing for objects than for faces. Children in the ESDM group displayed the opposite pattern of responses, responding both more quickly and with decreased α power and decreased θ power (indicative of increased attention and active cognitive processing) when viewing faces than objects. The pattern observed in the ESDM group was also observed in a typically developing control group (Dawson et al., 2012). Furthermore, children who received ESDM showed improved social behavior on the PDD-BI. Children's level of improvement in social behavior was correlated with their pattern of brain responses to social stimuli, with greater improvement associated with greater levels of brain activity while viewing social stimuli. This sample has now been followed up to age 6, 2 years after the cessation of active intensive early treatment. In this follow-up sample, the vast majority of children in the ESDM group (86 %) showed maintained or improved IQ scores (Estes et al., 2015). Assessments were conducted across multiple domains of functioning by clinicians naïve to previous intervention group status. The ESDM group, on average, maintained or increased improvements during the follow-up period in overall intellectual ability, adaptive behavior, symptom severity, and challenging behavior. No group differences in core autism symptoms were found immediately post-treatment, however, 2 years later, the ESDM group demonstrated improved core autism symptoms, as well as adaptive behavior and peer relations, as compared with the community-intervention-as-usual group.

The two groups received equivalent intervention hours during the original study but the ESDM group received fewer hours during the follow-up period. These results indicate sustained and, in some domains, enhanced long-term effects of early ASD intervention.

Both group- and individual-intensive ESDM delivery formats include simultaneous parent coaching in ESDM techniques. The inclusion of parents in children's treatment not only supports children's progress by increasing the number of learning opportunities throughout the day, but is also consistent with the recommendations of the National Research Council (National Research National Research Council, 2001). Several studies have now shown that parent use of ESDM techniques is associated with concurrent child change. The general P-ESDM coaching model is described earlier in this chapter. Results from both live, clinic-based and telehealth coaching procedures show that the majority of parents are able to successfully master these techniques by the end of treatment, often after as few as 6 weeks (Vismara et al., 2012; Vismara, Colombi, et al., 2009; Vismara, McCormick, et al., 2013). Three single subjects, multiple-baseline designs have investigated child change associated with this parent coaching program. These studies reported increases in infant social communication rates during active treatment (Vismara et al., 2012; Vismara, Colombi, et al., 2009; Vismara, McCormick, et al., 2013). The first of these single subject designs involved live, in person parent coaching (Vismara, Colombi, et al., 2009). In this investigation, the rate of spontaneous functional verbal utterances, number of imitative behaviors, and observed ratings of child engagement were used to monitor child changes associated with parent adoption of ESDM techniques. These measures demonstrated that children increased in the frequency and quality of these measures over the active treatment period, particularly once parents reached fidelity in their use of ESDM techniques. Importantly, these gains occurred gradually over the duration of treatment during interactions with both parents and the child's therapist, which suggests that rather than parents simply learning techniques for drawing out existing social communicative abilities, children were actually gaining these skills through interactions with their parents.

The last two single subjects studies involved parent coaching conducted via telemedicine technology (Vismara et al., 2012; Vismara, McCormick, et al., 2013). The first of these was a pilot of the telehealth procedure, and included nine families with a young child with ASD who received the 1-h, 12-week parent coaching program described above, but via an internet-based conference call in which parent and therapist could hear and see each other in real time. The materials (handouts, readings) that had been provided via hard copy in the traditional coaching program were provided via DVD, along with video examples of therapist-led ESDM sessions (Vismara et al., 2012). The second of these involved a similar telehealth approach, but included modifications based on the results of the 2012 study. These modifications included expansion of the session time from 1 h to 90 min, and the development of an integrated self-guided website, which included information, readings, videos, and a platform for messaging between parent and therapist (Vismara, McCormick, et al., 2013). In both studies, children increased in the frequency of spontaneous functional verbal utterances during the treatment phase.

Children also increased their spontaneous imitation, an outcome measure in the Vismara et al., 2012 study, and their initiation of joint attention and their vocabulary size, outcomes measures of the Vismara, Young, et al., 2013 study. Together, these single-subject studies demonstrated that children made gains in social communicative ability that co-occurred with parent implementation of ESDM techniques and thus support the use of P-ESDM as a low intensity treatment strategy for promoting child change.

The efficacy of P-ESDM in promoting children's development was tested more thoroughly in a large, multi-site, randomized controlled group trial which compared children's outcomes on standardized measures of developmental level and autism symptoms after receiving the P-ESDM coaching program versus a community treatment control group (Rogers, Estes, et al., 2012). Results from this study again indicated that children showed improvements after 12 weeks of treatment, with significant increases in MSEL Developmental Quotients (DQ) and decreases in ADOS Social Affect scores. However, it should be noted that children in both the P-ESDM and community treatment groups made significant improvements, and there were no group differences between them for either MSEL DQ or ADOS scores at the end of the 12 week active treatment period. Interpretation of these results is limited by the use of a community treatment control group, as children in this group received almost four times the treatment hours as children in the P-ESDM condition. These results highlight one area of need for future research on the efficacy of both P-ESDM and other treatment approaches: the direct comparison of two treatments equally well specified in terms of content, intensity, and quality, including measures of fidelity. An RCT comparing two P-ESDM coaching methods that will help to clarify some of these issues is currently underway at the University of Washington and UC Davis MIND Institute. Additional discussion of future research needs on parent-, group-, and therapist-implemented ESDM is included below.

Child Characteristics Associated with Positive Outcomes

The ESDM includes several features which contribute to a very tailored and individualized approach to treatment—the creation of specific learning objectives across multiple developmental domains based on children's unique skills and needs, the emphasis on following children's leads in terms of activity choice and theme, the incorporation of familial and cultural values in shaping children's treatment objectives and context for delivery, and the use of a decision tree to make modifications to a child's program when progress is not happening quickly enough. These features support learning in all children. There has also been a call to identify specific child characteristics that predict which children will respond best to a particular treatment, answering the question of what works for whom (Trembath & Vivanti, 2014). This question has been specifically addressed in two ESDM studies. The randomized controlled trial of P-ESDM (Rogers, Estes, et al., 2012) of toddlers 12–24 months analyzed associations between children's initial imitation, social orienting, social and developmental levels, treatment hours, and chronological age in predicting changes in MSEL and ADOS scores. Across both groups, a greater number of treatment hours and younger chronological ages were associated with significantly increased MSEL scores. Vivanti and colleagues (Vivanti et al., 2013, 2014) have investigated outcome predictors amongst children enrolled in group-based ESDM. They reported that in contrast to the Rogers, Dawson, et al. (2012) results, neither chronological age nor intensity of treatment were significant predictors of children's outcomes. However, children in the group-based programs were both slightly older and receiving more intensive services than children in the parent-implemented RCT, limiting the ability to draw strong conclusions on these particular factors. Vivanti et al. (2014) reported that children's ability to organize actions around goals were strong predictors of gains in verbal and non-verbal cognition. Specific predictors included children's spontaneous use of objects in a functional, goal-oriented manner, predictive looks towards the target of an actor's goal-oriented action (e.g., reaching), and spontaneous imitation of actions on objects. Initial symptom severity was a strong predictor of expressive language outcomes, explaining 40 % of the variance in gains on the MSEL Expressive Language subscale. Clearly, more work is needed to better understand which children are most likely to benefit from ESDM. Several ongoing research projects are actively investigating this question.

ESDM for High Risk Infants

Two studies have investigated the application of the ESDM in infants less than 12 months of age (Rogers et al., 2014; Vismara & Rogers, 2008). The first was a case study piloting P-ESDM procedures for "Robbie", a 9-month-old infant displaying clear and consistent symptoms of ASD, and his father (Vismara & Rogers, 2008). Robbie's father reached 85 % fidelity in his use of ESDM techniques by the eighth therapy session, which was maintained during a 3-month follow-up. Robbie demonstrated increases in social communication over the active treatment period that were maintained during follow-up as well. These included increases in the number of spontaneous functional verbal utterances, imitative behaviors, increased attentiveness to an adult interactive partner, and increases in the frequency of social initiations, and were observed during interactions with both his father and an interventionist.

More recently, a modified P-ESDM program (Infant ESDM) was developed and pilot tested with seven infants 7–15 months exhibiting early symptoms of ASD. These infants were referred from both an ongoing longitudinal study of high risk infant siblings of children with ASD as well as from the community. They were compared to other four other groups of infants constructed from the infant sibling study sample: high risk siblings identified as symptomatic at 9 months but who declined to participate in the intervention (DR), high risk siblings with existing 36-month outcome data who either met criteria for ASD at outcome (AO) or who did not meet criteria (HR), and low risk infants with no family history of ASD (LR). The final three groups had completed their participation in the larger infant sibling study, and thus were not eligible for participation in the intervention. They were matched to the IS group on the basis of 9-month autism symptoms measured via the Autism Observation Scale for Infants (AOSI, Bryson, Zwaigenbaum, McDermott, Rombough, & Brian, 2008), MSEL early learning composite, and gender. Although not formally diagnosed at 9 months, all seven infants in the IS group exhibited elevated AOSI scores on two separate occasions, scores in the risk range on the Infant-Toddler Checklist (ITC, Wetherby & Prizant, 2002), and concerns based on independent observations made by two expert clinicians.

Infant ESDM (I-ESDM) targets six symptom areas identified in the literature as particularly strong risk markers of autism in infancy: (1) unusual visual examination and fixations; (2) unusual repetitive patterns of object exploration; (3) lack of intentional communicative acts; (4) lack of age-appropriate phonemic development; (5) lack of coordinated gaze, affect, and voice in reciprocal social-communicative interactions; and (6) decreased eye contact, social interest, and engagement. Parent coaching focuses on techniques for targeting these six specific domains, as well as any other delays a particular infant may exhibit.

The results of this pilot study demonstrate that at the outset of treatment, infants in the treatment group exhibited significantly more autism symptoms and lower language ability than infants in the other groups. From 18 to 36 months, infants receiving I-ESDM exhibited significantly more autism symptoms than the LR and HR infants, but fewer symptoms than the DR and AO infants. A similar effect was observed for language ability, with infants receiving I-ESDM exhibiting no significant differences from LR and HR infants from 18 to 36 months. At 36 months of age, 2 of 7 I-ESDM infants and 3 of 4 DR infants received a clinical best estimate of ASD. These results suggest that identification and treatment of symptomatic infants in the first year of life is not only possible, but is associated with significant increases in infants' language abilities and decreases in both autism symptoms and diagnosis. While exciting, these results must be replicated within a larger, randomized, and well-controlled trial.

ESDM Dissemination Science

Therapist Training

While the ESDM materials (Manual and Curriculum Checklist) are publicly available, it is important to remember that the studies demonstrating the most significant child change at the group level have been conducted in an intensive format (15 or more hours per week) by certified therapists. The procedure for becoming a certified ESDM therapist is described earlier in this chapter, but generally involves a combination of reading, didactic instruction, hands-on training, self-evaluation, and feedback on treatment implementation and use of ESDM techniques. The dissemination process, feasibility, and implementation of ESDM have been evaluated in several studies that have generally supported the use of didactic workshops and ongoing supervision and feedback in reaching and maintaining high levels of therapist and program fidelity (Vismara, Young, et al., 2009, 2013; Vivanti et al., 2014). Vismara, Colombi, et al. (2009) evaluated the contribution of several features in training therapists to fidelity. These features included live vs. distance (telehealth) learning, and the use of self-instruction, didactic, and team supervision teaching techniques for both direct ESDM delivery and parent coaching. Results showed that learning occurred equally well for both live and distance learners and that fidelity of implementation significantly improved once therapists received didactic training and team supervision, features incorporated into the current certification procedure.

The workshop-based procedure now used to provide initial therapist training has also been evaluated. Vismara, Young, et al. (2013) analyzed therapists' fidelity in ESDM delivery directly following a training workshop as well as their understanding of the treatment techniques and overall satisfaction with the procedure. Significant increases in therapist fidelity in ESDM technique use were observed both during the workshop itself and at 4-month follow-up. Notably, the majority of professionals rated the procedure as highly satisfactory and all 24 attained full fidelity (80 %) by the conclusion of training. Despite their success in reaching fidelity by the end of the workshop, only half of the participants submitted post-workshop follow-up materials, though there are several possible explanations for this attrition rate, including lack of resources or support in their community organizations, or deciding not to adopt ESDM as the primary intervention approach. However, the professionals who submitted follow-up materials all maintained high levels of fidelity in ESDM implementation.

More detailed information regarding the community and organization supports necessary for providing group-based ESDM comes from the model programs recently implemented in Australia. Both the Sydney and Melbourne sites were established as part of the government-funded day-long childcare centers for children with autism (Autism Specific Early Learning and Care Centre, ASELCC). The ESDM Manual (Rogers & Dawson, 2010) provides specific guidelines for conducting ESDM treatment in a group-based delivery program. These will not be detailed here, but include recommendations for structuring the physical space, daily flow, and overall schedule for the classroom, organizing staff time and roles, strategies for addressing individual children's objectives into group activities, taking and maintaining accurate data on child learning, and other key features. Results from these two investigations demonstrate that children in these ESDM group-based programs make significant gains in cognitive, social, and adaptive skills and thus are effective programs for treating young children with ASD (Eapen et al., 2013; Vivanti et al., 2014). In terms of feasibility, Vivanti et al. (2014) evaluated several specific features: acceptability, demand, implementation, practicality, and adaptation and integration into the existing center system. The use of ESDM was supported on each of these dimensions. More than 90 % of parents indicated they found the program both suitable and satisfactory for their children, and more than 250 families requested placement in the program—far more than capacity. The program was also rated highly by government-led evaluations in terms providing service consistent with government regulations, collaboration with families and communities, and ease of integration into the existing childcare system. The most significant drawbacks identified by both the authors and the government evaluation is that demand far exceeded capacity, and thus, a large number of children were not receiving the same high quality of care and treatment (Vivanti et al., 2014).

Parent Coaching

Seven studies, including the modified infant version described earlier in this review, have evaluated the effectiveness of P-ESDM in terms of fidelity of implementation, acceptability, and effects on parental mental health, in addition to analyzing concurrent changes in children's behavior (Estes et al., 2014; Rogers et al., 2014; Rogers, Estes, et al., 2012; Vismara et al., 2012; Vismara, Colombi, et al., 2009; Vismara, McCormick, et al., 2013; Vismara & Rogers, 2008). These investigations have demonstrated that parents are able to successfully learn and apply ESDM techniques when interacting with their children. The majority of parents reach high levels of fidelity (e.g. 80 %) over the course of a short, low intensity, coaching process. Two studies have evaluated these features in a distance-learning program, with coaching sessions occurring via telehealth services, including web-based video conferencing and a self-guided website (Vismara et al., 2012; Vismara, McCormick, et al., 2013). These investigations reported similarly high levels of parent fidelity by the end of the active treatment period, with average group scores increasing significantly from baseline to ratings of 4.15 and 4.29 (of a possible 5) at post-treatment follow-up. Both live and distance parent coaching programs report that the majority of parents reach fidelity in less than 12 weeks, often after 6–7 weeks of training (Vismara et al., 2012; Vismara, Colombi, et al., 2009; Vismara, McCormick, et al., 2013; Vismara & Rogers, 2008).

In terms of acceptability, parents receiving P-ESDM training report both high satisfaction with the coaching procedure as well as strong working alliances with their therapist (Rogers et al., 2014; Rogers, Estes, et al., 2012; Vismara et al., 2012; Vismara, McCormick, et al., 2013). Compared to parents receiving treatment in the community, parents receiving P-ESDM coaching report significantly less parenting-related stress in the first 3 months after their child's diagnosis (Estes et al., 2014). This group difference in parental stress is driven by a significant increase in stress reported by the community treatment group; parents in the P-ESDM group reported no such changes during the same 3-month period.

The effectiveness of P-ESDM in promoting children's development has been described in earlier sections, and has consistently documented significant changes in children's language, social communication and developmental level using through both fine-grained behavioral coding analyses and scores on standardized measures. Both live and telehealth single-subjects designs have reported increases in children's frequency of vocalizations, imitations, social initiations, and social engagement (Vismara et al., 2012; Vismara, Colombi, et al., 2009; Vismara,

McCormick, et al., 2013; Vismara & Rogers, 2008). A randomized controlled trial comparing P-ESDM to community treatment found that both groups of children made significant gains on standardized measures of language and significant decreases in autism symptoms. While these results might seem to suggest a limited benefit of P-ESDM, these results are actually quite impressive considering children in the control group received nearly twice as many treatment hours as children in the P-ESDM group (Rogers, Estes, et al., 2012). Clearly, more work is needed to understand the effectiveness of P-ESDM, particularly when implemented in community practice and when compared to more intensive intervention formats. A follow-up P-ESDM randomized controlled trial is currently underway through the University of Washington and UC Davis MIND Institute sites, the results of which will help to answer questions about how best to coach parents in this model, mechanisms of change within both parents and children, and families for whom P-ESDM may be particularly effective. A fuller discussion of future research needs is included below.

Recommendations for Future Research

The existing body of ESDM research demonstrates that it is an effective treatment approach for young children with ASD, leading to significant developmental growth in children's cognition, language, social abilities, and adaptive functioning. These changes are observed both on an individual level and in group comparisons. There is also support for the training procedures for both therapist and parent models, demonstrating that both groups are able to learn the ESDM techniques and implement them with high fidelity. Despite these impressive results, there are several areas where additional research is likely to be particularly fruitful.

The first is in determining which treatments are most effective for which children, a current research need the field of intervention science as a whole (Trembath & Vivanti, 2014). This question cannot fully be answered without directly comparing two treatment programs that are both manualized (standardized), and delivered with the same quality and intensity. A large, multi-site randomized controlled trial is currently underway that will address this issue by comparing ESDM to a manualized discrete trial training program, which are also being evaluated at two intensity levels: 15 h per week versus 25 h per week.

The second area of research need is in comparing the outcomes of children in low-intensity ESDM (generally parent-implemented) models to the strong results observed in therapist-delivered formats (Dawson et al., 2010, 2012; Vivanti et al., 2014). While the results of several parent-implemented ESDM trials demonstrate significant gains in children's language, social communication, and developmental functioning, whether these gains are as strong as those obtained in intensive therapist-delivered ESDM formats is an open research question. There is initial evidence that P-ESDM is at least as effective as some high-intensity non-ESDM community treatment models (Rogers, Estes, et al., 2012). However, whether it is appropriate to expect parents to be the main provider of early intensive services is an important question for public policy. This question is directly related to the more general need for wider dissemination of evidence-based practices and for studies comparing the effectiveness of well-controlled, university-based studies with the real-world demands and limitations of the community setting. Even within established systems, many families experience issues of limited access due to long waiting lists or because intensive behavioral interventions are simply unavailable. Dissemination science will need to address these issues within both established systems and much more broadly in communities across the world where government-supported infrastructure does not exist and dissemination must be directly to families, without an intervening professional. A major focus of ESDM research going forward will be in developing and evaluating wider dissemination of this efficacious treatment.

Finally, the results from the pilot study of infant intervention are quite exciting, and suggest that intervening as soon as symptoms begin to appear may have particularly strong effects in reducing symptom severity and diagnostic rates and improving functional outcomes. This possibility has significant implications for public policy in terms of both screening, resource allocation, and the potential to significantly reduce the long-term costs associated with autism-related impairments (Ganz, 2015; Peters-Scheffer, Didden, Korzilius, & Matson, 2012).

Considerations for Practitioners and Families Interested in the ESDM

In terms of specific benefits to families over other treatment approaches, ESDM offers several positive features. First, the generalist model employed in the ESDM means that parents see only one primary therapist, who delivers a comprehensive treatment plan that addresses children's learning needs across all domains. This approach limits parents' need to integrate and reconcile potentially conflicting advice and plans from multiple professionals, which may contribute to the lower levels of parenting-related stress reported by parents receiving ESDM training (Estes et al., 2014). Second, the rigorous certification process for professionals ensures that treatment delivered by these therapists is of high quality and adheres to the manualized protocols. A list of certified trainers and certified therapists is maintained through the UC Davis MIND Institute website (http://www.ucdmc.ucdavis.edu/mindinstitute/research/esdm/), where families can search for certified therapists in their area. Third, the parent-training provided in the ESDM, whether in combination with therapist delivery or in the parent-implemented model, is consistent with the recommendations from the national research council to include parents in their child's treatment plan (National Research National Research Council, 2001). Parents who receive training in ESDM techniques report stronger working alliances with their therapists than parents whose children receive treatment in the community, suggesting the ESDM supports parents in playing an active role in their child's intervention (Rogers, Estes, et al., 2012). Finally, there is strong support for the efficacy of the ESDM in improving children's outcomes. This has now been demonstrated in both single-subjects designs and randomized controlled trials, across therapist-, parent-, and group-based treatment delivery. Gains in children's language, communication, adaptive, and cognitive abilities have been observed using both detailed behavioral coding of children's spontaneous behavior and on standardized behavioral measures such as the ADOS and MSEL. Long-term follow up of children who participated in a randomized controlled trial of ESDM as toddlers indicate that the developmental acceleration demonstrated during the toddler period is maintained for several years into early childhood, when core autism symptoms are reduced (Estes et al., in revision). These results suggest that the ESDM not only improves children's language and cognition, but results in deep, long-lasting changes in children's ability to both participate in and learn from social interactions.

References

Boyd, B. A., Hume, K., McBee, M. T., Alessandri, M., Gutierrez, A., Johnson, L., et al. (2014). Comparative efficacy of LEAP, TEACHH and non-model specific special education programs for preschoolers with autism spectrum disorders. *Journal of Autism and Developmental Disorders, 44*, 366–380.

Bryson, S. E., Zwaigenbaum, L., McDermott, C., Rombough, V., & Brian, J. (2008). The autism observation scale for infants: Scale development and reliability data. *Journal of Autism and Developmental Disorders, 38*, 731–738.

Cohen, I., & Sudhalter, V. (1999). Pervasive Developmental Disorder Behavior Inventory (PDDBI-C). *NYS Institute for Basic Research in Developmental Disabilities*.

Dawson, G. (2008). Early behavioral intervention, brain plasticity, and the prevention of autism spectrum disorder. *Development and Psychopathology, 20*, 775–803.

Dawson, G., Carver, L., Meltzoff, A. N., Panagiotides, H., McPartland, J., & Webb, S. J. (2002). Neural correlates of face and object recognition in young children with autism spectrum disorder, developmental delay, and typical development. *Child Development, 73*, 700–717.

Dawson, G., Jones, E. J. H., Merkle, K., Venema, K., Lowy, R., Faja, S., … Webb, S. J. (2012). Early behavioral intervention is associated with normalized brain activity in young children with autism. *Journal of the American Academy of Child and Adolescent Psychiatry, 51*, 1150–1159.

Dawson, G., Rogers, S., Munson, J., Smith, M., Winter, J., Greenson, J., … Varley, J. (2010). Randomized, controlled trial of an intervention for toddlers with autism: The Early Start Denver Model. *Pediatrics, 125*, 17–23.

Dawson, G., Webb, S. J., & McPartland, J. (2005). Understanding the nature of face processing impairment in autism: Insights from behavioral and electrophysiological studies. *Developmental Neuropsychology, 27*, 403–424.

DiClemente, C. C., & Marden Velasquez, M. (2002). Motivational interviewing and the stages of change. In W. R. Miller & S. Rollnick (Eds.), *Motivational interviewing* (2nd ed., pp. 201–216). New York, NY: The Guilford Press.

Eapen, V., Crnčec, R., & Walter, A. (2013). Clinical outcomes of an early intervention program for preschool children with Autism Spectrum Disorder in a community group setting. *BMC Pediatrics, 13*, 3.

Estes, A., Rogers, S. J., Greenson, J., Winter, J., & Dawson, G. (2015). Long-term outcomes of early intervention in 6-year-old children with autism spectrum disorder. *Journal of the American Academy of Child and Adolescent Psychiatry, 54*, 580.

Estes, A., Vismara, L. A., Mercado, C., Fitzpatrick, A., Elder, L., Greenson, J., … Rogers, S. J. (2014). The impact of parent-delivered intervention on parents of very young children with autism. *Journal of Autism and Developmental Disorders, 44*, 353–65.

Fulton, E., Eapen, V., Crnčec, R., Walter, A., & Rogers, S. J. (2014). Reducing maladaptive behaviors in preschool-aged children with autism spectrum disorder using the early start Denver model. *Frontiers in Pediatrics, 2*, 40.

Ganz, M. L. (2015). The lifetime distribution of the incremental societal costs of autism. *Archives of Pediatrics & Adolescent Medicine, 161*, 343–349.

Hanft, B. E., Rush, D. D., & Shelden, M. L. (2004). *Coaching families and colleagues in early childhood.* Baltimore, MD: Brookes Publishing.

Lord, C., Risi, S., Lambrecht, L., Cook, E. H., Leventhal, B. L., DiLavore, P. C., … Rutter, M. (2000). The autism diagnostic observation schedule-generic: A standard measure of social and communication deficits associated with the spectrum of autism. *Journal of Autism and Developmental Disorders, 30*, 205–23.

McGee, G. G., Morrier, M. J., & Daly, T. (1999). An incidental teaching approach to early intervention for toddlers with autism. *Research and Practice for Persons with Severe Disabilities, 24*, 133–146.

McGee, G. G., Paradis, T., & Feldman, R. S. (1993). Free effects of integration on levels of autistic behavior. *Topics in Early Childhood Special Education, 13*, 57–67.

Mullen, E. M. (1995). *The Mullen scales of early learning: AGS edition manual.* Circle Pines, MN: AGS.

National Association for the Education of Young Children. (2009). *Developmentally Appropriate Practice in Early Childhood Programs Serving Children from Birth through Age 8 (position statement). Young Children* (pp. 1–31).

National Research Council. (2001). *Educating children with autism.* Washington, DC: National Academy Press.

O'Neill, R. E., Jenson, W. R., & Radley, K. C. (2014). Interventions for challenging behaviors. In F. R. Volkmar, S. J. Rogers, R. Paul, & K. A. Pelphrey (Eds.), *Handbook of autism and pervasive developmental disorders* (4th ed., pp. 826–837). Hoboken, NJ: John Wiley & Sons.

Peters-Scheffer, N., Didden, R., Korzilius, H., & Matson, J. (2012). Cost comparison of early intensive behavioral intervention and treatment as usual for children with autism spectrum disorder in The Netherlands. *Research in Developmental Disabilities, 33*, 1763–1772.

Prochaska, J., Redding, C. A., & Evers, K. E. (2002). The transtheoretical model and stages of change. In K. Glanz, B. K. Rimer, & F. M. Lewis (Eds.), *Health behavior and health education* (3rd ed., pp. 99–120). San Francisco, CA: Jossey-Bass.

Rogers, S. J., & Dawson, G. (2010). *Early start Denver model for young children with autism: Promoting language, learning, and engagement.* New York, NY: The Guilford Press.

Rogers, S. J., Dawson, G., & Vismara, L. A. (2012). *An early start for your child with autism: Using everyday activities to help kids connect, communicate, and learn* (1st ed.). New York, NY: The Guilford Press.

Rogers, S. J., & DiLalla, D. (1988). A comparative study of the effects of a developmentally based instructional model on young children with autism and young children with other disorders of behavior and development. *Topics in Early Childhood Special Education, 11*, 29–47.

Rogers, S. J., Estes, A., Lord, C., Vismara, L. A., Winter, J., Fitzpatrick, A., … Dawson, G. (2012). Effects of a brief Early Start Denver model (ESDM)-based parent intervention on toddlers at risk for autism spectrum disorders: A randomized controlled trial. *Journal of the American Academy of Child and Adolescent Psychiatry, 51*, 1052–65.

Rogers, S. J., Herbison, J. M., & Lewis, H. C. (1984). An approach for enhancing the symbolic, communicative, and interpersonal functioning of young children with autism or severe emotional handicaps. *Journal of the Division for Early Childhood, 10*, 135–148.

Rogers, S. J., & Lewis, H. (1989). An effective day treatment model for young children with pervasive developmental disorders. *Journal of the American Academy of Child & Adolescent Psychiatry, 28*, 207–214.

Rogers, S. J., Lewis, H. C., & Reis, K. (1987). An effective procedure for training early special education teams to implement a model program. *Journal of the Division for Early Childhood, 11*, 180–188.

Rogers, S. J., Vismara, L. A., Wagner, A. L., McCormick, C., Young, G., & Ozonoff, S. (2014). Autism treatment in the first year of life: A pilot study of infant start, a parent-implemented intervention for symptomatic infants. *Journal of Autism and Developmental Disorders, 44*, 2981.

Rutter, M., Bailey, A., & Lord, C. (2003). *Social communication questionnaire*. Los Angeles, CA: Western Psychological Services.

Sparrow, S., Balla, D., & Cicchetti, D. (2005). *Vineland adaptive behavior scales* (2nd ed.). Circle Pines, MN: American Guidance Service.

Stahmer, A. C., & Ingersoll, B. (2004). Inclusive programming for toddlers with autism spectrum disorders: Outcomes from the children's toddler school. *Journal of Positive Behavior Interventions, 6*, 67–82.

Strain, P. S., & Bovey, E. H. (2011). Randomized, controlled trial of the LEAP model of early intervention for young children with autism spectrum disorders. *Topics in Early Childhood Special Education, 31*, 133–154.

Trembath, D., & Vivanti, G. (2014). Problematic but predictive: Individual differences in children with autism spectrum disorders. *International Journal of Speech-Language Pathology, 16*, 57–60.

Vismara, L. A., Colombi, C., & Rogers, S. J. (2009). Can one hour per week of therapy lead to lasting changes in young children with autism? *Autism: The International Journal of Research and Practice, 13*, 93–115.

Vismara, L. A., McCormick, C., Young, G. S., Nadhan, A., & Monlux, K. (2013). Preliminary findings of a telehealth approach to parent training in autism. *Journal of Autism and Developmental Disorders, 43*, 2953–2969.

Vismara, L. A., & Rogers, S. J. (2008). The early start Denver model a case study of an innovative practice. *Journal of Early Intervention, 31*, 91–108.

Vismara, L. A., Young, G. S., Stahmer, A. C., Griffith, E. M., & Rogers, S. J. (2009). Dissemination of evidence-based practice: Can we train therapists from a distance? *Journal of Autism and Developmental Disorders, 39*, 1636–1651.

Vismara, L. A., Young, G. S., & Rogers, S. J. (2012). Telehealth for expanding the reach of early autism training to parents. *Autism Research and Treatment, 2012*, 121878.

Vismara, L. A., Young, G. S., & Rogers, S. J. (2013). Community dissemination of the early start Denver model: Implications for science and practice. *Topics in Early Childhood Special Education, 32*, 223–233.

Vivanti, G., Dissanayake, C., Zierhut, C., & Rogers, S. J. (2013). Brief report: Predictors of outcomes in the Early Start Denver Model delivered in a group setting. *Journal of Autism and Developmental Disorders, 43*, 1717–1724.

Vivanti, G., Paynter, J., Duncan, E., Fothergill, H., Dissanayake, C., & Rogers, S. J. (2014). Effectiveness and feasibility of the early start Denver model implemented in a group-based community childcare setting. *Journal of Autism and Developmental Disorders, 44*, 3140–3153.

Wetherby, A. M., & Prizant, B. (2002). *Communication and symbolic behavior scales developmental profile* (1st ed.). Baltimore, MD: Paul H. Brookes.

Chapter 6
Prelinguistic Milieu Teaching

Nienke C. Peters-Scheffer, Bibi Huskens, Robert Didden, and Larah van der Meer

Introduction

During their first year of life typically developing children learn how to be effective communicators. While most children learn to communicate without formal teaching, children with developmental disabilities are often delayed in the use of first words and may need guidance to learn how to communicate. Long before they use words or signs, typically developing children interact with their caregivers through facial expressions, natural gestures, and vocalizations. Because prelinguistic communication is seen as a foundation for spoken word production, helping children to develop their prelinguistic communication may facilitate acquisition of spoken language.

This chapter explores Prelinguistic Milieu Teaching (PMT), an intervention designed to teach children to initiate nonverbal communication during social routines in their natural environment as a foundation for later spoken word production. First, we will discuss the theoretical background of PMT, which is typically viewed as a transactional model. Then, we will describe the implementation of PMT and review the available research. Finally, we will provide suggestions for further research and implications for practitioners.

N.C. Peters-Scheffer (✉) • R. Didden
Behavioural Science Institute, Radboud University Nijmegen,
P.O. Box 9104, 6500 HE Nijmegen, The Netherlands
e-mail: n.peters@pwo.ru.nl

B. Huskens
Dr. Leo Kannerhuis, Center for Autism, P.O. Box 62, 6865 ZH Doorwerth, The Netherlands

L. van der Meer
School of Education, Te Puna Akopai, Victoria University of Wellington,
Karori, Wellington 6147, New Zealand

R. Lang et al. (eds.), *Early Intervention for Young Children with Autism Spectrum Disorder*, Evidence-Based Practices in Behavioral Health,
DOI 10.1007/978-3-319-30925-5_6

Theoretical Background of PMT

Before children learn language, they use prelinguistic means to communicate with their caregivers. Almost immediately after birth, parents and infants engage in face-to-face interactions and communication begins to develop. During the first months of life, typically developing infants start to produce sounds, gestures, and facial expressions (Mundy & Willoughby, 1998). Between 3 and 5 months of age, infants are able to follow other peoples' gaze direction to nearby targets within their visual field and 1-year-old children follow other peoples' gaze to more remote targets (Corkum & Moore, 1995). At the same age, children also begin to point to objects and activities (Leung & Rheingold, 1981) and when infants are approximately 14 months old natural gestures (e.g., waving "bye-bye" or asking to be picked up by raising the arms) emerge (Acredolo & Goodwyn, 1988). Between 12 and 18 months of age, children begin to develop specific vocalizations with communicative intent that are recognizable to adults in their environment and first words appear (Vihman, 1996; Watt, Wetherby, & Shumway, 2006).

Early in an infant's development, a great deal of what is communicated may be unintentional. This means that communicative behaviors are not generated with the intent of transmitting a specific message and behaviors do not correspond to an explicit meaning. However, by behaving in a certain way (e.g., crying, smiling, turning away) children help others to interpret their wants and needs. Most caregivers perceive the infant's communicative acts as meaningful interaction and respond to the communicative behaviors (Wilcox, Kouri, & Caswell, 1990). The infant's behavior is communicative only because an adult interprets the child's behavior and assigns meaning to it.

When infants are approximately 6 months old, they begin to use non-verbal communication intentionally for behavioral regulation. For example, infants start to gesture or vocalize to request an object they desire. Later, infants direct their communicative behavior to a partner to share observations and experiences or to interact socially. As they continue to develop, more prelinguistic behavior become intentional meant to send a message to another person. Hence, they have a purpose and communicate to have that purpose fulfilled. The more children are able to communicate intentionally, the more they can express their feelings, wants and needs to others.

These early affective, communicative and social interactions fulfill a key purpose in the infant's development of communicative skills. Caregivers (e.g., parents and child care providers) respond to the infant's production and repetition of sounds. They also offer meaning, comment, and react to the infant's gestures, body movement, and vocalizations. Consequently, the child learns that his or her behavior has an effect on others and that his or her attempts serve a communicative purpose. In addition, these early social communication skills support lexical learning (i.e., learning new words), as such skills help the child to follow into and direct the attentional focus of the adult (Cress & Marvin, 2003; Tomasello, 1995, 1999).

From a transactional perspective, both children and parents play a role in determining the course of development. This is viewed as the result of an active environment and an active child adapting to and influencing the environment over time. Hence, parent behavior affects subsequent child behavior, but parent behavior itself is influenced by child behavior as well (Sameroff, 2009). The development of communication is a dynamic process, in which skills are developed over time during a series of interactions between the child and the parent in natural environments. Based on individual characteristics, both children and parents contribute to and influence this interaction and consequently the course of development (Sameroff, 2009). For example, Yoder and Munson (1995) showed that when children with developmental disabilities accompany their gestures with coordinated attention, their mothers are more likely to judge their children's prelinguistic behaviors as communicative. When parents recognize that a child communicates intentionally, they may respond by putting into words the presumed meaning of the child's communication act (linguistic mapping). Thus, responding to the adult's focus of attention or communicating intentionally allows a child to access linguistic information, which supports the process of early word learning (Yoder, Warren, McCathren, & Leew, 1998). This also shows that prelinguistic skills are seen as a necessary prerequisite for later symbolic language acquisition and when the transition from preintentional to intentional communication is delayed or does not occur; the development of symbolic communication may be negatively affected.

Children with developmental disabilities often show a delay in the acquisition and use of first words and some children may not develop the use of symbolic spoken language. Although communication delays are often not identified until children are 2 years old, these delays may have begun during the prelinguistic stage of development (Mundy & Crowson, 1997). Children with developmental disabilities use less prelinguistic communication and elicit fewer interactions from their caregivers. Even when they develop prelinguistic communication, their communication may be more difficult to interpret and less effective in expressing wants and needs than typically developing children. For example, certain movements or gestures may only be successfully interpreted by familiar communication partners but not by others (Carter & Iacono, 2002). As a result, caregivers respond less to the child's prelinguistic communication and provide the child with less additional linguistic input. When caregivers of children with developmental disabilities attend to their child's communicative attempts, they are also less likely to interpret and respond correctly than parents of children without developmental disabilities. Using communication to achieve goals may be more complex for children with developmental disabilities. This may delay the child in becoming an intentional communicator and may have a cascading effect on their language development (Tomasello, 1999). For example, Calandrella and Wilcox (2000) found that the rate of intentional nonverbal communication was a predictor of spontaneous word productions 1 year later in 25 toddlers with global developmental delay.

Some children with developmental disabilities do not develop symbolic spoken language and function on a prelinguistic communication skill level across their lifespan. Though prelinguistic communication may not facilitate the acquisition of spoken language, a consistent and clear set of prelinguistic communication skills can help increase the interpretability of communication and ability to interact successfully with environment. In addition, caregivers are more likely to respond correctly to clear recognizable prelinguistic communication.

When parents and professionals teach children to communicate, they often focus on symbolic communication based on objects, pictures, words, or signs. Yoder and Warren (2002) argue that children with developmental delays are more likely to benefit from language forms in their zone of proximal development (i.e., "the distance between the actual developmental level as determined by independent problem solving and the level of potential development as determined through problem solving under adult guidance or in collaboration with more capable peers"; Vygotsky, 1978, p. 86) rather than being taught word production. Therefore, these children may need help in developing their prelinguistic communication skills before they are ready to learn symbolic communication. Increasing the frequency of clarity of prelinguistic communication skills in young children may affect the responsiveness of caregivers in their environment. According to Yoder and Warren (2002), the parents' ability to interactively communicate with their child is the key to effective teaching.

Prelinguistic Milieu Teaching (PMT) is an intervention for children with language delays and facilitates the child's development of non-verbal communication as a foundation for later spoken word production. As children increase their rates of (nonverbal) communication, adults become more responsive, which in turn further increases the child's communication skills. Results of studies have shown that parent responsiveness is a critical factor in children's early language development (Brady, Marquis, Fleming, & McLean, 2004; Calandrella & Wilcox, 2000). After the child frequently uses intentional communication or when conventional symbols begin emerging, PMT can be followed by language intervention, such as milieu language teaching (MT; Hancock & Kaiser, 2006), forming a sequential approach referred to as milieu communication teaching.

Implementation of PMT

PMT has been developed to promote gestures, vocalizations, and eye gaze behavior in young children with delayed prelinguistic communication development. In MT several naturalistic procedures are combined and embedded within the context of everyday activities. Teaching episodes are child-initiated and child-paced; that is, teaching only occurs when a child shows interest (Allen & Cowan, 2008). Unlike MT which focuses on language, PMT focuses on nonverbal communication. In several studies, PMT has been combined with Responsivity Education (RE), constituting a two-component intervention, referred to as RE/PMT or RPMT (e.g. Yoder & Warren, 2002; Fey et al., 2006).

PMT is implemented in one-to-one natural play sessions by a teacher, speech-language pathologist (SLP), or other professional (Behavior Analyst). PMT is only appropriate for children who are not too advanced in prelinguistic communication skills and can be beneficial for children who do not use prelinguistic communication frequently by the age of 12–18 months. Specifically, PMT is designed for children that (a) produce less than ten words or signs, (b) understand less than 75 words, and/or (c) produce less than 1–2 spontaneous intentional communication actions per minute during social play (Warren et al., 2006).

Yoder and Warren (2004) identified parental responding as a predictor of language acquisition in children with developmental disabilities. By enhancing caregivers' responsiveness to the communication of the child, language development can be maximized. The RE component has been developed to teach parents to be highly responsive to the communication actions of their child (Yoder & Warren, 2002). More specific, RE teaches parents to (a) become more aware of the intentional and non-intentional communication of their child; (b) wait for their child to initiate motor or vocal behavior; (c) follow their child's focus of attention; and (d) provide appropriate contingent consequences to their child (Fey et al., 2006).

Professionals using PMT and parents in RE apply the same key principles, (a) arranging the environment, (b) following the child's lead, and (c) building in social routines. *Arranging the environment* is a strategy used to create communication opportunities (Warren et al., 2006). A teacher, for example, creates a communication opportunity for a child by placing a desired stuffed animal on a shelf, in sight but out of reach. Or, in the play room at home, the construction materials are kept in a clear box the child cannot open without the assistance of the parent. In both examples, the child is motivated to communicate, because s/he needs the adult to obtain the desired object. *Following the child's lead* is a strategy used to keep the child motivated and interested in activities and social interaction (Warren et al., 2006). Contingent upon a child's motor or vocal action the adult imitates the child. The adult has to adjust his/her behavior to the initiation rate of the child. For example, Tom likes to place toy cars in a row on the floor. When Tom places a car in a row on the floor, his mother contingently imitates him by placing a toy car in another row on the floor. *Building in social routines* can create communication opportunities when interrupted or modified (Warren et al., 2006). A social routine provides the child with a predictable structure. For example, Tom's mother starts to take turns by placing a toy car in his row instead of making her own row. After a couple of turns, she might wait before she starts with her turn. This change in routine might elicit Tom to initiate in requesting or commenting. A task analysis for building social routines is outlined in Table 6.1.

Warren et al. (2006) distinguished five hierarchical intermediate PMT goals to achieve the ultimate goal of clear and frequent intentional communication: (1) establish routines, (2) increase the frequency of nonverbal communicative acts (3) increase the frequency and spontaneity of coordinated eye gaze, (4) increase the frequency, spontaneity, and range of conventional and nonconventional gestures, and (5) combine components of intentional communication actions (i.e., eye contact with partner, vocalization, and gesture). Figure 6.1 provides a schematic overview of three PMT trials.

Table 6.1 Task analysis for building social routines

Given a child and professional are in a playroom
1. Child initiates a motor or vocal action
2. Professional imitates action of the child
3. Perform step 1 and 2 until a pattern of turn taking actions has been established
4. Professional ads an unexpected action into the routine
5. Professional waits for child to show interest by laughing or looking
6. Professional repeats the action of step 4
7. Child shows more interest
8. Perform step 6 and 7 until child imitates a part of the action
9. Professional completes the action

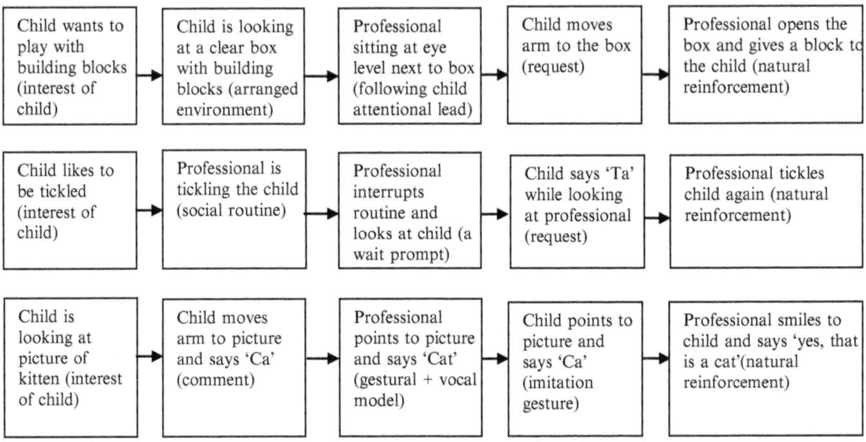

Fig. 6.1 Schematic overview of three PMT trials

Review of Intervention Research

To review the intervention research on PMT, three search strategies were used. First, literature searches of four electronic databases (MedLine, Psychinfo, Eric, and Google Scholar) were conducted using the keywords "prelinguistic milieu teaching". These searches resulted in 8, 15, 13, and 354 references, respectively. Studies identified through the database search were screened against inclusion criteria. Reference list and, finally, cited reference searches were conducted for selected studies. All empirical studies that evaluated the effectiveness of PMT and were published in English in a peer-reviewed journal before June 2014 were selected and

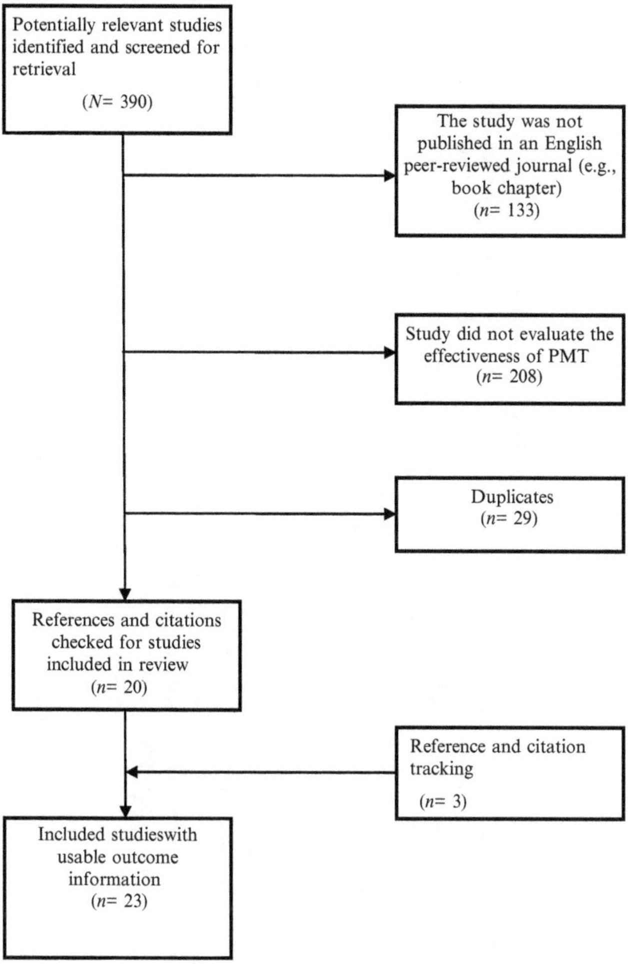

Fig. 6.2 Study identification, screening and selection

reviewed. Figure 6.2 gives an overview of the selection process. Twenty-three studies were included in the review (see Table 6.2).

Twenty studies were retrieved by database search, and reference and citation-tracking resulted in three additional studies. Eight studies employed a multiple baseline design (Brady & Bashinski, 2008; Franco et al., 2013; McCathren, 2000, 2010; Ogletree et al., 2012; Warren et al., 1993; Yoder et al., 1994; Yoder et al., 1995). Fourteen studies used a randomized group design of which nine compared PMT to another intervention, specifically the Picture Exchange Communication System (PECS; McDuffie et al., 2012; Yoder & Lieberman, 2010; Yoder & Stone, 2006a, 2006b) and Responsive Small Group (RSG) treatment (Yoder & Warren, 1998, 1999a, 1999b, 2001a, 2001b). In addition, comparisons between a high and low intensity PMT group were made (Fey et al., 2013; Yoder et al., 2014). Fey et al.

Table 6.2 Summary of included studies

Study	Design	Sample	Intervention	Outcomes
Brady and Bashinski (2008)	Multiple baseline design across participants.	Nine children between 3 and 7 years old with disabilities (ID, 6/9 children with moderate physical/motor challenges) with (a) adequate upper extremity mobility, (b) <3 symbolic communication acts, (c) complex communication needs, and (d) concurrent vision and hearing losses.	Three to four 30–60 min sessions a week for 2.5–8 months. An adapted version of PMT was used (e.g., activities that required vision or hearing were minimized, vestibular and tactile activities were emphasized, more physical and tactile prompts, other means than directed eye gaze).	Rates of initiated, intentional communication increased in all participants during the course of the intervention and each participant acquired new forms of natural gestures.
Fey et al. (2006)	A randomized group experiment comparing RPMT with a control group receiving no treatment.	51 children with ID (26 DS) with (a) a CA between 24 and 33 months, (b) a MDI < 70, (c) <10 spoken words/signs, (d) low risk of autism, (e) no hearing or visual impairment, and (f) adequate upper body motor skills.	Four 20 min sessions PMT per week by a trained therapist in the home and/or daycare center. In addition, the parents received 8 h sessions of responsive education. After 17–74 sessions of PMT 9 children (3 DS) moved to a word-oriented MT-program ($n = 25$).	After 6 months of intervention, the RPMT group produced more communicative acts than the no treatment group. No effects on outcomes due to the presence or absence of DS were found.

Fey, Yoder, Warren, and Bredin-Oja (2013)	A randomized group experiment comparing a low intensity group with a high intensity group.	64 children with intellectual and communication delay (35 DS; 4 premature; 1 seizures disorder; 1 cerebral palsy; 1 Beck-with-Wiedeman; 1 Shwachman-Diamond; 1 Dandy Walker; 1 Cornelia de Lange, 1 mitochondrial disorder, 1 chromosome 8; 1 septo-optic dysplasia) with (a) a CA between 18 and 27 months, (b) a MDI between 55 and 75 (one child with 80), (c) <20 expressive words or signs, (d) low risks of autism, (e) no hearing or visual impairment, (f) sufficient motor skills, and (g) English as primary language spoken in the home.	Treatment was conducted in the child's home or daycare center and comprised of nine sessions of responsivity education and PMT or milieu teaching. All, but one, children started with PMT. Three children moved from PMT to MT after 7, 23, or 32 sessions respectively. Over 9 months of treatment the low intensity group (n = 31) received one session of 60 min per week, while the high intensity group (n = 33) received five sessions of 60 min.	Across 9 months, the participants made growth related to the rate of behavior regulators, declaratives, intentional communication, and different words used and the number of words understood and spoken. There was no significant difference between the high and low intensity group, but there were moderate to large interactions between pre-treatment object interest and intensity level. Children who showed more object interest benefited more from the high than from the low intensity treatment on lexical measures.
Franco, David, and David (2013)	A multiple baseline design across participants.	Six nonverbal children with autism with (a) a CA between 5 and 8-years old and (b) few consistent interactions with others.	Fourteen PMT sessions implemented in the child's home by trained therapists.	All of the children showed an increase in the number of communicative interactions during play routines and their overall rate of initiated intentional communication.
McCathren (2000)	Multiple baseline design across behavior for both teacher and child.	A boy with severe communication and cognitive delays with a) a CA of 3.5 years old, b) a MDI < 50, and c) non-verbal.	Teacher implemented PMT during ongoing daily activities of a special education preschool classroom.	The teacher was able to implement PMT. Increases in the child's intentional communication, eye contact, vocalizations with consonants and conventional gestures were seen. In addition, progress in symbolic communication and symbolic play was seen.
McCathren (2010)	Multiple baseline design across adult behavior.	A mother with a tested IQ of 68 and her daughter with (a) a CA of 12 months, (b) a MDI of 62, and (c) no spoken or understood words.	Two sessions per week in which the researcher instructed the mother to implement PMT skills in her daughter.	The mother was able to implement PMT. The daughter's intentional communication increased.

(continued)

Table 6.2 (continued)

Study	Design	Sample	Intervention	Outcomes
McDuffie, Lieberman, and Yoder (2012)	A randomized group experiment comparing RPMT with PECS.	32 children with ASD (29 autism; 3 PDD-NOS) with (a) a CA between 18 and 60 months, (b) <10 expressive words, (c) no hearing impairment, (d) no sensory/motor impairments, and (e) English spoken in the home.	Three times a week RPMT (n=16) or PECS (n=16) of 20 min for 6 months implemented by trained therapists. The parent component of the RPMT condition involved teaching parents to use play routines to prompt and reinforce communication behaviors outside of the treatment setting. During PECS, parents observed the therapy sessions.	After RPMT, children showed greater increases in object interest than after PECS.
McDuffie and Yoder (2010)	Longitudinal correlation design.	32 children with ASD (29 autism; 3 PDD-NOS) with (a) a CA between 18 and 60 months, (b) <10 expressive words, (c) no hearing impairment, (d) no sensory/motor impairments, and (e) English spoken in the home.	Three times a week RPMT (n=16) or PECS (n=16) of 20 min for 6 months implemented by trained therapists. The parent component of the RPMT condition involved teaching parents to use play routines to prompt and reinforce communication behaviors outside of the treatment setting. During PECS, parents observed the therapy sessions.	Interventions did not moderate the predictive association between the parent variables and later spoken language. Parent verbal utterances that follow into the child's current focus of attention or respond to child verbal communicative acts may facilitate the process of early vocabulary acquisition by migiating the need for children with ASD to use attention following as a word learning strategy.

Ogletree, Davis, Hambrecht, and Wooten Philips (2012)	A multiple baseline design across four items.	7-year-old non-verbal boy with autistic disorder.	2 or 3 sessions of 30–45 min per week for 7 weeks of PMT to promote photograph exchange.	Although performance during intervention was variable, PMT was effective in promoting unprompted photograph exchange in three of four items trained.
Warren et al. (2008)	A randomized group experiment comparing RPMT with control group, receiving no prior PMT treatment.	51 children with ID (26 DS) with (a) a CA between 24 and 33 months, (b) a MDI < 70, (c) <10 spoken words/signs, (d) low risk of autism, (e) no hearing or visual impairment, and (f) adequate upper body motor skills.	During the 6 months immediately following implementation of RPMT (Fey et al., 2006) no project-based intervention was provided. However, after these 6 months, in both groups the children received one 45 min session of PMT per week and the parents six sessions of Responsive Education over the course of 6 months.	No long-term benefits of RPMT were detected 6 or 12 months after the conclusion of RPMT as conducted by Fey et al. (2006).
Warren, Yoder, Gazdag, Kim, and Jones (1993)	Multiple baseline design across training targets in experiment 1; Multiple baseline design across participants in experiment 2.	Experiment 1: A boy with DS of 20 months old Experiment 2: 4 children with developmental delay (1 DS, 1 micorcephaly, 1 agenesis of corpus collosum) with (a) a CA of 23–30 months, (b) a MA between 8 and 13 months, and (c) a MDI < 59.	Four staff implemented PMT sessions of 25 min each per week. In experiment 2, 37–61 sessions were provided.	Experiment 1 showed an increase in frequency of requesting, vocal imitation, and commenting. Experiment 2 showed increases in requesting for all participants; 1 child showed increases in commenting (not addressed in the other children). All participants demonstrated generalization from trainer to teacher and across settings, materials, and interaction style.

(continued)

Table 6.2 (continued)

Study	Design	Sample	Intervention	Outcomes
Yoder and Lieberman (2010)	A randomized group experiment comparing RPMT with PECS.	36 children with ASD (33 autism; 3 PDD-NOS) with (a) a CA between 18 and 60 months, (b) <10 expressive words, (c) no hearing impairment, (d) no sensory/motor impairments, and (e) English as primary language spoken in the home.	Three 20-min staff implemented PMT or PECS sessions per week for 6 months in a university clinic. During PMT parents were supported in the use of responsive play and communication strategies ($n=17$). The parent component in PECS involved demonstration and discussion of strategies to promote PECS use outside treatment ($n=19$).	Children receiving PECS training increased the number picture exchanges more than children receiving RPMT in a generalized context.
Yoder and Stone (2006a)	A randomized group experiment comparing RPMT with PECS.	36 children with ASD (33 autism; 3 PDD-NOS) with (a) a CA between 18 and 60 months, (b) <10 expressive words, (c) no hearing impairment, (d) no sensory/motor impairments, and (e) English as primary language spoken in the home	Three 20-min staff implemented PMT or PECS sessions per week for 6 months in a university clinic. During PMT parents were supported in the use of responsive play and communication strategies ($n=17$). The parent component in PECS involved demonstration and discussion of strategies to promote PECS use outside treatment ($n=19$).	In both groups, an increase in spoken communication was seen. After controlling for pre-treatment differences between groups a moderate treatment effect size favoring PECS was seen. However, PECS benefited children with high object exploration, while RPMT benefited children with lower object exploration.

Yoder and Stone (2006b)	A randomized group experiment comparing RPMT with PECS.	36 children with ASD (33 autism; 3 PDD-NOS) with (a) a CA between 18 and 60 months, (b) <10 expressive words, (c) no hearing impairment, (d) no sensory/motor impairments, and (e) English as primary language spoken in the home.	Three 20-min staff implemented PMT of PECS sessions per week for 6 months in a university clinic. During PMT parents were supported in the use of responsive play and communication strategies ($n=17$). The parent component in PECS involved demonstration and discussion of strategies to promote PECS use outside treatment ($n=19$).	RPMT facilitated the frequency of generalized turn taking more than PECS. For children with at least some pre-treatment IJA skills more generalized IJA was seen after RPMT than after PECS. However, PECS facilitated more generalized requesting than RMPT in children with very little pre-treatment IJA skills.
Yoder and Warren (1998)	A randomized group experiment comparing PMT with RSG.	58 children (4 DS; 4 prematurity, 3 failure to thrive, 2 pervasive developmental disorder, 1 Macrocephaly, 1 Microcephaly, 1 Duane's syndrome, 1 neonatal meningitis, 1 FAS, 1 tuberous sclerosis) with (a) a CA between 17 and 36 months, (b) a MDI between 35 and 85, (c) <5 words, (d) no severe visual or hearing impairment, and (e) the ability to hold an object while rotating the torso.	Children received four sessions of 20 min PMT ($n=28$) or RSG ($n=30$) per week for 6 months.	Treatment effects varied as a function of maternal responsivity. If mothers were responsive to the children's responsive acts, children in the PMT group used more frequent intentional communication than the RSG group. If mothers were less responsive, they used more frequent intentional communication after RSG than after PMT.

(continued)

Table 6.2 (continued)

Study	Design	Sample	Intervention	Outcomes
Yoder and Warren (1999a)	A randomized group experiment comparing PMT with RSG.	58 children (4 DS; 4 prematurity, 3 failure to thrive, 2 pervasive developmental disorder, 1 Macrocephaly, 1 Microcephaly, 1 Duane's syndrome, 1 neonatal meningitis, 1 FAS, 1 tuberous sclerosis) with (a) a CA between 17 and 36 months, (b) a MDI between 35 and 85, (c) <5 words, (d) no severe visual or hearing impairment, and (e) the ability to hold an object while rotating the torso.	Children received four sessions of 20 min PMT ($n=28$) or RSG ($n=30$) per week for 6 months.	The relationship between intentional communication and later language was mediated by maternal responses. There was no evidence that treatment assignment influenced the relationships examined in the present study.
Yoder and Warren (1999b)	A randomized group experiment comparing PMT with RSG.	58 children (4 DS; 4 prematurity, 3 failure to thrive, 2 pervasive developmental disorder, 1 Macrocephaly, 1 Microcephaly, 1 Duane's syndrome, 1 neonatal meningitis, 1 FAS, 1 tuberous sclerosis) with (a) a CA between 17 and 36 months, (b) a MDI between 35 and 85, (c) <5 words, (d) no severe visual or hearing impairment, and (e) the ability to hold an object while rotating the torso.	Children received four sessions of 20 min PMT ($n=28$) or RSG ($n=30$) per week for 6 months.	PMT facilitated self-initiated proto-imperatives and proto-declaratives directly following intervention and 6 months later. In families with high responsivity to children's communication acts at pre-treatment, PMT facilitated post-treatment increases in generalized use of self-initiated pro-imperatives and self-initiated proto-declaratives. In families with low responsivity to children's communication acts, the RSG intervention facilitated post-treatment increases in generalized use of self-initiated proto-imperatives. Weaker evidence at the 6 month follow up suggested some effects of RSG on self-initiated proto-declaratives.

Yoder and Warren (2001a)	A randomized group experiment comparing PMT with RSG.	58 children (4 DS; 4 prematurity, 3 failure to thrive, 2 pervasive developmental disorder, 1 Macrocephaly, 1 Microcephaly, 1 Duane's syndrome, 1 neonatal meningitis, 1 FAS, 1 tuberous sclerosis) with (a) a CA between 17 and 36 months, (b) a MDI between 35 and 85, (c) <5 words, (d) no severe visual or hearing impairment, and (e) the ability to hold an object while rotating the torso.	Children received four sessions of 20 min PMT ($n=28$) or RSG ($n=30$) per week for 6 months.	Treatment effects on maternal responses varied by pre-treatment maternal education level. Post-treatment intentional communication to mother was, at least in part, responsible for the effect on post-treatment maternal responses.
Yoder and Warren (2001b)	A randomized group experiment comparing PMT with RSG.	58 children (4 DS; 4 prematurity, 3 failure to thrive, 2 pervasive developmental disorder, 1 Macrocephaly, 1 Microcephaly, 1 Duane's syndrome, 1 neonatal meningitis, 1 FAS, 1 tuberous sclerosis) with (a) a CA between 17 and 36 months, (b) a MDI between 35 and 85, (c) <5 words, (d) no severe visual or hearing impairment, and (e) the ability to hold an object while rotating the torso.	Children received four sessions of 20 min PMT ($n=28$) or RSG ($n=30$) per week for 6 months.	6 and 12 months after treatment ended, treatment effect on children's receptive and expressive language varied as a function of pre-treatment maternal responsivity and educational level. Children whose mothers scored relatively high on responsivity and amount of formal education at pre-treatment benefited most from PMT, while children whose mothers scored relatively low on responsivity and amount of formal education benefited most from RSG. A growing effect with time was seen on the moderated treatment effect on lexical density.

(continued)

Table 6.2 (continued)

Study	Design	Sample	Intervention	Outcomes
Yoder and Warren (2002)	A randomized group experiment comparing RPMT with a control group receiving early intervention.	39 children with ID (17 DS; 2 Williams syndrome, 1 mild cerebral palsy, 1 encephalitis, 1 autism) with (a) a mean CA of 22 months, (b) a MDI < 70, (c) <10 words, and (d) no auditory impairment.	The RPMT group received 12 sessions of responsive education for parents combined with 3–4 sessions of 20 min PMT per week for 6 months (on average 71 sessions), while the control group received early intervention services from community providers.	RPMT facilitated parental responsivity. Although no main effect of RPMT was found, RPMT did accelerate growth in frequency of child initiated comments and requests and lexical density in particular subgroups of children. The effect of RPMT on growth rate of the child-initiated comments varied by pre-treatment child initiated comments, while the growth rate of requests varied by the presence or absence of DS. The effect on the growth of productive language varied by pre-treatment frequency of canonical vocal communication.
Yoder, Warren, and Hull (1995)	Multiple baseline design across participants.	8 children with developmental disabilities (3 DD, 3 DS, 1 microcephaly, 1 agenesis of the corpus callosum) with (a) a CA between 21 and 30 months, (b) a MA between 8 and 17 months, (c) a MDI below 59, (d) no auditory/visual impairment, and (e) no significant behavioral problems.	Three to four 20 min staff implemented PMT sessions per week (see Yoder, Warren, Kim, & Gazdag, 1994; Warren et al., 1993).	Pre-treatment play levels predict rate of change in prelinguistic intentional requesting during PMT in children with developmental disabilities.
Yoder et al. (1994)	Multiple baseline design across participants.	Four children with developmental disabilities (2 DS, 1 prematurity with DD, 1 DD) with (a) a CA between 21 and 27 months, (b) a MA between 10 and 17 months, (c) a MDI < 58, (d) absence of speech, and (e) delayed production of intentional requesting.	35–61 sessions of 25 min each (4 per week) implemented by two experienced trainers (university-based).	Increases in requesting for all 4 participants. This generalized to sessions with the children's mothers. Mothers were more likely to linguistically map their children's prelinguistic communication after PMT than before PMT. They were more likely to map intentional communication than pre intentional communication.

Yoder, Woynaroski, Fey, and Warren (2014)	A randomized group experiment comparing a low intensity group with a high intensity group.	64 children with intellectual and communication delay (35 DS; 4 prematurity; 1 seizure disorder; 1 cerebral palsy; 1 Beck-with-Wiedeman; 1 Shwachman-Diamond; 1 Dandy Walker; 1 Cornelia de Lange, 1 mitochondrial disorder, 1 chromosome 8; 1 septo-optic dysplasia) with (a) a CA between 18 and 27 months, (b) a MDI between 55 and 75 (one child with 80), (c) <20 expressive words or signs, (d) low risks of autism, (e) no hearing or visual impairment, (f) sufficient motor skills, and (g) English as primary language spoken in the home.	Treatment was conducted in the child's home or daycare center and comprised of nine sessions of responsivity education and PMT or milieu teaching. All, but one, children started with PMT. Three children moved from PMT to MT after 7, 23, or 32 sessions respectively.	Children without DS had more growth in spoken vocabulary than the DS group. When IQ was controlled for high intensity PMT led to greater spoken vocabulary growth in children with DS than low intensity PMT. Object interest moderated treatment effects.
			Over 9 months of treatment the low intensity group (n = 31) received one session of 60 min per week, while the high intensity group (n = 33) received five sessions of 60 min.	

Codes: CA: Chronological Age in months at onset of treatment; DS: Down Syndrome; ID: Intellectual Disability; IJA: initiating joint attention; MDI: Mental Development Index based on the Bayley Scales of Infant Development; MA: mental age; MT: milieu teaching; PECS: Picture Exchange Communication System; a communication intervention to teach children to communicate by giving a picture of a desired object to a recipient; PMT: prelinguistic milieu teaching; RPMT: combination of 6–12 sessions of responsiveness education and basic procedures of PMT; RSG: responsive small group; treatment in a small group of one teacher and three children who engaged in parallel play

(2006), Yoder and Warren (2002), and Warren et al. (2008) used a non-treatment (or treatment as usual) comparison group. Finally, one study utilized a longitudinal correlation design (McDuffie & Yoder, 2010).

Several studies used the same participants, resulting in 11 independent samples. Yoder et al. (1995) re-analyzed the participants from the Warren et al. (1993) and Yoder et al. (1994) studies. Yoder and Stone (2006a, 2006b) used the same participants and participants from Yoder and Lieberman (2010) were drawn from Yoder and Stone (2006a, 2006b). In addition, Yoder et al. (2014) is a reanalysis of Fey et al. (2013), while Warren et al. (2008) conducted a follow-up study of the participants from Fey et al. (2006). Yoder and Warren (1999b) is a reanalysis and extension of Yoder and Warren (1998) and these data are also used in Yoder and Warren (1999a), (2001a), and (2001b). Finally, McDuffie et al. (2012) and McDuffie and Yoder (2010) analyzed data on the same participants. Table 6.2 shows the demographic characteristics of the participants.

Participants

Each study included 1–64 participants who were 1 year, 5 months to 8 years old with most children under 3 years of age. Most participants were diagnosed with a developmental delay and etiologies, amongst others, were Down syndrome, prematurity, failure to thrive, autism spectrum disorder (ASD), cerebral palsy, Angelman's syndrome, Fragile X, and Fetal Alcohol Syndrome.

While most studies focused on nonverbal children between 2 and 5 years old and functioning at the 9–15 month communication level (Fey et al., 2006; Yoder & Stone, 2006a, 2006b; Yoder & Warren, 1998, 1999a, 1999b, 2001a, 2001b, 2002), some studies have been implemented in specific diagnostic groups, including Down syndrome (Fey et al., 2006; Warren et al., 2008), ASD (McDuffie et al., 2012) and children with complex communication needs (i.e., intellectual disability and concurrent vision and hearing loss; Brady & Bashinski, 2008).

Treatment

In general, participants received three to four PMT sessions of 20–60 min per week (e.g., McDuffie, Lieberman & Yoder, 2012; Ogletree et al., 2012; Yoder & Lieberman, 2010; Yoder & Stone, 2006a, 2006b; Yoder & Warren, 1998, 1999a, 1999b, 2001a, 2001b). However, the low intensity group and high intensity group in Fey et al. (2013) and Yoder et al. (2014) received 1 h or 5 h PMT per week, respectively. Warren et al. (2008) provided only 45 min of PMT per week. Their goal was to provide a follow-up training to participants who ended PMT treatment 6 months earlier. Treatment sessions lasted 7 weeks (Ogletree et al., 2012) to 9 months (Yoder et al., 2014).

Usually, treatment was conducted in the child's home, as well as in a daycare center (e.g., Yoder & Warren, 2002) and at a university clinic (e.g., Yoder & Stone, 2006a, 2006b; Yoder et al., 1994). Most PMT sessions were implemented by a trained therapist (e.g., Fey et al., 2006; Yoder & Stone, 2006a, 2006b). Studies of McCathren (2000, 2010) showed, however, that parents and teachers were also able to implement PMT during ongoing interactions with the child.

Some studies made slight adaptations to the treatment to address the specific needs of the target group (Brady & Bashinski, 2008). PMT was also used to teach specific forms of prelinguistic communication, such as photograph exchange (Ogletree et al., 2012). Yoder and Warren (1998, 1999a, 2001a) showed that high rates of parent responsivity were associated with better response to PMT by the child. Several studies (e.g., Fey et al., 2006, 2013; Yoder & Warren, 2002; Yoder et al., 2014) used a combination of 6–12 sessions of responsiveness education and basic procedures of PMT, which was referred to as RPMT.

Outcomes

Outcome variables varied across studies and included: (a) intentional communication (Brady & Bashinski, 2008; Franco et al., 2013; McCathren, 2000; McCathren, 2010; Yoder et al., 1994, 1995), (b) play skills (McCathren, 2000), (c) number of interactions (Franco et al., 2013), (d) exchange of photographs (Ogletree et al., 2012), and (e) object interest (McDuffie et al., 2012).

Several studies showed improvement in intentional communication during the intervention (Brady & Bashinski, 2008; Franco et al., 2013; McCathren, 2000; McCathren, 2010; Yoder et al., 1994, 1995). Improvement in symbolic communication (McCathren, 2000), symbolic play (McCathren, 2000), number of interactions during play routines (Franco et al., 2013), and exchange of photographs (Ogletree et al., 2012) were seen following PMT intervention.

Three studies (Fey et al., 2006; Warren et al., 2008; Yoder & Warren, 2002) compared PMT intervention to a control group receiving regular early intervention services from community providers. Yoder and Warren (2002) found that RPMT increased the frequency of child initiated comments and requests as well as lexical density in some children, but not in others. In contrast, Fey et al. (2006) found a main effect of RPMT; the RMPT group produced more communicative acts than the no treatment group. However, 6 and 12 months after termination of the RPMT no benefits of the intervention were detected (Warren et al., 2008).

Next, children receiving RPMT were compared to children receiving the same intensity of PECS or RSG. In general, children in the RPMT group did not outperform children who received RSG or PECS. However, treatment effects varied as a function of maternal responsivity or other pre-treatment variables, such as object interest or joint attention of the child. For example, children benefited more from PMT than from RSG if mothers were more responsive to their child, while children of less responsive mothers had better outcomes after RSG than after PMT (Yoder &

Warren, 1998, 1999b, 2001b). Yoder and Stone (2006a) found an increase in spoken communication in children with ASD who received RPMT or PECS. However, children with lower object exploration profited more from RPMT, while children with higher object exploration benefited more from PECS. For children who initiated joint attention before treatment, more generalized initiation of joint attention was seen after RPMT than after PECS. However, PECS facilitated more generalized requests than RMPT in children who showed very little initiating of joint attention during pre-treatment. PECS training resulted in a larger increase in picture exchanges than RPMT (Yoder & Lieberman, 2010), while after RPMT children displayed more generalized turn taking (Yoder & Stone, 2006b) and more interest in objects (McDuffie et al., 2012).

High intensity PMT (5 h per week) was compared to low intensity PMT (1 h per week). Overall, no significant differences between the high and low intensity group were found and all children made significant improvement related to intentional communication, different words used, and number of words understood and spoken. However, when IQ was controlled for, high intensity PMT led to greater spoken vocabulary growth in children with Down syndrome than low intensity PMT and children who showed more object interest benefited more from the high intensity than from the low intensity treatment on lexical measures (Fey et al., 2013; Yoder et al., 2014).

Although most studies were conducted with nonverbal children with global developmental delay, PMT was also effective in increasing object interest (McDuffie et al., 2012), communicative interactions (Franco et al., 2013), spoken communication (Yoder & Stone, 2006a), turn-taking (Yoder & Stone, 2006b), and photograph/picture exchange (Ogletree et al., 2012; Yoder & Lieberman, 2010) in children with ASD. Results on children with Down syndrome were mixed. In contrast to Yoder and Warren (2002) who found that Down syndrome was associated with a smaller growth rate on requests, others found no effects on child outcomes due to the presence or absence of Down syndrome (Fey et al., 2006; Warren et al., 1993).

Summary

PMT is a promising approach for increasing the communication of children with developmental disabilities. The first studies published used multiple baseline designs, which reported gains in requesting skills for all participants, while later studies compared PMT to other interventions such as PECS and RSG (Yoder & Warren, 1998, 1999a, 1999b, 2001a, 2001b). As several studies found that most progress was seen in children with responsive parents, 'responsivity education' was added to the PMT, resulting in RPMT. Studies comparing (R)PMT to PECS or RSG found that RPMT is effective in some children with developmental disabilities, but ineffective with others. RPMT seems most appropriate for children whose parents have high responsivity to their child's communication and in children who showed certain pre-treatment characteristics, such as lower object exploration (Yoder & Warren, 2001a, 2001b; Yoder & Stone, 2006a).

Suggestions for Future Research

Although the above studies show promising outcomes of PMT, results should be interpreted with caution given some methodological limitations (e.g., relatively small sample sizes, quasi experimental designs, lack of equivalent groups, lack of fidelity measures). In addition, participants of the studies were limited in terms of age ranges, disability categories, and level of severity of impairment. The degree to which differences between pre-treatment and post-treatment variables are clinically significant remains unclear. Furthermore, future research should address long term (maintenance) effects and assess the extent to which additional treatment is necessary to maintain treatment gains.

Due to unique child and family variables, no single intervention is appropriate for all children and outcome varies between and within studies. Therefore, future research should investigate how specific child, family, target behavior, and treatment variables influence treatment effectiveness. This may result in more effective individualized intervention protocols as well as approaches and guidelines regarding the intensity, duration, content, and quality of PMT necessary to achieve optimal outcome for different types of children.

Future research might evaluate what strategies should be adopted to further improve outcomes for non-responders. These children may need more intense PMT or perhaps technically very precise teaching to accelerate their development. Several studies showed that treatment effects varied as a function several pre-treatment child variables such as object interest and joint attention of the child. Perhaps children who do not respond to PMT enter PMT with key deficits that hinder the effectiveness and that are not readily remediable with routine PMT. Therefore, future studies should not only investigate which treatment variables predict response to treatment, but also if it is beneficial to address specific key deficits before commencing PMT.

In our review, participants were under 5 years old (with a vast majority under 3 years of age) and had mild to moderate intellectual disabilities. However, in clinical settings many children start treatment later than 3 years of age and a subset of children have more severe disabilities. Regardless of the type of treatment used, the prognosis for children with an higher IQ is better and lower chronological age at intake seems to be associated with better outcomes (Dietz, Swinkels, Buitelaar, van Daalen, & van Engeland, 2007; Granpeesheh, Dixon, Tarbox, Kaplan, & Wilke, 2009). Therefore, future studies should investigate the extent to which PMT is effective in older populations with more severe levels of developmental disability as this population is most likely to remain at the prelinguistic communication level over prolonged periods (Mundy & Crowson, 1997). Further research should also address the needs and outcomes of children with differing types of developmental disabilities. Studies should investigate how PMT programs can be tailored to accelerate language learning in children with distinctive profiles.

Although parents were involved in some studies by completing several sessions of responsivity education, in most studies PMT was implemented by professionals. When parents are instructed in PMT and are responsible for delivering part of the treatment, they might be able to assist in generalization and are better equipped to use the many opportunities they have to practice skills throughout their natural interaction with their child. It is likely that this changes the general interaction of the parents with their child and consequently has a collateral effect on the child's development because he/she is instructed during more waking hours. Therefore, future studies should investigate whether parents are able to implement PMT with their children and the outcome of these children should be compared to the outcome of the children who received PMT implemented by professionals.

Implications for Practitioners and Families

PMT can be beneficial for young children who function at the prelinguistic level of communication. It is important for practitioners to check that children have the skills that previous research suggests predicts best outcomes from PMT. For example, it is important to assess the child's object interest. As described in section "Review of Intervention Research", children with less object interest profit more from RPMT than from PECS, while children with higher object interest profit more from PECS than from RPMT. Therefore, PECS might be more suitable than RPMT for children with higher object interest (Yoder & Stone, 2006a).

Based on the research reviewed, PMT sessions can be provided by a practitioner on at least a weekly basis. With the exception of children with Down syndrome (where high intensity treatment of 5 h per week did lead to increased spoken vocabulary growth), the intensity of PMT does not appear to be related to the effectiveness of the treatment (Fey et al., 2013; Yoder et al., 2014).

Involving parents using responsivity education (RE) can be beneficial for children with developmental disabilities and with parents who are highly responsive to their child's communication. Because implementing the techniques at home can be difficult and even stressful for some parents, it is important to assess a parent's responsivity to the child's intentional communication. Parents who are less responsive to their child's communication could need more training sessions in RE with (video) modeling and feedback or their children could be referred to other interventions. For example, Yoder and Warren (1998, 1999b, 2001b) showed that children of less responsive mothers had better outcome after RSG than after PMT. Based on the literature reviewed, it might be suggested that a practitioner should monitor the progress of a child. After a child needs less prompting and displays approximately two communication acts per minute a child is ready for another language intervention.

References

Acredolo, L., & Goodwyn, S. (1988). Symbolic gesturing in normal infants. *Child Development, 59*, 450–466.

Allen, K. D., & Cowan, R. J. (2008). Naturalistic teaching procedures. In J. K. Luiselli, D. C. Russo, W. P. Christian, & S. M. Wilczynski (Eds.), *Effective practices for children with autism.*

Educational and behavioral support interventions that work (pp. 213–240). New York, NY: Oxford University Press.

Brady, N., & Bashinski, S. (2008). Increasing communication in children with concurrent vision and hearing loss. *American Journal of Speech and Language Pathology, 33*, 59–71.

Brady, N. C., Marquis, J., Fleming, K., & McLean, L. (2004). Prelinguistic predictors of language growth in children with developmental disabilities. *Journal of Speech, Language, and Hearing Research, 47*, 663–677.

Calandrella, A. M., & Wilcox, M. J. (2000). Predicting language outcomes for young prelinguistic children with developmental delay. *Journal of Speech, Language, and Hearing Research, 43*, 1061–1071.

Carter, M., & Iacono, T. (2002). Professional judgments of the intentionality of communicative acts. *Augmentative and Alternative Communication, 18*, 177–191.

Corkum, V., & Moore, C. (1995). Development of joint visual attention in infants. In C. Moore & P. Dunham (Eds.), *Joint attention: Its origins and role in development* (pp. 61–84). Hillsdale, NJ: Lawrence Erlbaum Associates.

Cress, C. J., & Marvin, C. A. (2003). Common questions about AAC services in early intervention. *Augmentative and Alternative Communication, 19*, 254–272.

Dietz, C., Swinkels, S. H., Buitelaar, J. K., van Daalen, E., & van Engeland, H. (2007). Stability and change of IQ scores in preschool children diagnosed with autistic spectrum disorder. *European Child Adolescent Psychiatry, 16*, 405–410.

Fey, M. E., Warren, S. F., Brady, N., Finestack, L. H., Bredin-Oja, S. L., Fairchild, M., … Yoder, P. J. (2006). Early effects of responsivity education/Prelinguistic milieu teaching for children with developmental delays and their parents. *Journal of Speech and Hearing Research, 49*, 526–547.

Fey, M. E., Yoder, P. J., Warren, S. F., & Bredin-Oja, S. L. (2013). Is more better? Milieu communication teaching in toddlers with intellectual disabilities. *Journal of Speech, Language, and Hearing Research, 56*, 679–693.

Franco, J. H., David, B. L., & David, J. L. (2013). Increasing social interaction using prelinguistic milieu teaching with nonverbal school age children with autism. *American Journal of Speech and Language Pathology, 22*, 489–502.

Granpeesheh, D., Dixon, D. R., Tarbox, J., Kaplan, A. M., & Wilke, A. E. (2009). The effects of age and treatment intensity on behavioral intervention outcomes for children with autism spectrum disorders. *Research in Autism Spectrum Disorders, 3*, 1014–1022.

Hancock, T. B., & Kaiser, A. P. (2006). Enhanced milieu teaching. In R. J. McCauley & M. E. Fey (Eds.), *Treatment of language disorders in children* (pp. 203–236). Baltimore, MD: Brookes.

Leung, E. H., & Rheingold, H. L. (1981). Development of pointing as social gesture. *Developmental Psychology, 17*, 215–220.

McCathren, R. B. (2000). Teacher-implemented prelinguistic communication intervention. *Focus on Autism and Other Developmental Disabilities, 15*, 21–29.

McCathren, R. B. (2010). Parent-implemented prelinguistic milieu teaching with a high risk dyad. *Communication Disorders Quarterly, 31*, 243–252.

McDuffie, A. S., Lieberman, R. G., & Yoder, P. J. (2012). Object interest in autism spectrum disorders: A treatment comparison. *Autism, 1*, 1–10.

McDuffie, A., & Yoder, P. (2010). Types of parent verbal responsiveness that predict language in young children with autism spectrum disorder. *Journal of Speech, Language, and Hearing Research, 53*, 1026–1039.

Mundy, P., & Crowson, M. (1997). Joint attention and early social communication: Implications for research on intervention with autism. *Journal of Autism and Developmental Disorders, 27*, 653–676.

Mundy, P., & Willoughby, J. (1998). Nonverbal communication, affect, and socio-emotional development. In A. M. Wetherby, S. F. Warren, J. Reichle, & M. E. Fey (Eds.), *Communication and language intervention series: Volume 7. Transitions in prelinguistic communication* (pp. 111–133). Baltimore, MD: Brookes.

Ogletree, B. T., Davis, P., Hambrecht, G., & Wooten Philips, E. (2012). Using Milieu Training to promote photograph exchange for a young child with autism. *Focus on Autism and Other Developmental Disabilities, 27*, 93–101.

Sameroff, A. J. (2009). *The transactional model of development: How children and contexts shape each other*. Washington, DC: American Psychological Association.

Tomasello, M. (1995). Joint attention as social cognition. In C. Moore & P. Dunham (Eds.), *Joint attention* (pp. 103–130). Hillsdale, NJ: Lawrence Erlbaum.

Tomasello, M. (1999). *The cultural origins of human cognition*. Cambridge, MA: Harvard University Press.

Vihman, M. M. (1996). *Phonological development: The origins of language in the child. Applied language studies*. Malden, MA: Blackwell Publishing.

Vygotsky, L. S. (1978). *Mind and society*. Cambridge, MA: Harvard University Press.

Warren, S. F., Bredin-Oja, S. L., Fairchild, M., Finestack, L. H., Fey, M. E., & Brady, N. C. (2006). Responsivity education/prelinguistic milieu teaching. In R. J. McCauley & M. E. Fey (Eds.), *Treatment of language disorders in children* (pp. 47–75). Baltimore, MD: Paul H. Brookes.

Warren, S. F., Fey, M. E., Finestack, L. H., Brady, N. C., Bredin-Oja, S. L., & Fleming, K. K. (2008). A randomized trial of longitudinal effects of low-intensity responsivity education/Prelinguistic milieu teaching. *Journal of Speech, Language, and Hearing Research, 51*, 451–470.

Warren, S. F., Yoder, P. J., Gazdag, G. E., Kim, K., & Jones, H. A. (1993). Facilitating prelinguistic communication skills in young children with developmental delay. *Journal of Speech and Hearing Research, 36*, 83–97.

Watt, N., Wetherby, A., & Shumway, S. (2006). Prelinguistic predictors of language outcome at 3 years of age. *Journal of Speech, Language, and Hearing Research, 49*, 1224–1237.

Wilcox, M. J., Kouri, T. A., & Caswell, S. (1990). Partner sensitivity to communication behavior of young children with developmental disabilities. *Journal of Speech and Hearing Disorders, 55*, 679–693.

Yoder, P. J., & Lieberman, R. G. (2010). Brief report: Randomized test of the efficacy of picture exchange communication system on highly generalized picture exchanges in children with ASD. *Journal of Autism and Developmental Disorders, 40*, 629–632.

Yoder, P. J., & Munson, L. J. (1995). The social correlates of coordinated attention to adult and objects in mother-infant interaction. *First Language, 15*, 219–230.

Yoder, P. J., & Stone, W. L. (2006a). A randomized comparison of the effect of two prelinguistic communication intervention on the acquisition of spoken communication in preschoolers with ASD. *Journal of Speech, Language, and Hearing Research, 49*, 698–711.

Yoder, P. J., & Stone, W. L. (2006b). Randomized comparison of two communication intervention for preschoolers with autism spectrum disorders. *Journal of Consulting and Clinical Psychology, 74*, 426–435.

Yoder, P. J., & Warren, S. F. (1998). Maternal responsivity predicts the prelinguistic communication intervention that facilitates generalized intentional communication. *Journal of Speech, Language, and Hearing Research, 41*, 1207–1219.

Yoder, P. J., & Warren, S. F. (1999a). Maternal responsivity mediates the relationship between prelinguistic intentional communication and later language. *Journal of Early Intervention, 22*, 126–136.

Yoder, P. J., & Warren, S. F. (1999b). Facilitating self-initiated proto-declaratives and proto-imperatives in prelinguistic children with developmental disabilities. *Journal of Early Intervention, 22*, 337–354.

Yoder, P. J., & Warren, S. F. (2001a). Intentional communication elicits language-facilitating maternal responses in dyads with children who have developmental disabilities. *American Journal on Mental Retardation, 106*, 327–335.

Yoder, P. J., & Warren, S. F. (2001b). Relative treatment effects of two prelinguistic communication interventions on language development in toddlers with developmental delays vary by maternal characteristics. *Journal of Speech, Language, and Hearing Research, 44*, 224–237.

Yoder, P. J., & Warren, S. F. (2002). Effects of prelinguistic milieu teaching and parent responsivity education on dyads involving children with intellectual disabilities. *Journal of Speech, Language, and Hearing Research, 45*, 1158–1174.

Yoder, P. J., & Warren, S. F. (2004). Early predictors of language in children with and without Down Syndrome. *American Journal on Mental Retardation, 109*, 285–300.

Yoder, P. J., Warren, S. F., Kim, K., & Gazdag, G. E. (1994). Facilitating prelinguistic communication skills in young children with developmental delays II: Systematic replication and extension. *Journal of Speech and Hearing Research, 37*, 841–851.

Yoder, P., Warren, S. F., McCathren, R., & Leew, S. (1998). Does adult responsivity to child behavior facilitate communication? In A. Wetherby, S. F. Warren, & J. Reichle (Eds.), *Communication and language intervention series: Volume 1. Causes and effects in communication and language intervention* (pp. 217–254). Baltimore, MD: Brookes.

Yoder, P. J., Warren, S. F., & Hull, L. (1995). Predicting children's response to prelinguistic communication intervention. *Journal of Early Intervention, 19*, 74–84.

Yoder, P., Woynaroski, T., Fey, M., & Warren, S. (2014). Effects of dose frequency of early communication intervention in young children with and without Down syndrome. *American Journal on Intellectual and Developmental Disabilities, 119*, 17–32.

Chapter 7
Enhanced Milieu Teaching

Terry B. Hancock, Katherine Ledbetter-Cho, Alexandria Howell, and Russell Lang

Introduction

Enhanced Milieu Teaching (EMT) is a behavioral language intervention that uses naturally occurring interactions to facilitate young children's language skills. EMT has been shown to be effective with a variety of children who are early language learners including toddlers with persistent language impairment (Roberts & Kaiser, 2012; Roberts, Kaiser, Wolfe, Bryant, & Spidalieri, 2014), preschoolers from low-income families who are high risk for developing language issues (Hancock, Kaiser, & Delaney, 2002; Peterson, Carta, & Greenwood, 2005), children with Down syndrome (Kaiser & Roberts, 2013; Wright, Kaiser, Reikowsky, & Roberts, 2013), children with cleft palate (Scherer & Kaiser, 2007; Scherer & Kaiser, 2010) and children who exhibit language delays (Hemmeter & Kaiser, 1994; Kaiser & Hester, 1994). However, more studies have been published on the efficacy of EMT with children with autism than any other diagnosis (Hancock & Kaiser, 2002, 2009, 2012; Kaiser, Hancock, & Nietfeld, 2000, Kasari et al., 2014; Kaiser & Roberts, 2013; Nunes & Hanline, 2007; Olive et al., 2007).

Although EMT has been effectively implemented by therapists and teachers (Hancock & Kaiser, 2002; Kaiser & Hester, 1994; Kasari et al., 2014; Olive et al., 2007; Wright et al., 2013) the majority of the research on EMT has investigated the effects of the intervention when implemented by parents with their children (Hancock et al., 2002; Hancock, Lang & Ledbetter-Cho, in progress; Hemmeter &

T.B. Hancock (✉) • K. Ledbetter-Cho • A. Howell • R. Lang
Texas State University Clinic for Autism Research Evaluation and Support, 601 University Dr., San Marcos, TX 78666, USA
e-mail: terryhancock@txstate.edu

R. Lang et al. (eds.), *Early Intervention for Young Children with Autism Spectrum Disorder*, Evidence-Based Practices in Behavioral Health,
DOI 10.1007/978-3-319-30925-5_7

Kaiser, 1994; Kaiser & Hancock, 2003; Kaiser, Hancock, & Hester, 1998; Kaiser et al., 2000; Kaiser, Hancock, & Trent, 2007; Kaiser & Roberts, 2013; Kasari et al., 2014; Nunes & Hanline, 2007; Peterson et al., 2005; Roberts et al., 2014). These studies provide evidence that parents can learn to implement EMT strategies with a high level of fidelity.

EMT includes three main areas of focus (i.e., connection, support and teaching). Connection strategies serve to facilitate a social connection between the adult and child and provide the foundation for conversational language learning (i.e., following the child's play/conversational lead, mirroring/mapping, matched turns, and environmental arrangement to promote connection). Support strategies focus on the development of children's language skills (i.e., language responsiveness and expansions). Teach strategies systematically teach children new language skills (i.e., language modeling, arranging the environment to promote requests and Milieu Teaching prompting procedures). EMT includes a number of evidenced-based strategies that parents can implement at the same criterion levels as trained therapists and teachers (Hancock & Kaiser, 2012; Hancock & Kaiser, 2009).

This chapter provides a detailed description of Enhanced Milieu Teaching beginning with the theoretical underpinnings of the intervention. Ten published studies investigating the effects of EMT are reviewed and the summaries of these research studies are included in Table 7.1. Next, each of the EMT strategies is described and clarifying examples are provided. Common issues when implementing EMT and possible solutions are discussed as considerations for practitioners and parents. Recommendations for effective EMT implementation are extrapolated from the overview of intervention research studies and future directions for EMT investigations are suggested to address areas in need of additional research.

Theoretical Support for EMT

One of the reasons that EMT may be such an effective language intervention is that it "cross-fertilizes" the key components of the two major language intervention approaches for children with autism: (a) naturalistic behavioral interventions, and (b) developmental social-pragmatic or relationship-based interventions (Ingersoll, 2010). Naturalistic behavioral interventions have been developed from applied behavior analysis and operant learning theory. Developmental interventions, on the other hand, are based on Piagetian developmental theory as well as the social-pragmatic language acquisition theory (Ingersoll, 2010). Tenets from each of these theoretical models were incorporated in the development and application of EMT. EMT strategies that connect the adult and child are derived from developmental theories of language based on observations of typical children and their parents. Social pragmatic interactionist theories have driven the EMT strategies that support language learning in children. Lastly, the EMT strategies that directly teach new or elaborated language forms are firmly based in learning theory and applied behavior analysis.

Table 7.1 Summary of published research studies on enhanced milieu teaching

Citation (in order of mention in Chapter)	Participants	Intervention procedures	Intervention outcomes
Hemmeter and Kaiser (1994)	*Children*: N=4 (3 males, 1 female); aged 25–49 months; with Down syndrome (N=1), with language delay and behavior problems (N=1), with PDD (N=1), and with cerebral palsy and seizure disorder (N=1); verbally imitative and had an expressive vocabulary of at least 5 words	*Intervention*: 45-min parent training sessions conducted twice per week for approximately 4 months; sessions conducted at a university-based research center; training sessions consisted of weekly home assignments, role-playing, modeling, coaching, and immediate and delayed feedback until the parent met criteria on environmental arrangement, followed by responsive interaction (feedback and modeling of the child's targets), and finally milieu teaching	*Spontaneous utterances*: increase for all 4 children; generalization to home and across communication partners
	Parents: N=4 (3 females, 1 male); education level: college degree—graduate degree	*Implementers*: NR for parent training; parents (EMT)	*Total use of targets*: increase for all 4 children; generalization to home and across communication partners
			Spontaneous use of targets: increase for all 4 children; all children generalized to home, 3 children generalized across communication partners
			Expressive communication: 3 children increased their scores
			Receptive communication: 2 children's scores increased; 1 child's score decreased
			MLU: no significant increase
			Environmental arrangement: all parents improved above baseline levels and met criterion; generalized to home setting
			Responsive feedback: all parents improved above baseline levels and met criterion; generalized to home setting

(continued)

Table 7.1 (continued)

Citation (in order of mention in Chapter)	Participants	Intervention procedures	Intervention outcomes
			Modeling targets: all parents improved above baseline levels and met criterion (decreasing trend for 2 parents observed); generalized to home setting
			Incidental teaching: all parents improved above baseline levels and met criterion; generalized to home setting
			MC: No. Gen: Yes. SV: Yes (parent and child enjoyment and parent satisfaction)
Kaiser and Hester (1994)	*Children*: N=6 (5 males, 1 female); aged 37–80 months; with developmental delays (N=2), with autistic-like symptoms (N=1), with autistic-like symptoms and developmental delays (N=1), with cerebral palsy and developmental delays (N=1), and with Down syndrome (N=1); verbally imitative and had an expressive vocabulary of 10 or more spontaneous words	*Intervention*: 15–20-min semi structured play activities conducted 4 days each week for a total of 35–47 intervention sessions; children with similar language goals were grouped into dyads; approximately half of the sessions were conducted in dyads and the other half were conducted in a one-to-one format; sessions conducted in various rooms in participant's school	*Total use of targets*: increase for all 6 children; 1 child maintained the increase during maintenance phase; decrease for 5 children during maintenance phase (but maintained above baseline levels)
	Parents: N=6 (5 mothers, 1 father); education level: some high school—college degree	*Implementers*: *EMT*-trained interventionists (N=3) (i.e., graduate students in special education who were receiving specialized training in early childhood education)	*Spontaneous use of targets*: increase for all 6 children; 2 children increased during maintenance phase; 4 children decreased during maintenance phase (but maintained above baseline levels)
	Peers: N=6 (4 males, 2 females); aged 42–89 months; with learning disabilities (N=3), with a language delay (N=1), and identified as environmentally at risk (N=1)		*Total utterances*: systematic increases for all 6 children; 4 children maintained increase during maintenance phase; 2 children decreased during maintenance phase (but maintained above baseline levels)

	Teachers: N=3 (3 females); experience: 7–18 years		*MLU*: modest increase for 5 children (sixth child showed increase during maintenance phase); increase for all 6 children above baseline levels during maintenance phase
			Diversity of words: increase for all 6 children; all 6 maintained increase during maintenance phase
			MC: Yes. Gen: Yes (evidence of generalization of some target behaviors across peers, teachers, and parents for all 6 children). SV: No
Hancock and Kaiser (2002)	*Children*: N=4 (3 males, 1 female); aged 35–54 months; with autism (N=2) and with PDD (N=2); verbally imitative and had an expressive vocabulary of at least 10 words	*Intervention*: 15-min sessions conducted twice per week for a total of 24 sessions; sessions conducted in a small playroom at a university-based clinic	*Total utterances*: increase for all 4 children; further increases at MC for 2 children; 2 children maintained at MC
		Implementers: trained interventionists (i.e., master's and doctoral-level students in special education or child psychology)	*Spontaneous utterances*: increase for 2 children; 1 child showed further increase at MC
			Total use of targets: increase for all 4 children; maintained at MC
			Spontaneous use of targets: increase for all 4 children, but minimal gains for 1 child; maintained at MC
			Diversity of words: increase for all 4 children; further increase for 3 children at MC
			MLU: increase for 3 participants
			Expressive communication: variable increases in score at MC
			Receptive communication: variable increases in score at MC

(continued)

Table 7.1 (continued)

Citation (in order of mention in Chapter)	Participants	Intervention procedures	Intervention outcomes
Kaiser et al. (2000)	*Children*: N=6 (6 males); aged 32–54 months; with autism (N=3), with PDD (N=2), and with Asperger's disorder (N=1); verbally imitative and had an expressive vocabulary of at least 10 spontaneous words	*Intervention*: 45-min parent training sessions conducted twice per week for a total of 24 sessions; sessions conducted in a small playroom at a university-based clinic; training sessions consisted of weekly home assignments, role-playing, modeling, and 15 min of practice and feedback with their child present; training sessions continued until the parent met criteria on environmental arrangement, followed by responsive interaction, and finally milieu teaching	MC: Yes. Gen: Yes (3 children generalized to home setting and with mother as communication partner). SV: Yes
			Spontaneous utterances: NR
	Parents: N=6 (6 mothers); aged 30–37 years; education level: some college education—graduate degree	*Implementers*: trained interventionists (N=2); with a PhD in special education (N=1) and a doctoral student in psychology (N=1) (parent training); parents (EMT)	*Total use of targets*: increase for all 6 children; all maintained at MC
			Spontaneous use of targets: increase for all 6 children; further increase for all 6 children at MC
			Diversity of words: 3 children increased during intervention; all 6 children increased at MC
			MLU: 3 children increased during intervention; all 6 children increased at MC
			Expressive communication: evidence of progress for 5 children
			Receptive communication: evidence of progress for 5 children
			Milieu teaching procedures: all parents showed systematic increases in accuracy; 5 parents met criteria; 5 parents maintained at MC
			Expansions: all parents increased above baseline levels; all maintained at MC
			Turn discrepancy: all parents improved from baseline; all maintained at MC

			Responsive feedback: all parents increased above baseline levels; all maintained at MC
			Pause errors: all parents improved from baseline; all maintained at MC
			Not following child's lead: all parents improved from baseline; all maintained at MC
			MC: Yes. Gen: Yes (for 5 children, to home setting; for 6 parents, to home setting). SV: Yes
Kaiser and Roberts (2013)	*Children*: N = 77 (57 males, 20 females); aged 30–54 months; with developmental delay (N = 43), with ASD (N = 16), and with Down syndrome (N = 18); with expressive vocabulary of at least 10 words and ability to verbally imitate at least 7 words; in 2 treatment groups: EMT with parent plus therapist (N = 39) or EMT with therapist only (N = 38); no significant differences in baseline characteristics between groups	*Intervention* (*EMT with therapist only*): 24 biweekly 30-min clinic sessions with 2 EMT-trained therapists and 12 20-min home sessions with 1 EMT-trained therapist; intervention lasted for approximately 4 months; clinic sessions were conducted at a university-based clinic	*Norm-referenced and parent report measures*: increase on all measures for both groups; no significant differences between groups

(continued)

Table 7.1 (continued)

Citation (in order of mention in Chapter)	Participants	Intervention procedures	Intervention outcomes
	Parents: N=77 (gender NR); M age=35 years; education level: high school—graduate degree; middle to upper-middle socioeconomic class; EMT with parent and therapist (N=39) and EMT with therapist only (N=38); no significant differences in baseline characteristics between groups	*Intervention* (*EMT with parent plus therapist*): 24 biweekly 30-min clinic play sessions with a parent and 2 EMT-trained therapists (one to work with the child and one to train the parent) and 12 20-min home sessions with a parent and a therapist serving as a parent trainer; intervention lasted for approximately 4 months; clinic sessions were conducted at a university-based clinic	*Frequency of unique targets*: increase for both groups; children in parent plus therapist group used a greater number of unique targets at 6 and 12-month MC
		Parent training: a 2–3 h interactive workshop on EMT prior to intervention and 36 1-h parent training sessions (24 sessions at the clinic, 12 sessions in the child's home); parent training sessions consisted of training on a specific EMT strategy, the therapist modeling EMT, the parent implementing EMT, and the therapist and parent reviewing the day's session and planning for the next session; as parents met mastery criteria for implementing a specific EMT strategy, they were introduced to a new EMT skill	*Percentage of target talk*: increase for both groups; children in parent plus therapist group used a significantly higher percentage of target utterances at 6 and 12-month MC
		Implementers: EMT-trained therapists with a minimum of a bachelor's degree in child development or special education (both EMT treatment groups and parent training); parents (EMT with parent and therapist group)	*MLU*: increase for both groups; children in parent plus therapist group had longer MLUs at 6 and 12-month MC
			Total number of different words: increase for both groups; children in parent plus therapist group used greater number of different words at 6 and 12-month MC

			Use of EMT strategies: parents in the parent and therapist group used significantly more responsive interaction, language modeling, expansions, and milieu teaching episodes in trained and untrained activities than parents in the therapist only group; these behaviors were maintained at a 6 and 12 month MC
			MC: Yes. Gen: Yes (across settings and activities for child and parent behaviors). SV: No
Peterson et al. (2005)	*Children*: N=3 (1 male, 2 females); aged 24–43 months; expressive communication delay of 7–11 months; receptive communication delay of 8–11 months	*Intervention*: 60-min parent training sessions in the home once per week for 21–25 weeks; all sessions were conducted in each family's apartment; parents were observed for the first 15 min, followed by the instructor describing and modeling the new skill, finally, the parent practiced with her child and received feedback; parents were taught environmental arrangement, responsive interaction skills, and incidental teaching techniques; parents were instructed to practice with their child twice a week for homework	*Verbal behavior*: increase for all 3 children following intervention; followed the pattern of the rate of their mother's milieu language teaching skills
	Parents: N=3 (3 females); age and education level NR; all received Temporary Aid for Needy Families; all faced 4 or more environmental risk factors (e.g., low income, poor mental health, domestic violence)	*Implementers*: NR	*MLU*: increase for all 3 children

(continued)

Table 7.1 (continued)

Citation (in order of mention in Chapter)	Participants	Intervention procedures	Intervention outcomes
			Receptive communication age: increase for all 3 children at faster than expected rates (as predicted by the proportional change index) *Expressive communication age*: increase for all 3 children at faster than expected rates (as predicted by the proportional change index)
			Milieu language teaching behaviors: increased following intervention; use of previously learned skills decreased slightly each time a new skill was introduced; all 3 parents maintained skills at 3-month MC; 1 parent maintained skills at 6-month MC (1 parent's skills decreased, the other was not available)
			MC: Yes. Gen: No. SV: Yes
Olive et al. (2007)	*Children*: N=3 (3 males); aged 45–66 months; with autism (N=2) and with PDD-NOS (N=1); all Caucasian	*Intervention*: 5-min play sessions conducted 4 times per week for a maximum of 19 sessions during a time period of 1 month; sessions conducted on the floor of the child's classroom	*VOCA use*: increase in prompted and independent VOCA use for all 3 children
		Implementers: EMT-trained teachers or assistant teachers (i.e., master's or doctoral-level students in special education)	*Spontaneous independent requests*: increase for all 3 children; 1 participant began vocalizing
			MC: No. Gen: No. SV: Yes (informal)
Hancock et al. (2002)	*Children*: N=5 (3 males); Aged 38–46 months; language delays (3) and rated behavior problems (5); African American (4), Caucasian (1); IQ score on WPPSI=63–79	*Intervention*: 30–45-min parent training sessions conducted twice per week for a maximum of 30 sessions; sessions conducted in an empty classroom or conference room at the child's daycare; training sessions consisted of providing information and feedback, role-playing, videotaped examples, modeling, and 15 min of practice and feedback with their child present;	*Percentage of child utterances 3 or more words*: two children doubled % of utterances 3 or more words end of intervention

	Parents: N=5 (5 females); ages 20–48; education level=8th grade—GED; Marital Status=4 single, 1 married; Annual income=$3000–$18,000	*Implementers*: Parent educators (3); early childhood educators (2 bachelor's degree, 1 masters); all Caucasian; completed 40 h of training in the intervention before the study	*MLU*: average baseline =2.25; average end of intervention=3.00; all children showed changes
			Diversity: average baseline=62.8; average end intervention=84.7
			Number of total utterances: 4 of 5 children increased from baseline to intervention
			Percentage of self initiated utterances: baseline average=67.2 %; average last 5 intervention sessions=86.1 %
			Noncompliance/negatives: all children decreased from baseline (3.7 per sessions) to last 5 intervention sessions (1.8 per session).
			Responsive feedback: all 5 parents reached criterion of 80 %; baseline average rate=59 %, end of intervention average rate=84 %
			Expansions: average baseline rate=18 %, average intervention rate=50 %, all reached criterion of 40 %
			Pause errors: average baseline rate=36 per session, average intervention rate=5 per session; all parents reached criterion of 5 or less per session
			Negatives: all parents decreased although some parents had relatively low observed negative behavior in baseline
			Praise: average baseline rate=3.6 per session, average intervention rate=12 per session

(continued)

Table 7.1 (continued)

Citation (in order of mention in Chapter)	Participants	Intervention procedures	Intervention outcomes
			Utterances including 4 or more words: baseline average rate 33 % per session; intervention average rate = 59.7 %
			Instructions = baseline average rate = 25 per session (13.3 % correct); intervention average rate = 4 per session (85 % correct)
			MC: Yes Gen: Yes, home. SV: Yes
Wright et al. (2013)	*Children*: N = 4 (2 males, 2 females); aged 23–29 months; with Down syndrome; expressive vocabulary between 1 and 15 words or manual signs; had ability to imitate placement and action of hand movements	*Intervention*: 20–30 min play-based treatment sessions were conducted twice weekly in a room at a pediatric therapy center; a total of 20 intervention sessions were conducted; therapist modeled and prompted 32 spoken words and manual signs using EMT and JASPER strategies; parents were given pictures and descriptions of their child's 32 signs, but no training on how to teach or use them	*Total signs*: increase for all 4 participants
	Parents: N = 4 (1 father, 3 mothers); aged 30–46 years; education level: college degree—graduate degree; middle to upper-middle socioeconomic class	*Implementers*: NR	*Unprompted number of different signs*: increase for all 4 participants
			Total words: gradual increase for all 4 participants, but no clear functional relation
			Unprompted number of different words: gradual increase for all 4 participants, but no clear functional relation
			Percentage of time in joint engagement: increase for the 3 participants whose videos were coded for joint engagement
			Percentage of time in symbol-infused joint engagement: small increase for the 3 participants whose videos were coded for symbol-infused joint engagement

			Use of signs: 3 parents displayed a systematic increase in signs used at home that was concurrent with the clinic intervention
			MC: No. Gen: Yes (to home with parents; all 4 participants generalized use of signs). SV: No
Kasari et al. (2014)	*Children*: N=61 (51 males, 10 females); aged 5–8 years; with ASD; used fewer than 20 different words during a 20 min observation period; had received at least 2 years of intervention; receptive language age of at least 24 months; began in 2 different treatment groups: JASP+EMT (N=30) or JASP+EMT+SGD (N=31); no significant differences in baseline characteristics between groups	*Intervention Stage 1* (*JASP+EMT*): Two 1-h naturalistic communication sessions per week for 12 weeks; sessions conducted in university clinic playrooms	*Total number of spontaneous communicative utterances* (*TSCU*): increase for both groups; however, the group that began with JASP+EMT+SGD increased significantly more (a moderate-to-large treatment effect size); out of participants that received an adapted intervention during stage 2, those that began in the JASP+EMT+SGD group and received additional sessions increased their TSCU the most, followed by participants that began in the JASP+EMT group who received the SGD during stage 2
		Intervention Stage 1 (*JASP+EMT+SGD*): Two 1-h naturalistic communication sessions per week for 12 weeks; sessions conducted in university clinic playrooms; identical to the JASP+EMT group except the addition of a SGD; interventionist used the SGD 50 % of the time he/she modeled language	*Total number of different word roots*: improvement for both groups; however, the group that began with JASP+EMT+SGD showed a larger increase (a small treatment effect size)

(continued)

Table 7.1 (continued)

Citation (in order of mention in Chapter)	Participants	Intervention procedures	Intervention outcomes
		Intervention Stage 2: children who were slow responders (i.e., did not have a 25 % or greater increase on at least half of the dependent variables) received an adapted intervention for an additional 12 weeks; children received either additional sessions of their current treatment (3 h per week as opposed to 2) or the addition of a SGD; children who were early responders continued to receive their original intervention for an additional 12 weeks; sessions were conducted in university clinic playrooms	*Total number of comments*: improvement for both groups; however, the group that began with JASP + EMT + SGD showed a larger increase (a small-to-moderate effect size)
		Implementers: speech clinician, special educator, or child psychologist who was trained to criterion on treatment fidelity (i.e., 90 % or greater accuracy)	MC: Yes. Gen: Yes (to home with parents). SV: Yes

Codes: N: total number of participants in study; PDD: pervasive developmental disorder; PDD-NOS: pervasive developmental disorder not otherwise specified; NR: not reported; MC: maintenance check; Gen: generalization; SV: social validity; IOA: inter-observer agreement; TF: treatment fidelity: JASPER: joint attention, symbolic play and emotional regulation

Theoretical Basis for EMT Strategies That Connect

The theoretical basis for the EMT strategies that connect the adult and child during communicative interactions (i.e., mirroring and mapping) derives from the patterns observed in interactions between typically developing children and parents that are believed to be foundational to effective language learning, such as joint attention and joint engagement (Bakeman & Adamson, 1984; Ratner & Bruner, 1978). Joint attention occurs naturally and early in the first year of a child's life with little additional adult support for children developing typically. Unfortunately, disruption in social communication development, especially joint attention, is an inherent characteristic of autism. Mirroring provides the adult with an approach to eliciting this joint attention for the child with autism and provides a foundation from which the child can connect with the adult and more effectively learn language from ongoing adult-child interactions.

Theoretical Basis for Supporting EMT Strategies

A social pragmatic interactionist perspective emphasizes the role of the transaction between a child and linguistically knowledgeable adult (Bruner, 1975) and serves as the guiding principle behind the EMT strategies that support children's language development (i.e., language responsiveness, expansions). The responsiveness of the adult to the child's communication attempts provides a foundation as the adult reads the child's communicative intentions and then provides language that maps the topic of the child's interest and focus. One of the overriding principles of this theoretical approach is that adults respond to all of the children's communication attempts as if they were purposeful and they adjust their linguistic input based on the child's current level of language understanding. Parents are often best suited to be a responsive language partner because they tend to understand their children's communicative intent more accurately than other adults (teachers and therapists). They also have the experience and ongoing context to more readily understand their children's communicative attempts, especially those utterances that are not clearly articulated; this relationship can make it easier for the parent to respond to their child with meaningful expansions.

Theoretical Basis for Teaching

Milieu Teaching procedures, used to prompt elaborated or new language forms, are derived from a behavioral model of language learning theories. These prompting episodes follow an ABC pattern (antecedent-behavior-consequence). The adult provides a prompt, which serves as an antecedent or discriminative stimulus for the child's language behavior. The adult then reinforces the child's communicative behavior by attending to the behavior in the form of providing attention, requested objects and contingent language responses. After these prompting episodes, children are to use these new/elaborated language forms because they have been contingently reinforced. The adult continues to shape the child's communicative behavior into more and more complex and independent use of language by providing prompts in a hierarchical, systematic manner (model, mand-model, time delay). In addition to the acquisition of language skills that the adult has facilitated through these prompting procedures, language learning in this behavioral paradigm also emphasizes the two other critical phases of learning: the generalization and maintenance of these newly learned forms. The Milieu Teaching component of EMT utilizes the core principles for promoting generalization that were outlined by Stokes and Baer (1977) including teaching multiple exemplars across various settings.

Review of Empirical Support for EMT

Currently, there are 12 published research studies investigating the effects of EMT. However, two of those studies are not discussed in detail in this chapter; one recent study was conducted and published in Spanish (Calleja, Rodríguez, & Luque, 2014) and the other study reported that the intervention was based on EMT but did not use the full array of EMT strategies (Roberts et al., 2014). The remaining ten studies are summarized in Table 7.1 and described more fully in this section. The first two research papers published on EMT investigated its effects with parents (Hemmeter & Kaiser, 1994) and therapists (Kaiser & Hester, 1994). The next several studies were conducted in the context of investigating the effects of therapists compared to parents implementing EMT (Hancock & Kaiser, 2002; Kaiser et al., 2000; Kaiser & Roberts, 2013). Other studies of EMT varied the targeted population (parents and children in multiple risk families instead of children with an identified diagnosis and significant language delay; Peterson et al., 2005) or the communication mode used (augmentative and alternative communication device instead of verbal communication; Olive et al., 2007). The last category of published EMT studies includes those that blend EMT with an additional intervention or approach to address issues that EMT alone has not previously addressed (Hancock et al., 2002; Kasari et al., 2014; Wright et al., 2013). The first published blended EMT approach was conducted by Hancock and her colleagues (2002) and investigated the effects of parents implementing EMT in addition to a behavioral intervention targeting the language and behavior of their preschool children. The latest generation of published blended EMT studies investigated the effects of EMT when blended with another evidenced based intervention (JASPER; Joint Attention, Symbolic Play, and Emotional Regulation; Kasari, Freeman, & Paparella, 2006). This blended intervention was implemented to teach alternative forms of communication in addition to verbal communication (signs, speech generating device) with child participants who had not been included in previous research of EMT (toddlers with Down syndrome; school aged children with autism who were minimally verbal) (Kasari et al., 2014; Wright et al., 2013).

First, a series of studies was conducted with parents implementing Milieu Teaching procedures versus Responsive Interaction strategies. Thirty-six preschool aged children with developmental disabilities and their parents were randomly assigned to either the Responsive Interaction condition ($N=18$) or Milieu Teaching ($N=18$). Almost all of the parents reached criterion levels for their assigned intervention at the end of 24 sessions. The data revealed that Responsive Interaction strategies were as effective as Milieu Teaching procedures on the language development of children (Kaiser et al., 1990). Analyzing the data by child characteristics revealed that children with a Mean Length of Utterance (MLU) of 1.8 or less showed more significant gains when Milieu Teaching was implemented and children with an MLU of 3.0 or greater showed more significant gains when Responsive Interaction strategies were implemented (Kaiser et al., 1990; Kaiser, Lambert, Hancock, & Hester, 1998). Given the strong effects of both interventions on children's language development (Responsive Interaction—connecting with the child and supporting language development; Milieu Teaching—direct teaching and prompting procedures) we blended these two intervention approaches and Enhanced Milieu Teaching was born.

Seminal Parent-Implemented EMT Study

The first published EMT study examined the effects of training four parents to use EMT with their preschool aged children who had developmental and language delays (Hemmeter & Kaiser, 1994). Parents (3 mothers, 1 father) implemented four EMT strategies (environmental arrangement, responsive language feedback, modeling child language targets, incidental prompting strategies) in sessions conducted twice per week for approximately 4 months at a university based clinic setting. A multiple probe design across two families, replicated across two additional families was used to evaluate the parents' implementation of the strategies on their children's communication skills. Although there was some variability in parents' use of the four EMT strategies, all parents reached criterion at the end of intervention and generalized their use of these strategies with their children to home settings. Parent implementation of EMT resulted in positive language outcomes for the children; specifically, after intervention all children showed increases in frequency of total and spontaneous target use. Increases in children's MLU in pre/post language samples were not greater than what would be predicted on their MLU at the beginning of the study. This first study of EMT did not assess maintenance of parent implementation over time (Hemmeter & Kaiser, 1994).

Seminal Therapist-Implemented EMT Study

The goal of the first published study of therapist-implemented EMT was to replicate the effects of the parent study in the classroom. The three therapists were female graduate students who were trained in EMT procedures before implementing the intervention with six preschool children who had significant language delays. EMT was implemented in 20-min play sessions in the children's classrooms 4 days a week with all children receiving at least 35 sessions of intervention. At the end of intervention, 5 of the 6 children doubled their use of targets from levels observed in baseline and increased their spontaneous utterances from pre to post intervention. Generalization of child language was assessed across conversational partners (teachers, parents and peers) and some generalization of language target use with these untrained partners occurred for all children.

Therapist and Parent-Implemented EMT

A number of studies conducted over a 15-year period by Kaiser and Hancock and their colleagues investigated the effects of EMT when implemented by parents or by therapists (Hancock & Kaiser, 2002; Kaiser & Hancock, 2000; Kaiser et al., 2000; Kaiser, Hancock, et al., 1998; Kaiser, Lambert, et al., 1998; Kaiser & Roberts, 2013). In one of the first group parent versus therapist comparison studies that was unpublished, Kaiser and Hancock (2000) randomly assigned 73 preschool aged children with significant cognitive and language delays to one of three intervention conditions: (a) parent-implemented Responsive Interaction (N = 18), (b) parent-implemented EMT (N = 19), or (c) therapist-implemented EMT (N = 18). Parents in the three groups did not differ significantly in age, education or family resources. All three approaches resulted in positive effects on children's language development assessed 6 months post-intervention (MLU, expressive language on the Sequenced Inventory of Communication Development, receptive vocabulary on the Peabody Picture Vocabulary Test). Children in either of the parent-implemented intervention groups (RI, EMT) performed better on expressive language measures 6 months post-intervention than the children in the therapist-implemented EMT group (Kaiser & Hancock, 2000). The published studies investigating parent versus therapist implemented EMT include (a) a multiple baseline study of therapist-implemented EMT with children with autism (Hancock & Kaiser, 2002), (b) a multiple baseline study of parent-implemented EMT with children with autism (Kaiser et al., 2000) and (c) a group comparison study of parent + therapist implemented EMT versus therapists only implemented EMT (Kaiser & Roberts, 2013). Data for both the single subject therapist-implemented study (Hancock & Kaiser, 2002) and parent-implemented study (Kaiser et al., 2000) described in this section below were selected from the longitudinal study described in this paragraph and the two single subject studies included those children with an autism diagnosis who were randomly assigned to one of those conditions and who had completed follow-up data; number of baseline sessions were pre-determined (5–7 sessions).

Therapist-Implemented EMT

A modified single subject design across four children with autism assessed the effects of EMT when implemented by trained therapists in 24 clinic based intervention sessions (Hancock & Kaiser, 2002). Observational time series data indicated that all four children showed positive changes for specific target language use (prompted and unprompted) at the end of intervention and these gains were maintained at the 6-month follow up observations. There were also increases in children's observed language complexity and diversity. Not surprisingly, the younger children whose language development was less delayed relative to their chronological age at the beginning of the study showed the greatest language gains at the end of the study. One of the most interesting findings in this study was that at the end of the intervention, 3 of the 4 children generalized these positive language gains to interactions at home with their mothers who had not been trained in EMT. These generalization gains with untrained parents did not maintain at the 6-month follow-up however. One of the limitations of this study was that participating children had to meet minimum criteria to qualify for the study (ability to imitate and at least ten productive words) so it was unclear if EMT would be effective with children who are functioning outside these criteria, for example, children who are not yet verbal.

Parent-Implemented EMT

This study examined the effects of parent-implemented EMT on the language development of preschool children with an autism diagnosis (Kaiser et al., 2000). The study used a modified single subject design across six parent-child dyads to assess parents' acquisition and maintenance of EMT strategies and their generalization of these strategies to a home setting. Parents learned and practiced the EMT strategies across 24 intervention sessions conducted in a university clinic. Five of the six parents implemented all of the EMT strategies to criteria by the end of intervention and generalized the use of these strategies to interactions at home with their child. Parents maintained their use of EMT at the 6-month follow-up in both the clinic and home settings, sometimes at levels higher than what had been observed for parents at the end of intervention. Parent-implemented EMT resulted in increases of spontaneous use of communication targets for all study children and for language complexity and word diversity for most of the children. All children showed positive changes from baseline to follow-up on standardized assessments of their language development with an average increase of 10 months on receptive language skills and an average increase of 9 months on expressive language skills on the Sequenced Inventory of Communication Development. The most significant language gain for the study children was 18 months from baseline to follow-up on expressive vocabulary skills as assessed by the Early One Word Picture Vocabulary Test (Kaiser et al., 2000). These observed and assessed language gains were consistent with those found when therapists implemented EMT with children with autism. Unlike the therapist-implemented EMT, parents were not implementing EMT at criteria until at least half way through the intervention so one of the limitations of including parents in intervention efforts is that it may take them longer to implement the intervention with fidelity (Hancock & Kaiser, 2002).

Parent Plus Therapist Compared to Therapist-Only EMT

Children in therapist-implemented EMT showed more rapid growth in language targets, MLU and vocabulary diversity during intervention sessions than children in the parent-implemented EMT study, but children in the parent-implemented EMT study continued to show increases in language development 6 months post intervention and better generalization to home settings (Hancock & Kaiser, 2012). The next generation of EMT studies investigated a parent+therapist-implemented EMT intervention developed to maximize the rapid target and language development support that therapists provide with the long term and generalized language effects that parent-implemented EMT supports. Kaiser and Roberts (2013) compared the effects of EMT when implemented by therapists and parents versus only therapists on the language skills of preschool children with language delays and intellectual disabilities. Seventy-seven children were randomly assigned to EMT intervention that included 36 intervention sessions provided by therapists and parents or by two therapists. In both groups, 24 of the training sessions were conducted in a university clinic setting and the remaining 12 sessions were conducted at the children's homes. A randomized group design was used to evaluate the effects of EMT on children's language development (both observed and assessed) at four time points (pre-intervention, at the end of intervention, 6 and 12 months post-intervention). There were no differences between the two intervention groups on children's language development at the end of intervention and no differences between groups on standardized language assessment results at any time period, but at the 6-month follow-up children in the parent+therapist group had longer and more complex utterances and used more targeted language forms in the trained activity at home than children in the therapist only group. As is true of the other parent-implemented EMT studies discussed in this section (Hemmeter & Kaiser, 1994: Kaiser et al., 2000, Kaiser & Hancock, 2000), parents in this study were highly-educated, middle class parents who had enough financial and time resources to participate in an intensive intervention which in this particular study included driving their child to clinic sessions every week for 6+ months (Kaiser & Roberts, 2013). This study provides results for EMT when implemented by a very homogenous parent group (predominantly middle class, Euro-American) and these results cannot be generalized to parents in other cultural or socio-economic groups.

EMT Variations

The next two published studies not only extended EMT to parent interventionists who varied from the sample found in the earlier studies (middle-class, Euro-American) but also to communication modes that were very different from the verbal mode investigated in all of the previous published EMT studies. Peterson et al. (2005) investigated the effects of EMT when implemented by low-income, minority status parents. Olive and her colleagues (2007) investigated the effects of EMT on the use of a voice output communication aid (VOCA). Both of these studies investigated variations of EMT that had not been previously researched.

EMT with High-Risk Families

A multiple baseline design across three preschool children and their mothers experiencing multiple risk factors (i.e., minority status, drug-use, single parent, low SES) was used to assess the effects of parent-implemented EMT on the verbal language development of their children (Peterson et al., 2005). Parents received EMT training in their apartment once a week for between 21 and 25 sessions. The project also provided a play material (book, puzzle or toy) to the family each week for their permanent use. Two of the three families participated in 3- and 6-month follow-up sessions; the remaining family moved with no forwarding information before these follow-up sessions could be conducted. Results indicated that parents experiencing multiple risks could learn and implement EMT strategies and both parents who completed follow-up sessions maintained the use of these strategies at 3-months post-intervention; only one of the parents continued to maintain her use of these strategies at the 6-month follow-up. Children increased their use of verbal comments when parents were taught Responsive Interaction strategies and increased their correct verbal responding when parents were taught to use Milieu Teaching prompting strategies. Additionally, all children increased the length of their sentences and their language scores on the Sequenced Inventory of Communication Development from pre to post-intervention. While parents in this study were able to learn and somewhat maintain their implementation of EMT over time, the project interventionists needed to provide additional scaffolding beyond EMT training during the study to support parents regarding issues of domestic abuse, housing disruptions, mental health problems, and financial assistance (Peterson et al., 2005). While the positive effects of this study are promising, clinicians and projects providing EMT training to families with multiple risk factors may need to also have the resources to provide comprehensive and possibly intensive social work services as well.

EMT Using a VOCA

Olive et al. (2007) used a multiple probe design across participants to investigate the effects of teacher-implemented EMT when combined with a Voice Output Communication Aid (VOCA) on the communication skills of three children with autism. The study children received an EMT play-based intervention delivered by their teacher or teacher assistant in their classroom for 5 min a day for no more than 19 sessions. None of the children used the VOCA during baseline sessions but all three children learned to request using the VOCA during the EMT intervention. The children showed increases in their frequency of independent (not prompted) gestures, vocalizations and VOCA use during intervention, although only one of the child participants actually was observed vocalizing during the intervention portion of the study. While this research holds promise of using EMT procedures with children with autism who need communication modes other than verbal communication, it is important to note that the teachers in this study were graduate students who were comprehensively trained in both communication interventions in general and EMT specifically. Additionally, while this intervention study was very time efficient (less than month), no data were collected on the maintenance or generalization of these effects (Olive et al., 2007).

Blended EMT Interventions

Three published studies to date have blended EMT with another intervention or approach to provide support to children who have not traditionally benefited from the implementation of EMT alone (Hancock et al., 2002; Kasari et al., 2014; Wright et al., 2013). The first study that utilized a blended approach investigated the effects of teaching parents from low-income families to implement EMT with a positive behavioral intervention on their children's language skills and observed/rated behavior issues (Hancock et al., 2002). While the children in this study did not have significant language delays as had been the case in all of the previous EMT studies, they did have significant behavior issues that might have made it difficult for them to interact in ways with their parents that would have supported positive language gains. The other two blended EMT studies investigated the effects of combining EMT with JASPER (Kasari et al., 2014; Wright et al., 2013). JASPER (Joint Attention Symbolic Play Engagement and Regulation; Kasari, Gulsrud, Wong, Kwon, & Locke, 2010) "is a naturalistic behavioral intervention focused on the development of prelinguistic gestures (joint attention, requesting) and play skills within the context of play-based interactions as a means to increase joint engagement between an adult and child with ASD" (Kasari et al., 2010, p. 636). Wright and her colleagues used this blended EMT+JASPER intervention with toddlers who have Down syndrome; since JASPER had been developed for and previously implemented only with children with autism this was a novel sample for JASPER implementation. The most recently published EMT study blended with another intervention (JASPER) was novel in its participation selection (children with ASD who were minimally verbal and had "failed" in previous language interventions) and its adapted approach to revising the intervention when children did not respond effectively to the first phase of the intervention (Kasari et al., 2010).

Blended EMT and Behavior Intervention

Hancock et al. (2002) used an AB single-subject design replicated across five participants to evaluate the effects of an EMT and behavior intervention that taught parents to support their preschool children's communication skills and manage their behavior. Parents from low SES backgrounds completed 30 individual sessions at their child's preschool. They were taught to be responsive to their child's communication and to provide contingent consequences for their child's behavior. Generalization to interactions at home and maintenance of intervention effects every month for 6 months were assessed. Results indicated that parents were able to learn the intervention strategies (EMT + behavioral), generalize these strategies to interactions with their child at home, and maintain these positive changes 6 months after the intervention ended. Study children showed positive changes in language development and behavior during the intervention, but maintenance and generalization of these effects were more variable. For example, on standardized measures of behavior (Child Behavior Checklist/4–18), all five children were rated by their parents as having lower externalizing and internalizing score from pre-intervention to 6-months post intervention and 4 of those 5 children moved from clinical/subclinical levels of behaviors before the intervention to within normal limits 6 months after the intervention ended. Children's observed non-compliance and negative behavior decreased from an average of 3.7 occurrences per session in baseline to an average of 1.8 during the last five intervention sessions; this decreased rate of negative behavior maintained with an average rate of less than 1 episode per session during the follow-up observations. The results of both observed and tested language skills was much more variable. For example, all children showed increases in their average MLU from baseline (2.25) to the end of intervention (3.00), but at the end of the 6-month follow-up the average MLU was 3.04, approximately the same MLU observed at the end of intervention. Parents in this study showed more modest and less consistent changes during the intervention, more variable generalization to interactions at home and fewer changes maintained during the follow-up period then previous parent applications of EMT (Hemmeter & Kaiser, 1994; Kaiser et al., 2000). There were some notable differences in this study from those previous parent-implemented EMT studies including that most of the parents in this study were single mothers who were low SES and very stressed by their everyday life. Additionally, all of the parents were African-American and all of the parent trainers were Euro-American (Hancock et al., 2002). It is difficult to determine from this initial blended EMT intervention study if these factors were more responsible for the variable implementation of EMT strategies by the study parents or if the EMT strategies were more difficult to learn and implement because the intervention was more complex with the addition of learning positive behavioral strategies as well.

Blended EMT and JASPER with Toddlers with Down Syndrome

Using a multiple baseline design across participants, Wright et al. (2013) investigated the effects of blending EMT with JASPER to teach verbal language and manual signs to young children with Down syndrome. Four toddlers (ages 23–29 months) completed 20 play-based EMT+JASPER intervention sessions with a therapist; each session lasted 20–30 min and occurred twice weekly. EMT strategies used by the therapist included: (a) following the child's lead, (b) responding to child communication with language rich talk, (c) mirroring and mapping, (d) expanding communication attempts, (e) modeling target signs, and (f) time delay. JASPER strategies used by the therapist included: teaching new play actions and sequences by modeling and expanding children's play. The therapist used these EMT+JASPER strategies to teach 32 signs paired with spoken words to each child. Generalization of child language to interactions with their parents at home was also assessed. All children demonstrated an increase in their rate of signing and the diversity of signs used spontaneously during intervention sessions (0–2 spontaneous different signs during baseline; 0–9 spontaneous different signs during intervention). Rate of spoken words though varied across the study children with results showing a gradual increase across sessions but no clear functional relationship between the blended intervention strategies and the children's use of spoken words. All children generalized their use of signs when interacting with their parents at home. While this was the first published study using EMT strategies to teach children signs (in addition to verbal language) and specifically targeting only children with Down syndrome (other studies have included children with Down syndrome but not targeted children with Down syndrome, see Kaiser & Roberts, 2013), this study was not able to provide information about the value of the JASPER component added to EMT in this blended intervention (Wright et al., 2013).

Blended EMT and JASPER with School-Aged Children with Autism

Kasari et al. (2014) investigated the effects of EMT blended with JASPER on the spontaneous communicative utterances of minimally verbal school-aged children with autism. To be included in the study, children had to have less than 20 spontaneous different words observed during a language sample and at least 2 years of previous language intervention as reported by the parent. The researchers utilized a SMART design that included two stages of treatment and randomly assigned 61 children ages 5–8 to 1 of 2 interventions. In the first stage, children received EMT + JASPER twice a week for 3 months with half of the children receiving the intervention with a speech-generating device (SGD) and the other half receiving intervention without the SGD. At the end of this phase, children who were making progress (defined as 25 % or greater change on at least half of 14 pre-selected communication variables) continued with their phase 1 intervention for an additional 12 weeks. For slow responders, the second stage of the intervention was adapted for the next 12 weeks and children were randomly assigned to treatment with an increased number of sessions from two to now three a week or assigned to treatment adding a SGD to the intervention. Results of the study indicated that children in the initial SGD group showed more improvement in spontaneous communicative utterances, novel words and comments than the children in the initial condition without the SGD. Additionally, among the two interventions adapted in the second stage (increased sessions versus including SGD) for children who were in the initial no SGD condition and were slow responders, including a SGD lead to greater total socially communicative utterances than increasing the number of sessions per week. The study found that beginning intervention with SGD combined with the blended EMT + JASPER was more effective for children's spontaneous communication than beginning the blended EMT + JASPER intervention targeting spoken words only. The researchers concluded that the study children who were minimally verbal at the beginning of the study made rapid and significant gains in spontaneous spoken language possibly because of the combination of strategies that included a focus on supporting children's joint attention and engagement in addition to the language strategies of systematic modeling and prompting (Kasari et al., 2014).

Implementing EMT

EMT is a naturalistic, child-directed intervention approach using a set of conversation-based strategies for supporting the language and communication skills of young children. While EMT has traditionally included both responsive interaction and milieu teaching strategies (Hemmeter & Kaiser, 1994) sometimes it has been described as having three components (environmental arrangement, responsive interaction, milieu teaching; Hancock & Kaiser, 2009) or four components (environmental arrangement, responsive interaction, language modeling, milieu teaching; Hancock & Kaiser, 2012). Most recently, as seen in Table 7.2, the authors have used a framework to discuss EMT that includes three major components that are taught sequentially: (a) strategies that connect, (b) strategies that support, and (c) strategies that teach (Hancock et al., in progress).

Table 7.2 Enhanced milieu teaching components

Current framework	Strategy	Traditional component
Connecting	Following child's lead	RI
	Environmental arrangement to connect	EA
	Mirroring and mapping	RI
	Matched turns	RI
Supporting	Language responsiveness	RI
	Limit questions and instructions	RI
	Expansions	RI and LM
Teaching	Modeling child's target level	RI and LM
	Environmental arrangement for requests	EA
	Prompting strategies	MT

Codes: RI: Responsive Interaction; EA: Environmental Arrangement; LM: Language Modeling; MT: Matched-Turns

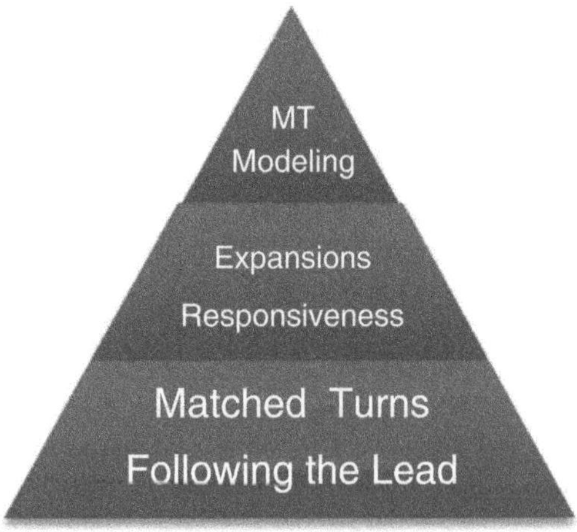

Fig. 7.1 EMT triangle illustrating the emphasis of and relationship between EMT strategies

EMT Strategies That Connect

The EMT strategies that connect the adult with the child and the child with the adult (environmental arrangement to connect, following the child's lead, and matched turns) are foundational to the effectiveness of all of the other EMT strategies (see Fig. 7.1). Language is learned in relationship and interactions with the important people in our lives—our family. This process of language learning is generally seamless and occurs naturally with very little thought given to this process unless there are issues with learning language. This process is often disrupted when children have autism, which makes it difficult for them to learn language incidentally from people in their environment. These first three strategies help the adult meet and connect with the child where he/she is. In joining with the child, the adult is more able to understand the child's world and what he may be trying to communicate. The adult uses this understanding to translate the world of language for the child in ways that are functional and make sense to the child. Additionally, when adults use these strategies, the child experiences an acknowledgement of his communication attempts, which in turn reinforces him to attempt more communication acts with this adult. These strategies first provide specific ways for the adult to connect to the child and in those moments, the child is then able to connect with the adult thus providing the foundation for the child to learn language.

Environmental Arrangement to Connect

Before the adult-child interaction takes place, it is important to carefully consider the environment to optimize opportunities and make it easier for the child to connect with the adult. When we have a connected conversation with another adult we generally think about a conversation that is face to face, with fairly equal contributions by both partners and with no competing distractions that keep us from fully listening and attending to the conversational topic (no cell phones!). So how can we set the stage for that same type of connected conversation with a child, especially when that child is highly distractible? First, set up the space so there are as few distractions as possible. It is difficult to have a connected conversation with the television blaring in the background or when the child is engrossed in an activity on an I-pad. Limit the number of toys or materials so the child is not overwhelmed by visual distractions in the environment. Choose toys and activities (conversation topics) that the child enjoys and about which he is knowledgeable and skilled so he is more likely to be an equal conversational partner. Finally, arrange the environment to facilitate face-to-face interactions. This could be setting up carpet squares or a child-sized table in the corner of a room to help provide the child with a physical boundary for the interaction. There are also contained environments across the day (bathtub, car, highchair) that allow for naturally occurring face-to-face interactions. Many children enjoy bath time so this can be an effective moment for a connected conversation. Some of the best conversations I had with my children as they were growing up occurred while they were "contained" in our car going from one place to another. Considering how an environment can be set up or managed to facilitate a physical connection provides a canvas that is prepped for a conversational connection to take place.

Following the Child's Lead

Following the child's lead is a core strategy of EMT that distinguishes it from other "naturalistic" language intervention approaches. Adults frequently approach communicative interactions with children fully in charge of the topics that are discussed and the part they want children to play in that interaction (answer my questions). When we follow the child's lead, we first carefully observe the child's actions including what interests him (play and talk topics), how he is communicating (gestures, eye contact, vocalizations, words) and what he is attempting to communicate (request for attention, request for a tangible item, request for assistance, social bid, comment about a shared activity). The importance of this observation time cannot be overstated since adults tend to preemptively strike in interactions with children, anticipating what the child might need or want to say which then diminishes the child's opportunities and capacity to communicate. When the adult actively observes the child's behavior and asks with each behavior, "What is this child trying to communicate?" the adult is much better positioned to translate that behavior into communication that is more functional and better resonates with the child's meaning. After carefully observing the child's communicative behavior, the adult joins the child's play or conversational topic, follows the child's lead on that topic while focusing on what the child is trying to communicate. While following the child's lead and interacting with the child, we coach adults to use the "child's voice" in interactions. For example, a child is playing with a puzzle and the adult tries to help him position the puzzle piece in the board correctly. Without looking at the adult, the child places one of his hands on the adult's hands, which appears to be a blocking motion. The adult is asked by the EMT coach, "What do you think he is trying to communicate?" The adult answers, "that he doesn't want me to touch the puzzle piece; that he wants to do the puzzle himself." We suggest to the adult that she respond to the child using this message in the child's voice; what the child would say if he had the ability and skill to do so. The next time the child places his hand on the adult's hands the adult says, "I want to do it myself." For the first time in the interaction, the child looks up at the adult and says, "myself!" As the interaction continues, when the adult picks up a puzzle piece or tries to help the child adjust the piece, the child looks at the adult and is able to use a verbal message, "myself" without using only the non-verbal message of pushing the adult's hand away. The adult followed the child's lead in this interaction ("I don't want your help with this puzzle"), acknowledged the child's message and provided him with functional language to communicate in future interactions ("myself"). Children have only so much energy (brain processing power) each day to focus, learn and process the world. When adults ask children to join their topics and to follow their lead, children have to use all of their available processing power to understand the adult's topic and what part the adult wants the child to play in the conversation. There is little available cognitive energy left to integrate the language the child is hearing in the environment and make it his own. When the child leads the play and the conversations, it allows him to initiate and practice play and talk topics, establishes him as competent conversational partner and frees him to integrate the communication skills the adult is providing him.

Matched Turns

Most adults believe that it is important to provide a language rich environment when children are learning to talk but often this results in inundating the child with an endless stream of language modeling. This is even more probable when children are not talking and adults begin to fill in the gap taking their turn and the child's turn. This can result in the child tuning out the adult because there is too much language for the child to process. Think about the analogy of learning another language. When you are first learning to understand and speak another language, it is very helpful if the teacher says one short sentence and then pauses to provide you with an opportunity to process what has been said and then practice saying it. If the teacher recites a long story without taking a break, it would probably be very difficult for you to understand everything that is being said and it would be impossible to repeat the entire story word for word. This is often how it feels when adults are modeling lots and lots of language to a child who is an early language learner. It can be overwhelming to the child and result in the child tuning out the adult and the opportunity to learn language from that adult. When adults pace their language with the child's language level and match children's communicative turns, it allows the child time to process the adult's language models and integrate this language so the child can then use parts of this in functional ways.

There are two ways for adults to match their conversational turns with children by: (a) mirroring and mapping and (b) equal verbal turn taking. When children are not talking, adults can use mirroring and mapping as a way to connect and match their communicative turns. When children are verbalizing then adults can pace their verbal turns so they are matched to the child's turns. Every time the child communicates (verbally or non-verbally), the adult matches that child turn by verbally responding. If the adult does not verbally respond to a child communicative utterance, that is considered an unmatched turn. If the adult says more than one thing after a child communicative turn, then each utterance is counted as a turn not matched with the child. The goal for matched turns is that the adult's utterances be matched 75 % with the child's communicative attempts.

The EMT strategy mirroring and mapping involves the adult specifically imitating the actions the child is completing while providing verbal descriptions (mapping) of the child's actions. When mapping, the adult verbalizes as if the child was talking for himself as discussed in the Following the Child's Lead section above. If the child is racing cars on a track, the adult would mirror and map this play action by racing another car on the track next to the child's car and saying, "I race my car." It is important for the adult to imitate the child's action as close in space and time proximity as possible. We as adults do not imitate children's actions very often so what tends to happen when we imitate is the child seems a little surprised by the action and his attention is now turned to the adult. The power of this mirroring strategy is it facilitates joint engagement/joint attention with the child when we imitate his actions. With joint engagement/attention comes fertile ground for children's language learning (Bruner, 1975) so after the adult mirrors the child's action, she provides a verbal description or maps language onto that action. Given that the child is often actively engaged with and attending to the adult at that moment, it is much more likely that he will be able to cognitively process this language and integrate it into his language repertoire. Recently when we asked one of our parents learning EMT about how mirroring and mapping was working with her son she related that when she was mirroring his play actions and he would look up at her (joint attention) "I realize it's like at that moment he has turned on his video recorder and I everything I say is being recorded in his memory!" This is a great analogy for the language learning mechanism triggered by mirroring a child's actions and mapping that behavior. Since mirroring and mapping powerfully reinforces the child's behavior by imitating the child's actions explicitly, it is important for the adult to only mirror and map positive acceptable actions. The adult would not mirror and map destructive actions (throwing large objects), aggressive or self-harming behaviors. Mirroring and mapping is a very effective strategy to use when a child is not yet verbal or is not talking very much during an activity.

When the child is actively communicating during an activity, it's very important for the adult to pace her verbal responses so they are equitable with the child's communication attempts. This means the adult waits for the child to communicate, responds with one utterance and then pauses to provide a window/opportunity for the child to communicate again. It is important that the adult verbally respond every time the child communicates to reinforce these communication attempts. Communication can include words, sounds or gestures requesting attention, assistance or a tangible object. The adult tries to determine the child's message in each of these communicative attempts and then responds using the words the child would use. Responding contingently to every child communication attempt reinforces that attempt and increases the likelihood that the child will continue to practice communication. We coach adults to envision this verbal turn-taking strategy as a tennis match or game of catch. The child hits the ball to the adult (communicative attempt), the adult lobs the ball back to the child (one verbal response) and waits for the child to return the ball. The ultimate goal is for the adult and child to keep the conversational ball going as long as possible; learning to take multiple turns provides the child with a framework of how conversational interactions work.

EMT Strategies That Support Language

When adults and children are connected in interactions, the EMT support strategies of language responsiveness and expansions become much more effective. Adults are connected to children in ways that help them translate the child's communicative meaning. When learning the EMT connecting strategies, the only coaching/feedback adults are provided about the content of their language responses is to try their best to capture the child's meaning and say what the child would say if he had the words. It is interesting that many adults provided with that feedback and who connect with the child seem to naturally revise their language so it is language rich and it expands the child's communication attempts. When adults use the EMT connecting strategies, children often increase the frequency of their communicative utterances. When adults begin implementing language responsiveness strategies and using expansions, children's language learning is supported and often their language becomes more complex, both in sentence length (MLU) and diversity (number of vocabulary).

Language Responsiveness

Language responsiveness is providing "rich" vocabulary when interacting with children. It is important when being language responsive with children that we are somewhat restrained and our responses are within the boundaries of matched turns so we don't barrage children with so much language that they opt out of the interaction and are no longer equitable conversational partners. When we define language responsiveness, we often describe all of the elements that are not considered to be language responsiveness: (a) yes/no questions, (b) test questions, (c) praise statements, (d) instructions, and (e) "fillers." There are times when it is important to receive information quickly from children using a yes/no question format ("Do you need to go to the bathroom?"), but we tend to overuse these questions as a prompt to get children to take their turn in the conversation. Children's only response to this question format is a one word "yes" or "no" which depresses their language complexity (diversity, MLU). The same issues are true when adults use "test" questions in their interactions with children. A test question is one in which the adult knows the answer to the question but is quizzing the child's knowledge. Unlike open-ended questions, test questions generally elicit a one-word answer ("blue," "three," "square"). Not only do the use of test questions tend to break the connection between the adult and child (Let me just give you a pop quiz while we are having fun playing) and imbalance the conversational partnership between the adult and child (the adult is now taking the lead in the topic and the role the child will play in the interaction), but once again it potentially depresses the complexity of the child's response. Yes/no and test format questions can be very seductive for adults to use especially when the child is not an active partner in the interaction. It cues the child to take a turn in the interaction, which can be very reinforcing to the adult and makes it seem that there is a conversation taking place between the child and adult but the truth is this approach results in a very one-sided interaction and does not provide the child with an opportunity to be an equal conversational partner. The adult response that usually follows a correct answer to a test question is praise—"good answer," "great job," "yeah," "way to go." The problem is if the goal is to have multiple turn conversations with children, praise statements tend to end the conversation abruptly. What can the child say in response to being praised by the adult? There are times that adults need to provide instructions to children ("Get off the top of the refrigerator!"), but adults can overuse instructions in play interactions when children's behavior is not problematic. These instructions can seem innocuous on the surface ("Throw the ball to me." "Put your train on the track." "Give the baby a bottle."), but they avert the child's attention from learning and processing language to understanding what action the adult is asking the child to complete. Instructions also position the adult in the lead during these interactions and the child loses the opportunity to initiate conversations with the adult. Lastly, adults are not being language responsive when they use "filler" words or phrases. Responses like "uh-huh," "okay," "yeah," "hmm," and "oh" allow adults to take a conversational turn but they are often not carefully listening or present in the interaction when they are using these "fillers." What is left when adults limit questions, instructions, praise statements and fillers is descriptive talk, which provides children with rich language models. We ask that adults respond with descriptive talk to at least 80 % of the communication children attempt.

Expansions

Expansions are the most effective and powerful EMT language strategy adults can use to support children's language complexity (diversity of vocabulary, MLU). When adults expand, they simply add more words to a child's utterance or correct the child's utterance. The most basic kind of expansion is to add a word or words to what the child said. For example, if the child said "car" while pointing to a car on a shelf the adult could expand this with "want car," "my car," "I want the car," "please give me the car." Adding one or two words to the child's utterances can facilitate a child from using one word to communicate to using two or three word sentences. Expansions are a very effective support strategy for early language learners (MLU of 1.00–3.00) and are less effective as a language-learning tool when children are communicating in more complex sentences. Additionally, depending on the diversity of the words the adult is adding to expand the child's utterance, expansions can facilitate vocabulary development. Expansions in EMT can also correct the articulation of a child's response (correcting "ghetti" to "spaghetti") or the grammar (correcting "I runned" to "I ran"). Expansions are a powerful language learning strategy because they connect the child's communication (what he is trying to communicate, what is important to him) and bridge this to new words and thoughts. The child does not need to use as much cognitive processing to integrate these words and more complex sentences because they are attached to his own words. Repeating what the child said and adding more information to that utterance, not only reinforces the child's communication attempts because he hears his own words repeated by the adult, but it also provides a model of more complex language which helps move the child to the next language level. Expansions are a very effective support strategy for early language learners (MLU of 1.00–3.00) and are less effective as a language-learning tool when children are communicating in more complex sentences. The criterion level we have set for expansions is that the adult expands at least half of the child's communication attempts.

EMT Strategies That Teach Language

The last set of EMT strategies that adults learn are those that directly teach the child new language forms. The three components of these EMT teaching strategies are: (a) language modeling, (b) environmental arrangement to set up requesting, and (c) prompting strategies. For maximum effectiveness, it is very important that these strategies are implemented in the context of also using the EMT connecting and support strategies discussed previously. If these teaching strategies are implemented when the child is not connected to the adult, the child will have a difficult time integrating any information from the language models that the adult is providing, will most likely not make overt request communication acts toward the adult when the environment is arranged, and may not respond to the prompts the adult provides for more elaborated language.

Language Modeling

Language modeling provides children with salient, specific models of targeted language forms in interactions with adults. These language models are slightly ahead of the child's current language production. For example, if the child is an early one-word communicator, then the adult would model language using one or two words. If the child consistently puts two words together then the adult would model language using 3–4 words. Depending on the child's expressive language skills, language modeling can include semantic targets (vocabulary, word knowledge), syntactic targets (combining words into sentences) or pragmatic targets (social use of language). For early language learners (MLU = 1.00–2.00) and some children with autism, we ask adults to use "I" when modeling language as if they are speaking in the child's voice to offset their frequent issues with pronoun reversal. For example, when the adult is mirroring and mapping the child's action while playing with playdoh, the adult can model "I make a playdoh snake!" When the child makes a nonverbal request to the adult by trying to take the train the adult is holding, she can model "I want your train mama!" The criteria for language modeling is that at least half of what the adult says in interactions with the child should be at the child's targeted language level.

Environmental Arrangement for Requests

The environmental arrangement that was discussed earlier in this chapter involved arranging the environment to promote connection between adults and children. Adults can also arrange the environment to promote child requesting. Child requests present the adult with opportunities to scaffold that communication into more elaborated forms because the child's motivation for communicating is potentially the highest when he wants something from the adult (attention, tangible, assistance). When adults set up the environment for requests they are making themselves an important component in the interaction with the child, which makes it easier for the child to connect with the adult when communicating. Environmental arrangement can increase the child's engagement with his environment, including the adult, which then can provide more opportunities for the adult to communicate with the child, elicit communicative responses from the child, to model appropriate language forms and to respond contingently to verbal and nonverbal communication attempts.

Environmental arrangement includes selecting, arranging or managing toys and materials in ways that set up opportunities for the child to request that the adult be included in the interaction by providing attention, a tangible object or assistance. Adults can provide children with an opportunity to initiate a request by selecting toys or materials that require assistance to open the packaging (top off the playdoh can), help with the toy (blowing bubbles) or help putting the toy together so they can play with it (connecting train tracks). Additionally, the adult can select toys that are more fun with a partner or require a partner participate (throwing and catching a ball, board or card games). Adults can use environmental arrangement when arranging materials by having items where children can see the item but can't reach it (on a counter, shelf) and need the adult's assistance. The adult can also store materials in clear bins with locking tops or Ziploc bags that require adult help to open. Lastly, the adult can manage toys or materials in ways that set up opportunities for possible child requests by not providing all of the items at once (one piece of candy, one crayon, one car) or only providing half of what a child needs to complete a favorite activity (potato head and no body parts, paper but no markers, shape sorter with no shapes).

The adult needs to be judicious with the use of these environmental arrangement strategies to set up requesting opportunities since these are demands placed on the child to elicit more elaborated communication forms. Using too many of these strategies in a short period of time could be experienced by the child as roadblocks and could disrupt the adult-child connection that is foundational to accelerated language learning.

Prompting Strategies

The last EMT strategy is Milieu Teaching (the MT in EMT), which includes strategies to prompt children to use more elaborated or new language forms. Milieu Teaching strategies have been discussed in detail in many previous publications (see for example, Hancock & Kaiser, 2009) so this chapter will briefly summarize the most important considerations when implementing Milieu Teaching. To ensure this teaching strategy is consistent with the responsive nature of the intervention (the E in EMT), adults should only prompt in response to child-initiated requests (gestural or verbal), which has been termed incidental teaching (Hancock & Kaiser, 2009). Incidental teaching allows the child to be in charge of the interaction by initiating a request to the adult and ensures that the child is motivated and interested before the adult prompts for more elaborated communication.

For Milieu Teaching to be the most effective, adults should have specific information about the child's projected target language level because those language (or communication) forms become the content of the prompt. If the child initiates a request that is at this target level, the adult responds to the child's request with the assistance, object or attention needed and expands the child's communication form. If the child's request is below this targeted level, the adult can use a Milieu Teaching prompt to support the child in using a more elaborated form either at the targeted level or closer to the targeted level. These prompts are sequenced from a most-to-least hierarchical support (model, questions/mands to talk, time delay) so that children are progressing from imitating the adult (model) to independently initiating (time delay) targeted communication forms. The adult can provide the child with a model prompt to imitate ("say Mama look"). The adult can provide a question prompt ("do you want juice or milk?") or a mand to talk prompt ("tell me what you want") as a way to cue the child that more elaborated communication is important. Lastly, the adult can use a time delay prompt by actively waiting (eye contact with the child, holding the item the child requested) to signal that the adult expects the child can make a more linguistically complex request. The prompting sequence should be brief and always end with the child receiving the requested item/assistance and the adult providing targeted language modeling or expanding the child's communication. In previous descriptions of Milieu Teaching, for the prompting sequence to be counted as correct implementation, the adult needed to provide a specific number of prompts when the child was not responding to the adult prompt with a targeted level form. To use Milieu Teaching strategies in a more responsive individualized manner, the adult can determine how many prompts to use based on the child's ability and attention. Additionally, these prompting procedures need to be used very judiciously so as not to disrupt the adult-child connection or imbalance the equality of the interaction. To illustrate the relationship of the EMT strategies, we use a triangle that shows Following the Lead is foundational to the intervention and should be used frequently and that Milieu Teaching is used very infrequently and only when all of the other strategies are in place (see Fig. 7.1).

Considerations When Implementing EMT

EMT is a complex intervention so even when parents and therapists are provided with specific definitions of EMT strategies and multiple implementation examples, it can be difficult to implement with fidelity. Most of the published (and unpublished) studies investigating EMT (see Review of Empirical Support for EMT section in this chapter) were conducted with English speaking children who were between 2.5 and 5 years of age, had a base vocabulary of at least ten words and were verbally imitative. More recent studies are beginning to investigate the clinical use of EMT with children outside of this narrow range (children who are non-verbal, school aged, or Spanish speakers) but currently there is very little practical information about how to adapt EMT in these situations so if children do not meet these criteria it can be very challenging to implement EMT. Currently, the authors are developing and evaluating an EMT model that can be implemented statewide with parents and their children who have been diagnosed with autism. In the process of investigating the feasibility and effectiveness of a statewide EMT system, the authors have included in the project all parents and their children who were interested in participating with no consideration to entry criteria other than an autism diagnosis (Hancock et al., in progress). This has broadened the types of children for whom EMT is being implemented and has provided opportunities for us to review and better understand the entry level skills that children may need before EMT can be successfully implemented including play, behavior and imitation skills.

While EMT can be implemented across the routines in a child's day (dressing, eating, bathing) it has been primarily used during adult-child play interactions. One of the unstated criteria for successful EMT implementation is that the child has the ability and desire to engage in functional play skills. It can be problematic to effectively implement EMT strategies when (a) children do not engage in play because of age or skill level or (b) their stereotypical behavior limits their ability to play functionally with objects. Without this foundational skill of play, it is very difficult to have a platform from which to build joint attention/joint engagement, which is a critical element of the EMT intervention. If children do not have foundational play skills or stereotypical/challenging behavior limits their ability to play in a functional manner, adults may want to consider implementing a play intervention similar to the one described by Lang and his colleagues (2010) that not only taught children specific play skills but also simultaneously decreased children's stereotypy and challenging behavior as a result of the play skills instruction. Additionally, toy play may not be the most developmentally appropriate framework for implementing EMT with older children. Given our current efforts of developing a statewide model delivery system to provide EMT services to children with autism who range in age from 3 to 15 years, we are investigating the use of EMT outside of toy play for older children (7–15 years of age). EMT may be effective with this age range when implemented in activities that include arts and crafts, board and card games, indoor/outdoor sports and other hobbies. One last consideration related to play interactions is that some adults may not be naturally skilled play partners, which may limit the effectiveness of EMT. When this is the case, supporting adults to be more engaging in their play and providing them with ideas for a richer play repertoire may be necessary. Creating play theme kits that adults can borrow (all of the materials in one box with multiple specific ideas for play activities), developing parent-to-parent play groups, or providing access to creative social media supports like Pinterest boards that are organized by toy/play schema possibilities may be important for adults to successfully implement EMT within a play framework.

Future Research Directions for EMT

There is a solid body of research investigating EMT over the last 20 years that demonstrates it is an effective language intervention when implemented by therapists and teachers (Hancock & Kaiser, 2002; Olive et al., 2007) or parents (Hancock et al., 2002; Hemmeter & Kaiser, 1994; Kaiser et al., 2000; Kaiser & Roberts, 2013) with preschool children who have significant language delays, children with diagnoses like Down syndrome and autism (Kaiser & Roberts, 2013), as well as young children who are at high risk for developing language delays (Hancock et al., 2002; Peterson et al., 2005). Despite this strong evidence base, research on EMT has been generally limited to intervening with preschool aged children (2½–5 years of age) who are early language learners (imitative, at least ten spontaneous words) and have significant language delays/disorders; intervention has been conducted following specific training procedures in English by therapists or parents over 20–36 sessions (Hancock & Kaiser, 2009; Hancock & Kaiser, 2012). To date, very little is known about the effects of EMT with children outside the preschool aged sample (younger than 2½ years; older than 5 years of age) who may have different entry language skills than previously researched (no verbal language or tested language within typical limits for children with autism). Very little research on EMT has included families other than those who are Euro-American or has been delivered in a language other than English. Parent-implemented EMT has generally followed a prescribed protocol including 20–36 individualized training sessions in the clinic (Kaiser & Hancock, 2003; Kaiser, Hancock, et al., 1998; Kaiser et al., 2007) with very little known about the effects of implementing EMT in a more efficient manner (fewer sessions, group parent sessions) using a variety of instructional methods (for example, remote learning at home using technology). The limits of EMT have not been tested or reported.

Diverse Families

Except for one recent study with teachers implementing EMT in Spanish with their preschool students (Calleja et al., 2014) there have been no published studies of EMT implemented in Spanish. A next logical step for EMT would be to test its use with Spanish speaking Hispanic families since they are the fastest growing minority population (U.S. Census Bureau, 2010) and Hispanic children are the largest culturally distinct ethnic group in the United States (Lopez & Velasco, 2011). While the number of Spanish-speaking Hispanic families with a child with autism spectrum disorder (ASD) is increasing (Coo et al., 2008; Magaña, Parish, Rose, Timberlake, & Swaine, 2012); to date, there are no empirically validated language interventions for this population (Kingsdorf, 2014). Hispanic children with ASD and language deficits raised in Spanish-speaking homes face a number of challenges not represented in samples used in previous research involving early language interventions for ASD (Hancock & Kaiser, 2002; Kaiser et al., 2000; Kingsdorf, 2014), including research published on EMT. Interventions and procedures (like EMT) evaluated with non-Hispanic participants should not be assumed effective with this population (e.g., Lang et al., 2011; Rispoli et al., 2011). Given the paucity of language intervention research with this population and a call for increased efforts to validate interventions to meet the needs of families from diverse cultural, linguistic, and socioeconomic backgrounds (Machalicek, Lang, & Raulston, 2015), it is imperative that interventions like EMT be tested to determine if they are sensitive to the cultural and linguistic diversity of Hispanic children with ASD (Rodriguez, 2009). The authors have recently submitted an application for a federal grant to investigate the effects of EMT with Spanish-speaking Hispanic parents and their children who have been diagnosed with ASD as a first step in understanding if EMT is effective, culturally sensitive and socially valid with this population.

More Efficient Delivery Models

Parents of children with autism often experience significantly higher levels of stress than parents of typically developing children and children with other developmental disabilities. These stressors include time pressures related to intense caregiving responsibilities and the time spent supporting their children in a variety of educational and therapeutic interventions (Karst & Van Hecke, 2012). In most published studies of EMT to date, the intervention was implemented by therapists and/or parents across a number of sessions ranging from a low of 20 sessions to the highest number being 36 sessions (Hancock & Kaiser, 2009, 2012). Not surprisingly, the parents who participated in the most EMT sessions displayed the highest fidelity of implementation data, including their ability to maintain the strategies over time and generalize across settings (clinic to home) and across untrained routines (snack, book reading) (Kaiser & Roberts, 2013). A limitation noted in almost every published parent implemented EMT study has been the significant investment of time that parents make when they participate in the project. While parents report in social validity measures of EMT that the positive outcomes for their children far outweighed the time devoted to training and practice (Hancock & Kaiser, 2012), many parents are not in a position to attend training with their child twice a week for 2–4 months. It is important given that EMT is considered a naturalistic language intervention, to investigate ways that EMT can contextually fit a family's needs and priorities through more efficient applications of this intervention.

The first step in developing EMT as a more efficient intervention model may be to examine dosage dependent effects by varying the number of sessions parents complete and measuring parent and child outcomes by number of sessions (Fey, Yoder, Warren, & Bredin-Oja, 2013; Machalicek et al., 2015). The authors have preliminary data on teaching parents EMT in six sessions (once a week for

Table 7.3 Parent criteria at intervention 6 on EMT strategies in the responsive interaction parent training project

Strategy	Criterion level (%)	Parent A	Parent B	Parent C
Matched turns	≥75	Yes	Yes	Yes
Responsiveness	≥80	Yes	Yes	Yes
Expansions	≥50	Yes	No	Yes
Target talk	≥50	Yes	Yes	No
Prompting	≥80	Yes	Yes	Yes

6 weeks) that show promising results in terms of parents being at criteria on the EMT strategies they are learning by the sixth session (see Table 7.3; Hancock, Lang & Ledbetter-Cho, in progress). While these preliminary data are promising in terms of parents being able to implement EMT at criteria in relatively few sessions, more research is needed on this brief approach to determine if parents can maintain their use of these strategies over time or if there are longer-term positive language effects for children.

To develop EMT into a more efficient and accessible language intervention, the next step may be to test different models of teaching parents EMT strategies including group training (Kaiser, Hemmeter, Ostrosky, Alpert, & Hancock, 1995) and distance learning options (for example, online access with Skype or video feedback). While there is no research on training parents in EMT strategies in a group format and only limited research on training parents in any communication intervention within a group setting, research on interventions like Pivotal Response Training show positive results not only in terms of parents learning the communication intervention strategies to fidelity within a group format, but also additional benefits like decreased parenting stress at the end of training (Minjarez, Mercier, Williams, & Hardan, 2012). Other formats for training parents of children with ASD, for example distance learning models, have been found to be effective in disseminating evidenced based practices to parents (Wainer & Ingersoll, 2013) and hold promise for parents learning EMT concepts and strategies in more time and personnel efficient ways.

It is important in the next generation of EMT research to test ways to adapt this intervention to include more non-traditional implementation methods that will allow families who have not previously been included in EMT research to access this intervention. These adaptations include but are not limited to making EMT available to culturally and linguistically diverse families (Spanish implementation with Hispanic families), families who live in rural locations (distance learning EMT) as well as families who may have limited time resources because of work or other family commitments (group training). While testing these un-traditional models of EMT, it will be important to determine under which contexts parents can implement EMT at sufficient levels of fidelity to positively impact their children's long-term language and communication development.

References

Bakeman, R., & Adamson, L. (1984). Coordinating attention to people and objects in mother-infant and peer-infant interaction. *Child Development, 55*, 1278–1289.

Bruner, J. S. (1975). The ontogenesis of speech acts. *Journal of Child Language, 2*, 1–19.

Calleja, M., Rodríguez, J. M., & Luque, M. L. (2014). La utilidad del procedimiento del Milieu Teaching Mejorado en bebés con severos problemas de comunicación y lenguaje en el contexto clínico. *Revista de Investigación en Logopedia, 4*, 28–47.

Coo, H., Ouellette-Kuntz, H., Lloyd, J. E. V., Kasmara, E. L., Holden, J. J., & Lewis, M. E. (2008). Trends in autism prevalence: Diagnostic substitution revised. *Journal of Autism and Developmental Disorders, 38*, 1036–1046.

Fey, M. E., Yoder, P. J., Warren, S. F., & Bredin-Oja, S. (2013). Is more better? Milieu communication teaching in toddlers with intellectual disabilities. *Journal of Speech, Language, and Hearing Research, 58*, 679–693.

Hancock, T. B., Lang, R., & Ledbetter-Cho, K. (in progress). The effects of a brief EMT-based intervention when implemented by parents of children with autism.

Hancock, T. B., & Kaiser, A. P. (2002). The effects of trainer-implemented enhanced milieu teaching on the social communication of children who have autism. *Topics in Early Childhood Special Education, 22*, 39–54.

Hancock, T. B., & Kaiser, A. P. (2009). Enhanced milieu teaching. In R. McCauley & M. Fey (Eds.), *Treatment of language disorders in children*. Baltimore, MD: Paul Brookes.

Hancock, T. B., & Kaiser, A. P. (2012). Implementing enhanced milieu teaching with children who have autism spectrum disorders. In P. Prelock & R. McCauley (Eds.), *Treatment of autism spectrum disorders: Evidence-based intervention strategies for communication & social interaction*. Baltimore, MD: Paul Brookes.

Hancock, T. B., Kaiser, A. P., & Delaney, E. M. (2002). Teaching parents of preschoolers at high risk: Strategies to support language and positive behavior. *Topics in Early Childhood Special Education, 22*, 191–212.

Hemmeter, M. L., & Kaiser, A. P. (1994). Enhanced milieu teaching: Effects of parent-implemented language intervention. *Journal of Early Intervention, 18*, 269–289.

Ingersoll, B. (2010). Teaching social communication: A comparison of naturalistic behavioral and development, social pragmatic approaches for children with autism spectrum disorders. *Journal of Positive Behavior Interventions, 12*, 33–43.

Kaiser, A. P., Alpert, C. L., Fischer, R., Hemmeter, M. L., Tiernan, M., & Ostrosky, M. (1990). *Analysis of the primary and generalized effects of milieu and responsive-interaction teaching by parents*. Paper presented at the annual meeting of the Division of Early Childhood, Albuquerque.

Kaiser, A. P., & Hancock, T. B. (2000). *Supporting children's communication development through parent-implemented naturalistic interventions*. Presented at the 2nd annual conference on Research Innovations in Early Intervention (CRIEI), San Diego.

Kaiser, A. P., & Hancock, T. B. (2003). Teaching parents new skills to support their young children's development. *Infants and Young Children, 16*, 9–21.

Kaiser, A. P., Hancock, T. B., & Hester, P. P. (1998). Parents as co-interventionists: Research on applications of naturalistic language teaching procedures. *Infants and Young Children, 10*, 1–11.

Kaiser, A. P., Hancock, T. B., & Nietfeld, J. P. (2000). The effects of parent-implemented enhanced milieu teaching on the social communication of children who have autism. *Journal of Early Education and Development, 4*, 423–446.

Kaiser, A. P., Hancock, T. B., & Trent, J. A. (2007). Teaching parents communication strategies. *Early Childhood Services: An Interdisciplinary Journal of Effectiveness, 1*, 107–136.

Kaiser, A. P., Hemmeter, M. L., Ostrosky, M. M., Alpert, C. L., & Hancock, T. B. (1995). The effects of group training and individual feedback on parent use of milieu teaching. *Journal of Childhood Communications Disorders, 16*, 39–48.

Kaiser, A. P., & Hester, P. P. (1994). Generalized effects of enhanced milieu teaching. *Journal of Speech, Language, and Hearing Research, 37*, 1320–1340.

Kaiser, A. P., Lambert, W., Hancock, T. B., & Hester, P. P. (1998, March). *The effects of naturalistic intervention on vocabulary growth.* Paper presented at the 32nd Annual Gatlinburg Conference on Research and Theory in Mental Retardation and Developmental Disabilities, Charleston, SC.

Kaiser, A. P., & Roberts, M. Y. (2013). Parent-implemented enhanced milieu teaching with preschool children who have intellectual disabilities. *Journal of Speech, Language, and Hearing Research, 56*, 295–309.

Karst, J. S., & Van Hecke, A. V. (2012). Parent and family impact of autism spectrum disorders: A review and proposed model for intervention evaluation. *Clinical Child and Family Psychological Review, 15*, 247–277.

Kasari, C., Freeman, S., & Paparella, T. (2006). Joint attention and symbolic play in young children with autism: A randomized controlled intervention study. *Journal of Child Psychology and Psychiatry, 47*(6), 611–620.

Kasari, C., Gulsrud, A. C., Wong, C., Kwon, S., & Locke, J. (2010). A randomized controlled caregiver mediated joint engagement intervention for toddlers with autism. *Journal of Autism and Developmental Disorders, 40*, 1045–1056.

Kasari, C., et al. (2014). Communication interventions for minimally verbal children with autism: A sequential multiple assignment randomized trial. *Child and Adolescent Psychiatry, 53*(6), 635–646.

Kingsdorf, S. (2014). Do you speak my language? Are behavior analysts considering the needs of learners on the autism spectrum? *Childhood Education, 90*, 143–147.

Lang, R., O' Reilly, M., Sigafoos, J., Machalicek, W., Rispoli, M., Lancioni, G., … Fragale, C. (2010). The effects of an abolishing operation intervention component on play skills, challenging behavior and stereotypy. *Behavior Modification, 34*, 267–289.

Lang, R., Rispoli, M., Sigafoos, J., Lancioni, G., Andrews, A., & Ortega, L. (2011). Effects of language of Instruction on response accuracy and challenging behavior in a child with autism. *Journal of Behavioral Education, 20*, 252–259.

Lopez, M. H., & Velasco, G. (2011). *The toll of the great recession childhood poverty among Hispanics set records, leads nation*. Washington, DC: Pew Hispanic center. Available at http://www.pewhispanic.org/files/2011/10/147.pdf.

Machalicek, W., Lang, R., & Raulston, T. J. (2015). Training parents of children with intellectual disabilities: Trends, issues and future directions. *Current Developmental Disorder Report, 2*, 110–118.

Magaña, S., Parish, S. L., Rose, R. A., Timberlake, M., & Swaine, J. G. (2012). Racial and ethnic disparities in quality of health care among children with autism and other developmental disabilities. *Intellectual and Developmental Disabilities, 50*, 287–299.

Minjarez, M. B., Mercier, E. M., Williams, S. E., & Hardan, A. Y. (2012). Impact of pivotal response training group therapy on stress and empowerment in parents of children with autism. *Journal of Positive Behavior Interventions, 15*, 71–78.

Nunes, D., & Hanline, M. F. (2007). Enhancing the alternative and augmentative communication use of a child with autism through a parent-implemented naturalistic intervention. *International Journal of Disability, Development and Intervention, 54*, 177–197.

Olive, M. L., de la Cruz, B., Davis, T. N., Chan, J. M., Lang, R. B., O'Reilly, M. F., Dickson, S. M. (2007). The effects of enhanced milieu teaching and a voice output communication aid on the requesting of three children with autism. *Journal of Autism and Developmental Disorders, 37*, 1505–1513.

Peterson, P., Carta, J. J., & Greenwood, C. (2005). Teaching enhanced milieu language teaching skills to parents in multiple risk families. *Journal of Early Intervention, 27*, 94–102.

Ratner, N., & Bruner, J. (1978). Games, social exchange, and the acquisition of language. *Journal of Child Language, 5*, 391–401.

Rispoli, M., O'Reilly, M., Lang, R., Sigafoos, F., Mulloy, A., Aguilar, J., & Singer, G. (2011). Effects of language of implementation on functional analysis outcomes. *Journal of Behavioral Education, 20*, 224–232.

Roberts, M. Y., & Kaiser, A. P. (2012). Assessing the effects of a parent-implemented language intervention for children with language impairments using empirical benchmarks: A pilot study. *Journal of Speech, Language, and Hearing Research, 55*, 1655–1670.

Roberts, M. Y., Kaiser, A. P., Wolfe, C. E., Bryant, J. D., & Spidalieri, A. M. (2014). Effects of the teach-model-coach-review instructional approach on caregiver use of language support strategies and children's expressive language use. *Journal of Speech, Language, and Hearing Research, 57*, 1851–1869.

Rodriguez, D. (2009). Culturally and linguistically diverse students with autism. *Childhood Education, 85*, 313–317.

Scherer, N., & Kaiser, A. (2007). Early intervention for children with cleft palate. *Infants and Young Children, 20*, 355–366.

Scherer, N., & Kaiser, A. (2010). Enhanced milieu teaching/Phonological emphasis: Application for children with cleft lip and palate. In L. Williams, R. McCauley, & S. McLeod (Eds.), *Speech sound disorders in children* (pp. 427–452). Baltimore, MA: Brookes.

Stokes, T. F., & Baer, D. M. (1977). An implicit technology of generalization. *Journal of Applied Behavior Analysis, 10*, 349–367.

U.S. Census Bureau. (2010). *Overview of race and Hispanic origin*. Washington, DC: U.S. Census Bureau. Retrieved from http://census.gov/prod/cen2010/briefs/c2010br-02.pdf.

Wainer, A. L., & Ingersoll, B. R. (2013). Disseminating ASD interventions: A pilot study of a distance learning program for parents and professionals. *Journal of Autism and Developmental Disorders, 43*, 11–24.

Wright, C. A., Kaiser, A. P., Reikowsky, D. I., & Roberts, M. Y. (2013). Effects of a naturalistic sign intervention on expressive language of toddlers with Down syndrome. *Journal of Speech, Language, and Hearing Research, 56*, 994–1006.

Chapter 8
Training Parents to Implement Early Interventions for Children with Autism Spectrum Disorders

Traci Ruppert, Wendy Machalicek, Sarah G. Hansen, Tracy Raulston, and Rebecca Frantz

Introduction

Early Intervention (EI) for young children with disabilities such as autism spectrum disorder (ASD) is heavily influenced by ecological and family systems theories (Brofenbrenner, 1986; Bruder, 2000). At the crux of these theories are the empirically demonstrated bidirectional and transactional interactions within family units and their dynamic effects on children and their families (Sy, Gottfried, & Gottfried, 2013). Interventions addressing any part of the family unit (e.g. parent or child skill acquisition) may result in more positive child outcomes (Bailey, Raspa, & Fox, 2012; Guralnick, 2011) and/or improved parent and family outcomes (Dunst, Bruder, & Espe-Sherwindt, 2014; Espe-Sherwindt, 2008). Family-centered EI that includes parent education has been linked to improved child outcomes, more positive parent perceptions of child behavior, and greater perceptions of parental self-efficacy (Noyes-Grosser et al., 2014; Strauss et al., 2012). Moreover, federal legislation (i.e., PL 99-457; Individuals with Disabilities Education Act, 2004) supports family-centered practices in EI (e.g. active family participation in Individualized Family Service Plans (IFSPs); Beckman & Bristol, 1991; Bruder, 2000).

Accordingly, EI for young children with or at risk for ASD includes family-centered capacity building and helpgiving practices in natural contexts such as family homes (Bailey et al., 2012; Friend, Summers, & Turnbull, 2009; Mahoney et al., 1999). Increasingly, research indicates that earlier, more intensive intervention for young children (infants and toddlers) with or at risk for ASD delivered by trained

T. Ruppert • W. Machalicek (✉) • S.G. Hansen • T. Raulston • R. Frantz
Department of Special Education and Clinical Sciences, University of Oregon, Eugene, OR 97403-1235, USA
e-mail: wmachali@uoregon.edu

R. Lang et al. (eds.), *Early Intervention for Young Children with Autism Spectrum Disorder*, Evidence-Based Practices in Behavioral Health,
DOI 10.1007/978-3-319-30925-5_8

and supervised therapists improves outcomes (Dawson et al., 2012; Peters-Scheffer, Didden, Korzilius, & Sturmey, 2011; Wallace & Rogers, 2010). However, parents of children with ASD have a pivotal role in EI as care providers, interventionists, and early language and play partners (Kasari, Lawton, Shih et al., 2014). In keeping with other EI services, early intensive behavior intervention (EIBI) (McConachie & Diggle, 2006) and focused, targeted behavioral interventions (e.g. Nefdt, Koegel, Singer, & Gerber, 2010; Schertz, Odom, Baggett, & Sideris, 2013) for young children with ASD oftentimes involves parents as interventionists or parent-mediated EI.

However, the appropriateness of expecting parents to be their child's teacher in EI has been questioned (Mahoney et al., 1999). Specific criticisms have included undue burden on parents (Rosenberg & Robinson, 1988) and tacit responsibility of the parent for their child's current state of developmental delays (Turnbull & Turnbull, 1990). Additionally, the outcomes of parent-mediated intervention may suffer from a parent's lack of time to implement and manage the intervention, barriers to accessing resources and technical knowledge, and difficulties adapting to the teacher role (Bagner & Graziano, 2012). Moreover, expecting parents to deliver large amounts of intervention could add significant stress to a population already at risk for stress and depression (Hodge & Runswick-Cole, 2008). While parenting any young child is both stressful and rewarding, parenting a young child with ASD has been shown to be potentially more stressful than a child who is typically developing, or even a child with another disability or developmental delay (Benson, 2006; Davis & Carter, 2008). High levels of parent stress can interfere with treatment adherence, reduce the likelihood the parent uses new skills, and decrease positive child outcomes (Osborne, McHugh, Saunders, & Reed, 2008). Despite these cautions, an extensive and growing body of literature suggests mostly positive effects from training and supporting parents to implement interventions to address the core symptoms of their child's ASD (Oono, Honey, & McConachie, 2013; Strauss, Mancini, the SPC Group, & Fava, 2013).

Myriad studies indicate that EIBI can reduce core deficits in ASD such as social communication and language delay, rigid and repetitive behaviors and interests, and common comorbidities such as challenging behavior (Howlin, Magiati, & Charman, 2009; Makrygianni & Reed, 2010; Matson & Konst, 2013; McConachie & Diggle, 2006). Importantly, more positive child outcomes are seen with intensive (i.e. 20–40 h per week) services (Matson & Konst, 2013; Warren et al., 2011). Trained and supported parents and other caregivers can help to meet this high dosage (i.e. hours of direct intervention) of EIBI by delivering intervention during everyday family routines. Parent training for the implementation of EIBI is also cost effective, allows intervention to take place in the natural setting and increases opportunities for intervention and generalization of learned skills (Diggle, McConachie, & Randle, 2002).

Parents are uniquely able to intervene within common routines (e.g. bedtime, meals) and in an array of natural settings (e.g. home, playground, grocery store) and are often highly motivated to learn new strategies for supporting their child's development as the gains directly impact them. Gains made with parent interventionists in the natural environment can allow for easier generalization than skills taught exclusively in a clinic or school setting (Makrygianni & Reed, 2010; McConachie & Diggle, 2006). Moreover, parent's routine involvement in intervention planning and implementation can provide interventionists with important opportunities to individualize a child's treatment plan, and can increase the acceptability and feasibility of interventions (Kaiser & Hancock, 2003; Mahoney et al., 1999; Woods, Kashinath, & Goldstein, 2004). Research on parent-mediated intervention in a variety of settings and intervention modes has shown that when trained with fidelity, parents can be effective interventionists (Kaminski, Valle, Filene, & Boyle, 2008). With support from professionals, parents can effectively assess, intervene, and monitor their child's progress (Benzies, Magill-Evans, Hayden, & Ballantyne, 2013; Patterson, Smith, & Mirenda, 2012). The efficacy of parent-mediated intervention has been shown with a variety of skills, such as Discrete Trial Teaching (DTT; e.g. Lafasakis & Sturmey, 2007), Pivotal Response Training (PRT; e.g. Coolican, Smith, & Bryson, 2010) and packaged interventions (e.g. Oono et al., 2013).

A number of recent reviews have summarized the procedures and outcomes of parent-mediated early intervention with young children with ASD (e.g. Oono et al., 2013; Singer, Ethridge, & Aldana, 2007) and there are numerous topical reviews discussing the results of research addressing the core symptoms of ASD which include parents among other adult change agents as interventionists (Fettig & Barton, 2014; Meadan, Ostrosky, Zaghlawan, & Yu, 2009; Patterson et al., 2012; Roberts & Kaiser, 2011; Strauss et al., 2013; White et al., 2011). For instance, Lang, Machalicek, Rispoli, and Regester (2009) examined the available literature on training parents to implement communication interventions. Results indicated a range of research on parent-mediated communication intervention with a variety of strategies including PRT, Enhanced Milieu Training (EMT) and Early Start Denver Model (ESDM). Barton and Fettig (2013) conducted a review on attempts to incorporate parents into function-based interventions on challenging behavior, and showed several successful coaching strategies for the training of parents to implement interventions with fidelity. The literature on parent implemented EIBI for children with autism has also been reviewed more broadly, showing positive results for a range of formats and specific targets (Oono et al., 2013) However, the literature is vast, scattered across multiple disciplines and peer-reviewed journals, and varies in quality.

The purpose of the current chapter is to selectively summarize research related to parent-mediated EI for young children, ages 12–60 months, with or at risk for ASD, and to offer suggestions for practice and future research. The remainder of this chapter is organized into the seven sections of (a) overview of parent involvement in early intervention; (b) targeted parent skills and desired outcomes; (c) parent education and training methods; (d) training parents to address core symptoms of ASD; (e) summary and suggestions for future research; (f) implications for practice; and (g) conclusion.

Overview of Parent Involvement in Early Intervention

Parent involvement is EI and EIBI for young children with ASD is commonplace and well supported by the inclusion of family-centered practices in federally funded EI services (Bailey et al., 2012; Beckman & Bristol, 1991; Bruder, 2000; IDEA, 1990, 1997; IDEIA, 2004) and the provision of private insurance funding for medically necessary applied behavior analysis (Autism Speaks, 2015). Additionally, recent reviews of interventions involving parents of children with developmental disabilities including ASD validates the ubiquitous involvement of parents in EI (Brookman-Frazee, Stahmer, Baker-Ericzèn, & Tsai, 2006; Diggle et al., 2002; Hastings, Robertson, & Yasamy, 2012; Lang et al., 2009; McConachie & Diggle, 2006; Oono et al., 2013; Patterson et al., 2012; Roberts & Kaiser, 2011; Strauss et al., 2013). Parents have been involved in EI and EIBI by: (a) implementing intervention, (b) providing input about intervention procedures, (c) collaborating on the development of a behavior intervention plan, (d) informing a functional behavior assessment (FBA) or participating in an experimental functional analysis to determine the consequences maintaining challenging behavior, (e) taking data, (f) answering questions about the feasibility and acceptability of the goals, procedures, and outcomes of the intervention, and (g) teaching others intervention strategies (Machalicek et al., 2014).

Despite parents' documented participation in EI and in research efforts in this area, we know relatively little about how well currently utilized interventions work to reduce the symptoms of ASD for diverse participants. In the literature, there is a worrisome absence of participant demographic information such as ethnicity/race, socio economic status, and severity of ASD diagnosis and adaptive behavior profiles. Additionally, intervention setting and the format (e.g. group based, one to one, online) of parent training are inconsistently reported. These gaps in the literature make it difficult to determine for whom parent training strategies and parent implemented interventions are most effective, Nevertheless, we can state some general known facts about the children and parents who have participated in parent-implemented early intervention research over the last 18 years (Machalicek et al., 2014). Although exceptions exist (Elder, Valcante, Won, & Zylis, 2003), mothers are more commonly interventionists in parent-implemented intervention for children with intellectual and developmental disabilities such as ASD (Flippin & Crais, 2011). This finding is not restricted to ASD and occurs across disability category (Fabiano, 2007; Tiano & McNeil, 2005). When reported, the ethnicity/race of participating parents is more often White or Hispanic/Latino than another ethnicity/race (Machalicek et al., 2014). This finding is not restricted to parent implemented intervention and likely reflects a larger problem of lack of diverse participant recruitment in special education research (Artiles, Trent, & Kuan, 1997; Vasquez III et al., 2011).

Parents of children with ASD have been effectively taught to implement a variety of focused interventions to increase their child's social communication skills (e.g. Roberts & Kaiser, 2011) and to decrease challenging behavior (e.g. Brookman-Frazee et al., 2006; Fettig & Barton, 2014). Parents have also been taught to implement one or more components of early intensive applied behavior analysis focused on all educational and behavioral needs related to ASD (EIBA; e.g. Strauss et al., 2012). The focus of parent education programs on improving child social communication and on decreasing challenging behavior is well-aligned with the core diagnostic criteria of ASD. However, outside of EIBA programs, few parent-implemented interventions exist in the areas of functional life or self-help skills (e.g. dressing, bathing), feeding (see Najdowski et al., 2010), toileting (see Kroeger & Sorensen, 2010; Rinald & Mirenda, 2012) and sleep interventions (see Malow et al., 2014).

Group-based parent education is more commonly used than one-to-one parent training and the use of online technology (e.g. online learning modules, use of telecommunication technology such as laptop computers with wireless headset and videoconferencing software) to facilitate the delivery of parent education is rapidly growing, but until relatively recently, has been absent in the literature. A number of parent education interventions have been delivered via online technology (e.g. Machalicek et al., in press; McDuffie et al., 2013; McDuffie, Bullard, Nelson, Machalicek, & Abbeduto, in press).

Targeted Parent Skills and Desired Outcomes

Parent involvement in EI is typically focused on capacity-building interventions that support the parent to implement interventions addressing the core characteristics of ASD. However, EI also involves helpgiving interventions such as respite care, case management, and helping the parent to access existing social supports and community resources (Dunst, Trivette, & Hamby, 2006, 2007, 2008; Dunst, Trivette, Humphries, Raab, & Roper, 2001). This chapter focuses on the role of parents as interventionists rather than recipients of helpgiving interventions, but we also acknowledge the oftentimes necessity of using a team-based approach to moderate the impact of parent mental health symptoms. Although it is well-understood that both family-centered capacity-building and helpgiving practices positively influence child and family outcomes, most behavioral interventions for children with ASD focus exclusively on child outcomes, with an emphasis on managing the child's behavior (Blackledge & Hayes, 2006). Considering that parents of children with ASD experience greater levels of parental stress and depression than parents of either typically developing children or children with other developmental disabilities (Falk, Norris, & Quinn, 2014), which may in turn influence less positive intervention outcomes, it is critical to target parental mental health outcomes in behavioral interventions for children with ASD. Therefore, in this section, we discuss both interventions aimed at teaching parents new skills (i.e. parent skill acquisition) to use with their children and interventions aimed at decreasing stress and depression of parents.

Parent Education and Training Delivery Methods to Increase Parent Skills

As previously discussed, parents of young children with ASD have successfully implemented both individualized and packaged interventions to improve their child's social communication (Mahoney & Perales, 2005; Vismara & Rogers, 2008) and to decrease challenging behavior (Moes & Frea, 2002). Parents have also effectively implemented interventions to teach their child other adaptive behavior skills including school-readiness skills (Lafasakis & Sturmey, 2007), and age appropriate functional life skills such as making a simple snack (Shipley-Benamou, Lutzker, & Taubman, 2002). Consequently, much research is concentrated on increasing parent skill acquisition. This body of parent skill acquisition research can be categorized into three main categories based on the format and delivery modality of parent education: (a) Group-based parent education and training, (b) Individualized parent education and coaching, and (c) Internet-based parent training.

Parent training components across these three categories of parent education and training provide information through (a) didactic or written means (i.e. handouts, manual); (b) in-vivo modeling or video modeling the procedures; (c) involving the parents in role plays; and (d) providing corrective feedback while the parent practices targeted intervention strategies with their child. Past research suggests that performance feedback is the essential component in behavioral parent training that improves adult use of evidence-based strategies (Alvero, Bucklin, & Austin, 2001; Barton & Fettig, 2013; Hattie & Timperley, 2007; Sprick, Knight, Reinke, Skyles, & Barnes, 2010). Common elements in performance feedback protocols include: (a) positive feedback for strategies implemented correctly, (b) corrective feedback for strategies not implemented correctly, and (c) ensuring understanding of corrective feedback by asking questions or asking the individual to repeat corrective feedback (O'Reilly et al., 1992; Parsons & Reid, 1995). The reader can refer to Table 8.1 for a concise, defined list of common evidence-based components of parent education and training programs.

Group-Based Parent Education and Training

Group-based behavioral parent education programs deliver manualized material based on social learning principals to small groups of parents (i.e. 8–12 participants) over weekly sessions. They typically use randomized control group trials with wait-list control groups to evaluate outcomes. Group-based programs take a public health perspective to family intervention. They explicitly recognize the role of the broader ecological context for human development by changing the community context of parenting (Biglan, 1995; National Institute of Mental Health, 1998; Sanders, 1999). The larger system of intervention aims to change this broader ecological context of parenting by normalizing parenting experiences (particularly the

Table 8.1 Glossary of parent education, training, and coaching terms

Term	Operational definition
Behavior skills training (BST)	Includes a combination of individual or group instruction with modeling, role-play or behavioral rehearsal with performance feedback, and parent demonstration of a set of skills to a specified mastery criterion.
Behavioral rehearsal	Practice of a complex skill under simulated conditions with performance feedback including praise and correction. Often includes modeling and role-play
Delayed coaching/ performance feedback	Involves a parent coach or other professional providing verbal and/or nonverbal (e.g. gestures, facial expressions) information after a parent has performed a skill. The time between the parent performing the skill and receiving feedback from a professional varies. Information includes praise for correct demonstrations of skills and correction for incorrect demonstrations. Delayed coaching and performance feedback can be delivered in different methods including in person or through teleconsultation. Delayed teleconsultation often involves a parent coach and parent viewing a video of the parent and child while the coach delivers performance feedback.
Discussion	A trainer presents information to an audience (individual or group) and guides conversation to promote learning.
Immediate coaching/ performance feedback	Involves a parent trainer or coach providing verbal and/or nonverbal (e.g. gestures, facial expressions) information during or immediately after a parent is performing a skill. The information includes praise for correct demonstrations of skills and correction for incorrect demonstrations. Coaching and performance feedback can be delivered in different methods including in person or through teleconsultation.
In vivo modeling	A teaching strategy wherein a parent trainer or coach demonstrates a skill live, often in the family's home, with the intention of the parent imitating it immediately afterward or later. Modeling is showing the parent how to perform a skill.
Lecture	Includes didactic based delivery of information in an individual or group format to promote procedural or conceptual learning.
Role play	A type of behavioral rehearsal that includes the parent practicing the targeted skill with a confederate.
Video modeling	Video demonstrations of a skill intended to teach or cue a parent to perform/imitate the skill. Video modeling can include another person performing the skill or the parent performing the skill, which would be video self-modeling.

Note. Definitions include information from "Behavior Analysis for Lasting Change" by G. R. Mayer, B. Sulzer-Azaroff, and M. Wallace

process of participating in parent education), breaking down parents' sense of social isolation, increasing social and emotional support from others in the community, and to validate and acknowledge publicly the importance and difficulties of parenting (Sanders, 1999). This method of parent education has its advantages.

Group-based programs may require more resources to implement, but they are still more cost efficient than individually delivered interventions (McIntyre & Phaneuf, 2007). Not only is there a low individual training cost when used in groups, but also the possibility of mass dissemination (Webster-Stratton, 2001). Another advantage is the support and kinship available from other participants, which could lead to increased parental engagement with the intervention and the children's early education programs (McIntyre & Phaneuf, 2007).

The majority of group-based parent education programs for parents of children with autism have been adapted from research-based programs for parents of children with behavioral difficulties or other developmental disabilities. They have focused on teaching parents to acquire behavior management skills.

For example, Webster-Stratton's *Incredible Years* (Webster-Stratton, 2001) is a video-based parent intervention for parents of children ages 0–13 years. They offer four separate age range programs that includes age-appropriate video examples (i.e. infant (0–1 years), toddler (1–3 years), preschool (3–6 years), and school age (6–13 years)). The program procedures consist of a lead therapist showing video vignettes of modeled parenting skills to groups of 8–12 parents. The videos demonstrate social learning and child development principles and serve as the stimulus for focused discussions, problem solving, and collaborative learning. Depending on child age, 8–20 weekly sessions of 2-h in length are held. The efficacy has been demonstrated in numerous published randomized control group trials (RCT) by the program developer et al. (Reid, Webster-Stratton, & Hammond, 2007; Webster-Stratton, 1984; Webster-Stratton & Hammond, 1997; Webster-Stratton, Hollinsworth, & Kolpacoff, 1989; Webster-Stratton, Kolpacoff, & Hollinsworth, 1988; Webster-Stratton, Reid, & Hammond, 2004). In all of these studies, the program has been shown to improve parental attitudes and parent-child interactions. It also reduces harsh discipline and child conduct problems compared with both wait-list control groups. A treatment component analysis indicated that the combination of group discussion, trained therapist, and video modeling produced the most lasting results compared with treatment that involved only one training component (Webster-Stratton et al., 1988, 1989).

Sanders's *Triple P-Positive Parenting Program* (Sanders, 1999) is a multilevel, preventively oriented parenting and family support strategy that aims to prevent severe behavioral, emotional, and developmental problems in children by enhancing the knowledge, skills, and confidence of parents. There are five levels of intervention on a tiered continuum of increasing strength for parents of children from birth to age 16 (Sanders, Cann, & Markie-Dadds, 2003). Level 1 provides universal parent information about parenting through print and electronic media, as well as user friendly parenting tip sheets and videotapes which demonstrate specific parenting strategies. Level 2 is one- to two-sessions and provides early anticipatory developmental guidance to parents of children with mild behavior difficulties. Level 3 is four-sessions and includes active skills training for parents with children who have mild to moderate behavior difficulties. Level 4 is up to 12, 1-h intensive sessions that are delivered individually or in a group-based parent training format for children with more severe behavioral difficulties. Level 5 is up to 11, 60–90 min sessions for enhanced behavioral family intervention program for families where parenting difficulties are complicated by other sources of family distress (e.g. marital conflict, parental depression, or high levels of stress). The multilevel strategy was designed to maximize efficiency, contain costs, avoid waste and over-servicing, and to ensure the program has wide reach in the community (Sanders, 1999). In a meta-analysis and review of articles (Thomas & Zimmer-Gembeck, 2007), it was found that participation in Triple-P improved parenting (i.e. improving parental warmth, decreasing parental hostility, increasing parental self-efficacy, and reducing parental stress) and reduce negative child behaviors (i.e. aggression and extreme tantrums and opposition).

Individualized Parent Education and Coaching

The most common package used to train parents in a one to one fashion is behavioral parent training (BPT; Serketich & Dumas, 1996; Van Camp et al., 2008). BPT is based on the empirical and applied concepts of behavior modification and the principles of social learning theory (Maughan, Christiansen, Jenson, Olympia, & Clark, 2005). BPT is one of the most successful and well-researched approaches used in the treatment and prevention of child problem behavior with a large body of empirical support for its clinical utility (see Shaffer, Kotchick, Dorsey, & Forehand, 2004). BPT is often designed and implemented by someone considered an expert in parent training in a clinic or home setting. The education is focused on training the parents how to define behavior problems accurately, implement assessment measures that further define the problem and its intensity, and teach parents in the treatment plan that would be appropriate for the problems within their individual context (Briesmeister & Schaefer, 1998). BPT typically involves describing behavioral procedures, modeling of the procedures, including parents in role plays, and providing corrective feedback while the parent practices targeted intervention strategies with their child. One advantage of BPT is training parents who have more frequent influence on the child in their natural environment to manage the challenging behaviors will increase the likelihood that behavior change will occur, generalize, and maintain treatment gains (Maughan et al., 2005). Another advantage is addressing the parent's ability to deal with the challenging behaviors displayed by a child will decrease parental stress and increase parental confidence in the ability to manage the child (Baker-Ericzèn, Brookman-Frazee, & Stahmer, 2005). Due to the shortage of mental health professionals, there may not be enough qualified therapists to treat all children individually; therefore, training parents also provides greater economy and cost-effectiveness (Maughan et al., 2005).

There is a vast and growing literature related to behavioral parent training for parents of children with ASD (Brookman-Frazee et al., 2006; Kaminski et al., 2008; Matson, Mahan, & LoVullo, 2009; Matson, Mahan, & Matson, 2009). The majority of studies have focused on (a) challenging behavior, (b) social communication (i.e. picture exchange communication system (PECS), (c) pivotal response training (PRT), (d) functional assessment, and (e) early intervention (i.e. Early Intensive Behavioral Intervention (EIBI); Early Start Denver Model (ESDM)).

For example, Butter (2007) used a manualized parent training program to reduce noncompliant behavior and enhance adaptive behavior in children with ASD. During the 24-week study, parents were seen weekly for 75–90-min training visits until week 14 and then for a home visit (week 17) and booster sessions (weeks 18, 20, and 22). An initial home visit was also conducted between week 2 and 3's session. The program targeted irritability, tantrums, aggression and self-injury. The package included 11 required sessions covering topics such as prevention strategies, schedules, reinforcement, planned ignoring, compliance training, functional communication training, teaching techniques (task analysis, chaining, and prompting), and generalization. Additionally, there were up to four optional sessions including time-out, contingency contracting, imitation training, and crisis management that could be implemented at the clinician's discretion. Parent training sessions included a structured curriculum and clinician script, video vignettes depicting various skills to be taught to the parents, worksheets, and parent handouts. Children were required to participate in portions of up to eight sessions, which allowed for direct observation of parent-child interactions demonstrating the interventions introduced in sessions. Parents had high attendance to sessions, satisfaction with the program, and adherence to assignments. The program was implemented with high treatment integrity. Parent-reported rates of noncompliance were reduced by 39 %, irritability was reduced by 34 %, and daily living skills were enhanced by 19 %.

In a study about training parents to increase communication, Park, Alber-Morgan, and Cannella-Malone (2011) trained mothers to teach their child with ASD independent communication with PECS. A formal preference assessment was conducted at the beginning of this study to identify potential reinforcers for each child. A training session was implemented with each parent at their home without the child prior to baseline and each phase of PECS training. Each session lasted for 40–60 min. For Phases 1 and 2, the mother was trained to serve as the communication partner and was trained to initiate each trial by presenting preferred items and pictures, provide the appropriate consequence (e.g. allowing access to the item, naming the item, praising, conducting error correction procedures), and then ending the trial. The first experimenter provided the mother with written guidelines for each phase, explained the details of how to conduct each step in each phase, modeled the procedures, and showed a video clip in which adult models conducted the procedures. The mother was asked to practice the procedures until she reached at least 90 % accuracy across three consecutive trials. During the practice sessions, the experimenter took the child's role, observed the mother, and provided feedback when necessary. During PECS training, the mother taught her child Phases 1 through 3B as described in the PECS manual (Frost & Bondy, 2002). Specifically, the child was taught how to exchange a picture (Phase 1), spontaneously exchange a picture for requesting despite the increased distance from both the communication partner and the book (Phase 2), and discriminate a correct picture and exchange it when a preferred and a nonpreferred item or activity were presented (Phase 3A) and when two preferred items or activities were presented (Phase 3B). During sessions where the mother was training her child, the experimenter provided a prompt or feedback on the mother's implementation of the training procedures. The parents implemented the procedures with high fidelity and all three children successfully acquired independent picture exchanges that were generalized to a different communication partner and maintained for at least 1 month. Vocalizations across participants showed limited or no improvement.

Parent training in PRT has also shown to enhance the communication skills of children with autism. For example, Coolican et al. (2010) evaluated the effects of a brief parent training in PRT for parents of preschool children with ASD. Parents received three separate 2-h training sessions over 2 consecutive weeks. Prior to the first session, parents were provided with 'How to teach pivotal behaviors to children with autism: A training manual' (Koegel et al., 1989). The first two parent training sessions were conducted in a clinical lab setting and the third session was conducted in the family home. Parents were introduced to basic PRT principles, and the trainer modeled the techniques with the child during the initial session. The second and third sessions consisted mainly of in-vivo feedback for the parents while implementing the PRT techniques with their child, as well as problem solving issues that arise since the previous session. PRT was taught in the context of play with the child. Overall, children's communication skills, namely functional utterances, increased following training. Parents' fidelity in implementing PRT techniques also improved after training, and generally these changes were maintained at follow-up.

Stokes and Luiselli (2008) examined the effects of a consultant teaching two sets of parents to conduct a functional analysis (FA) under simulated condition with a graduate student in their homes using verbal, written, and video performance feedback. Each simulated session lasted 5 min and consisted of the social disapproval, demand, or play condition. During sessions, one parent from each family interacted with the student. There were three sessions per day (17 total sessions), implemented in random order, and scheduled over a 1-week period. The participants first received verbal and written feedback for each step in the form of praise or correction immediately following each FA session. The trainer met with each participant for 3–5 min. The trainer used a flow chart to discuss each step comprising the FA condition that had been implemented. Video feedback was added next. The participants viewed a videotape that had been made of them conducting each of the three FA conditions. The trainer watched the videotape with each participant, using verbal feedback (praise and correction) as each step of the FA condition was reviewed. The parents FA skills improved when family members received verbal and written feedback, and their performance was enhanced further after observing themselves on videotape. The parents were able to learn quickly how to implement a functional analysis and generalize implementation with their child in the home environment.

In another study, Rogers et al. (2012) examined the efficacy of a 12-week, low intensity, parent-delivered intervention for toddlers at risk for ASD. Parent-delivered Early Start Denver Model (P-ESDM) consists of 12 consecutive sessions that each last 1-h in length. The intervention sessions were conducted in a clinic setting. In session one, the children's learning objectives were developed. Session 2–10 parents were introduced the new topic each week through verbal description and written materials from the manual and briefly modeled the interaction skill with the child in play. Parents were coached in each of ten intervention techniques: increasing child's attention and motivation; using sensory social routines; promoting dyadic engagement and joint activity routines; enhancing nonverbal communication; building imitation skills; facilitating joint attention; promoting speech development; using antecedent–behavior–consequence relationships ("ABCs of learning"); using prompting, shaping, and fading techniques; and conducting functional assessment of behavior to develop new interventions. Sessions 11 and 12 focused on maintenance after treatment and review of progress. Both groups of parents improved interaction skills, and both groups of children demonstrated progress.

Joint attention is another area of focus for children with ASD. Kasari, Gulsrud, Paparella, Hellemann, and Berry (2015) compared the effects of two parent-mediated interventions on joint attention. Parent-child dyads received 10 weeks of hands-on parent training in a naturalistic, developmental behavioral intervention (joint attention, symbolic play, engagement and regulation (JASPER)) or a parent-only psychoeducational intervention (PEI). PEI provided one-on-one interventionist meetings with the parents in informational sessions of 1-h per week for 10 weeks. Sessions covered content of the manualized intervention which included information on autism, details of specific behavioral impairments, principles of managing behavior, strategies for teaching new skills, improving social interaction and communication, service availability, managing parental stress, and sibling, family, and community responses to autism. JASPER is a manualized treatment for toddlers and preschoolers with a primary focus on sustaining periods of joint engagement and increasing joint attention gestures and play skills. Intervention sessions were based on developmental and behavioral principles consistent with JASPER. Parents were first taught to recognize the child's current developmental level of play and use of social-communication gestures. Parents provided opportunities for the child to initiate interest in a toy/activity and to establish jointly engaged play routines. Parents used a number of strategies to keep children engaged while also improving their frequency of social communication gestures, spoken words, and play acts. PEI intervention was effective in reducing parenting stress associated with child characteristics. All secondary effects were generally small to moderate. JASPER intervention had significant effects on the primary outcome of joint engagement. The treatment effect was large and maintained over the 6-month follow-up. JASPER also had significant effects on the secondary outcomes of play diversity, highest play level achieved, and generalization to the child's classroom for child-initiated joint engagement.

Internet-Based Parent Training

There is a reported shortage of healthcare, educational, and medical services for children diagnosed with an ASD and their families (World Health Organization [WHO], 2007). This is especially true for families who live in rural areas due to a lack of specialized training and professionals, the distance to and transportation of services, and the increased expense of providing services (Graeff-Martins et al., 2008). This situation has created a significant gap between the intensive service requirements for children with a disability and service providers' availability (Baharav & Reiser, 2010). Telepractice (also called 'telehealth' and 'telemedicine')—"the application of telecommunications technology to deliver professional services at a distance by linking clinician to client, or clinician to clinician for assessment, intervention, and/or consultation" (American Speech-Language Hearing Association [ASHA], 2005) has shown to be a cost-effective service-delivery model in bridging this gap in service delivery (e.g. Barretto, Wacker, Harding, Lee, & Berg, 2006; Machalicek et al., 2010; Vismara, Young, Stahmer, Griffith, & Rogers, 2009).

For example, Vismara, Young, and Rogers (2012) piloted a 12, 1-h per week parent intervention program using telehealth delivery with nine families with ASD. The parents became skilled at using teachable moments to promote children's spontaneous language and imitation skills. They were pleased with the support and ease of telehealth learning, so the pilot was followed-up with a randomized control trial contrasting the telehealth intervention to an online control group. The study reported on the first eight families who used a telehealth program consisting of two-way, live video conferencing and a self-guided website to conduct the 12-week parent training in the homes of families of young children with ASD. Parents' intervention skills and engagement with the website, as well as children's verbal language and joint attention skills were assessed and the preliminary results suggests that parents were able to implement the intervention strategies with fidelity and alter their engagement styles to be more attentive and responsive to their children after the hybrid telehealth programs. Furthermore, children in both studies demonstrated gains in important social communicative behaviors (e.g. language, imitative behaviors) as their parents participated in the telehealth programs.

In another study, Wacker et al. (2013a) examined behavior consultants' use of telehealth consultation to coach parents to conduct functional analyses (FA) with 20 young children with ASD between the ages of 29 and 80 months who displayed problem behavior and lived an average of 222 miles from the tertiary hospital that housed the behavior consultants. The children's parents conducted all procedures during weekly telehealth consultations in regional clinics located an average of 15 miles from the participants' homes. Parent assistants were briefly trained by the behavior consultants and were on-site to provide support for families during consultations. The FA identified environmental variables that maintained problem behavior for 18 of the 20 cases, as a result, this suggest that behavior analysts can conduct FA effectively and efficiently via telehealth. Wacker et al. (2013b) followed-up with a study investigating behavior consultants' coaching parents of 17 young children with ASD who displayed problem behavior via telehealth to conduct FAs with telehealth consultation and then conducted functional communication training (FCT) that was matched to the identified function of problem behavior. All procedures were conducted at regional clinics located an average of 15 miles from the families' homes and the behavior consultants were located an average of 222 miles from the regional clinics. Parent assistants located at the regional clinics supported the families during the clinic visits. The FCT conducted by the parents reduced problem behavior by an average of 93.5 %. These results suggest that when experienced applied behavior analysts provide consultation, FCT can be conducted by parents via telehealth.

Suess et al. (2014) examined a retrospective, descriptive evaluation of the fidelity with which parents of three children with ASD conducted FCT in their homes. All training was provided to the parents via telehealth by a behavior consultant. FCT trials coached by the behavior consultant were conducted during weekly 1-h visits. Parents made video recordings of treatment trials in which they conducted the procedures independent of coaching. Levels of fidelity were evaluated during both coached and independent trials and the results showed no consistent differentiation between the coached and the independent trials. All children showed substantial reductions in problem behavior during the final treatment trials and especially during the coached trials. These results suggest that behavior analysts can use telehealth to train parents to implement FCT with acceptable fidelity and achieve substantial reductions in children's problem behavior.

Psychosocial Interventions to Decrease Parent Mental Health Symptoms

Parent training can potentially result in improved parental mental health outcomes through support and advice, but most programs are not designed to support parental mental health. There is some evidence to suggest that psychological interventions can remediate parental stress in parents of children with ASD (Hastings & Beck, 2004). Cognitive Behavioral Therapy (CBT) is one type of psychological intervention to decrease parent stress. CBT teaches parents coping skills and muscle relaxation techniques to handle stressful situations and cognitive strategies to modify dysfunctional thoughts. For example, Tonge et al. (2006) used a group-comparison design to examine the effectiveness of (a) a behavioral management intervention using early intervention and CBT for parents compared to (b) a parent education program on improving parental mental health. They found that both treatments contributed to improved mental health outcomes at follow-up, but the behavior management intervention (early intervention and CBT) was more effective in alleviating anxiety, insomnia, somatic symptoms and family dysfunction. A meta-analysis examining the effects of parenting and stress management interventions for parents of children with developmental disabilities in six studies (Singer, 2006), suggests that CBT has small, but consistent positive outcomes on parental stress.

Acceptance and Commitment Therapy (ACT) is another type of psychological intervention that has been used with parents of children with ASD that appears particularly applicable to the experiences of this population, in which the challenges faced by raising a child with ASD are unlikely to change (Blackledge & Hayes, 2006). ACT is an alternative approach to traditional cognitive and emotional change strategies that focuses on challenging the content of difficult and invalidating thoughts and feelings (Blackledge & Hayes, 2006). ACT emphasizes acceptance of unpleasant moments, diffusion from difficult thoughts, clarification of the parent's personally held values and corresponding goals, and enhancement of the parent's effectiveness in moving toward those goals and values (Blackledge & Hayes, 2006).

Blackledge and Hayes (2006) conducted a within-subject, repeated measures design to examine the effects of a 2-day (14 h) group ACT workshop for parents and guardians of children with ASD. Findings suggested that participation in the ACT workshop lead to improved parental mental health outcomes, including positive outcomes on Beck Depression Inventory-II (BDI-II) and the Global Severity Index (GSI) of the Brief Symptom Inventory (BSI). Most of the gains achieved were retained at 3-month follow-up. It should be noted that this study had several limitations, including a small sample size and no comparison group. Although these findings are promising, more research is needed to evaluate the effectiveness of ACT on parent mental health outcomes.

Mindfulness-based interventions have also been used with parents of children with ASD. Mindful parenting involves applying the practices of paying attention in an intentional and non-judgmental way to the child (Kabat-Zinn & Kabat-Zinn, 1997). Mindfulness training teaches parents to modify maladaptive cognitive schemata, habits, and reinforcement patterns, while using a gentle, compassionate, and self-reflective parenting approach (Cachia, Anderson, & Moore, 2015). For example, Neece (2014) examined the effectiveness of a group-based Mindfulness-Based Stress Reduction Program on depressive symptoms and stress in parents of children with autism, using a randomized group design. Parents in the intervention group experienced a significant decrease in stress and a significant decrease in depressive symptoms. Cachia et al. (2015) systematic literature review on the efficacy of mindfulness-based interventions in reducing stress and increasing psychological well-being in children with ASD found that mindfulness-based interventions may have long-term positive effects on parental mental health outcomes, with positive effects maintaining or even increasing up to 3 months post-training. These findings corroborate previous evidence from the literature that mindfulness training reduces stress in parents of children with a range of disabilities (Cachia et al., 2015; Dabrowski & Pisula, 2010). In addition, mindful parenting also impacts child behavior, including decreased aggressive and maladaptive behavior and increased social behavior (Singh et al., 2007).

Training Parents Acros Autism Symptomology

Children with ASD present with delayed social communication skills and rigid and repetitive behaviors and interests (RRBIs) (American Psychiatric Association, 2013). Children also often present with comorbid diagnosis of ADHD, ODD, anxiety and mood disorders, as well as challenging behaviors such as aggression and self-injury, sleep disorders and feeding issues (Babbit et al., 1994; Machalicek et al., 2016; Richdale, 1999). This section will present research evaluating parent-implemented interventions to address social communication deficits, RRBIs, challenging behavior, pre-academic skills, and functional life skills. Parent involvement in intervention research addressing sleep disorders, feeding issues and comorbid mental health diagnoses is not covered in this chapter (interested readers see Binnendyk & Lucyshyn,

2009; Malow et al., 2014; Machalicek et al., in press; Weiskop, Richdale, & Matthews, 2005). Comprehensive EIBI models of EI (Leaf, Taubman, McEachin, Leaf, & Tsuji, 2011), such as the UCLA Young Autism Project (Lovaas et al., 1981), address multiple symptoms of ASD at once, but utilize focused, individualized interventions to address specific areas of need. Learning sessions are provided in a one-to-one discrete trial (DTT) format, focusing on the systematic teaching of measurable behavioral units, repetitive practice, and structured presentation of tasks from the simplest to the more complex. Table 8.2 cross references a select number of studies evaluating parent implemented focused intervention for young children with ASD against the categories of EIBI, Social communication, restricted and repetitive patterns of behaviors and interests (RRBIs), challenging behavior, functional life, and pre-academic skills. Within this section, we summarize the goals, procedures, and outcomes of two illustrative single-case research studies evaluating the effects of parent-implemented intervention on social communication, RRBIs, challenging behavior, functional life skills, and pre-academic skills.

Social Communication

Social communication is a core deficit in ASD (Williams White, Koenig, & Scahill, 2007). Examples of important social communication skills targeted in EI for children with ASD include joint attention, functional communication including mands (requests) and tacts (labeling), and social pragmatic skills like entering and sustaining play (Williams White et al., 2007). Parents are often a child's earliest communication partners; for that reason, parent-mediated interventions on pivotal social skills, language, and early play skills for children with ASD is a rich area of research.

Social communication skills are of particular importance to parents because of their role in facilitating every day routines, as well as in allowing for sharing positive experiences with their child. Early social skills, such as joint attention, may be pivotal to later successful social communication. Parent-mediated interventions on social communication have covered a range of skills and include parent training on the use of teaching strategies such as DTT and visual supports (Crockett et al., 2007). In one such study, Rocha et al. (2007), taught parents to intervene on joint attention skills in a single-case concurrent multiple baseline design across participants. Joint attention is a dynamic shift in attention between someone who points out an object or event and the object. In this study, parents used strategies including DTT and elements of PRT to teach three preschool age children to respond to parent joint attention bids. Parents were taught to train children to respond to increasing levels of difficulty of joint attention bid using most to least prompting. For example, parents began by putting their hand on the object, and faded prompts until the child could respond to a gaze shift from parent towards an object. Data indicated parents were able to learn to teach these joint

Table 8.2 Targeted child outcomes in parent implemented early intervention for young children with autism spectrum disorder

Citation	EIBI	Social communication	RRBI	Challenging behavior	Functional life	Pre-academics
Barretto et al. (2006)				X		
Batu (2014)					X	
Boyd, McDonough, Rupp, Khan, and Bodfish (2011)			X			
Butter (2007)				X	X	
Coolican et al. (2010)	X					
Crockett, Fleming, Doepke, and Stevens (2007)						X
Dawson et al. (2010)	X					
Dawson et al. (2010)	X					
Dunlap, Ester, Langhans, and Fox (2006)				X		
Eikeseth (2011)	X					
Howlin et al. (2009)	X					
Ingersoll and Gergans (2007)		X				
Kaiser and Hancock (2003)		X				
Kaiser, Hancock, and Nietfeld (2000)		X				
Kaiser and Roberts (2013)		X				
Kashinath, Woods, and Goldstein (2006)		X				
Lafasakis and Sturmey (2007)						X
Leaf et al. (2011)	X					
Lucyshyn et al. (2007)				X		
Machalicek et al. (in press)				X		

(continued)

Table 8.2 (continued)

Citation	EIBI	Social communication	RRBI	Challenging behavior	Functional life	Pre-academics
Mahoney and Perales (2005)		X				
Moes and Frea (2002)				X		
Park et al. (2011)		X				
Reid et al. (2007)		X				
Rickards, Walstab, Wright-Rossi, Simpson, and Reddihough (2009)	X					
Roberts and Kaiser (2011)		X				
Rocha, Schreibman, and Stahmer (2007)		X				
	X					
Sallows and Graupner (2005)	X					
Sears, Blair, Iovannone, and Crosland (2013)				X		
Shipley-Benamou et al. (2002)					X	
Smith et al. (2010)	X					
Smith (2001)	X					
Stokes and Luiselli (2008)				X		
Suess et al. (2014)				X		
Vismara et al. (2012)	X					
Vismara and Rogers (2008)		X				
Wacker et al. (2013b)				X		

Codes: EIBI: Early Intensive Behavioral Intervention; RRBI: Restricted and Repetitive Patterns of Behaviors and Interests attention skills with fidelity across participants. Additionally, child data indicated that responses to parent bids for joint attention increased for all three children as a result of participation in this intervention.

Kaiser and Roberts (2013) investigated the benefits of adding parent training to interventionist-led Enhanced Milieu Training (EMT) to increase child language use and functional play skills in a randomized control trial. 77 participants were randomly selected to either the EMT condition or the EMT plus parent training condition. Children in the EMT condition received interventionist led EMT and children in the EMT plus parent training condition received the same amount of EMT delivered by a therapist as well as simultaneous EMT delivery by a parent. Results indicated while both groups showed improvement in targeted language, there was significantly greater improvement in those children whose parents were also trained to implement the strategies.

Restricted and Repetitive Behaviors and Interests (RRBIs)

In addition to social communication deficits, children with ASD experience behavioral excesses, which include the presence of restricted and repetitive patterns of behavior and interests (RRBI) (American Psychiatric Association, 2013). RRBIs are a core feature of ASD and encompass a variety of behaviors such as repetitive motor movements, speech, or use of objects (e.g. motor stereotypies, lining up objects, echolalia, idiosyncratic speech), often referred to as stereotypy. RRBIs also include a need for insistence on sameness, fixed adherence to routines, or ritualized patterns of verbal or nonverbal behavior, which often entail significant distress during minor activity changes or transitions. RRBIs also involve highly restricted, fixated interests of abnormal focus or intensity such as preoccupation with peculiar objects or remarkably circumscribed or perseverative interests. Finally, hyper- or hypo-sensory related reactions or unusual interactions to sensory aspects of the environment (e.g. indifference to pain, extreme responses to particular sounds, textures, or smells, visual attraction to lights or movement) are also observed in children with ASD (American Psychiatric Association, 2013, Machalicek et al., in press). RRBIs are often divided into two categories: (a) lower order, which consist of stereotypies including repetitive motor movement, object manipulation, and repetitive self-injurious behavior; and (b) higher order, which include insistence on sameness, repetitive language, perseverative interests, and rigidity (Boyd, McDonough, & Bodfish, 2012; Machalicek et al., in press, Patterson, Smith, & Jelen, 2010).

RRBIs can be observed in young children with ASD (Kim & Lord, 2010); however, there remains a lack of consensus in the literature regarding the use of RRBIs during the diagnostic process for an ASD (Stronach & Weatherby, 2014). One of the reasons for this could be that typically developing young children engage in repetitive behaviors especially between the ages of 2 and 4 years old (Evans et al., 1997;

Richler, Biship, Kleinke, & Lord, 2007). For example, it is common for an infant to bang toys and objects repetitively or body rock (Arnott et al., 2010) and for a toddler to request the same book be read over and over again, insist on a familiar bedtime routine or certain clothing, or carry around a special object of high interest. These aforementioned examples are a part of normal infant and toddler development, which may be a reason RRBIs have received less attention in the literature (Arnott et al., 2010). However, research has shown that repetitive patterns of behavior are highly elevated in children who later go on to receive ASD diagnoses (Wolff et al., 2014). Repetitive behaviors have been shown to be strongly correlated with comorbid conditions such as mood and behavior problems in children with ASD and are also associated with increased parent stress levels (Boyd, McDonough, & Bodfish, 2011). Thus, there is a need to train parents to address this core symptom of ASD.

When compared to the abundant collection of available focused and comprehensive interventions to address social communication skills (e.g. joint attention, language), evidence-based practices aimed at RRBIs currently represent a scant piece of literature (Boyd et al., 2011). An even smaller part of that is devoted to parent-implemented interventions. Boyd et al. (2011) trained parents of five preschool aged children with ASD to implement the *Family Implemented Treatment for Behavioral Inflexibility* (*FITBI*). The FITBI involved training parents to implement response interruption and redirection (RIRD; Martinez & Betz, 2013) for lower order repetitive behavior (e.g. spinning objects, lining up objects) and/or differential reinforcement of variability (DRV) for higher order RRBIs (e.g. repeatedly watching the same movie, perseveration with cars). Parents were trained to address two RRBIs with their child. RIRD is a common intervention used with individuals with developmental disabilities to decrease stereotypy and other challenging behavior (Boyd et al., 2011) that entails physically or verbally blocking or interrupting a targeted inappropriate behavior and redirecting (sometimes with prompts) the child to engage in a different, or alternative, behavior. Boyd et al. (2011) taught a parent to use RIRD to decrease a child's "object attachment" with sticks by redirecting the child to hold other objects in his hand. DRV is a strategy that is primarily used with higher order RRBIs that are non-functional (e.g. perseveration with certain toys), and it involves using behavioral shaping to gradually increase the variety of a child's behavior by using reinforcement (Boyd et al., 2011). In this study, Boyd et al. (2011) trained a parent to decrease a child's perseveration with cars by teaching the child new play routines with the car, therefore, increasing the child's varied behavior while engaged with the toy cars. The method of training the parents involved 12 weekly clinic-based sessions (60–120 min) with parent education and training, which included teaching trials wherein the triggering stimuli (i.e. item that evoked the RRBI) was present in the clinic room and the child was prompted to refrain from engaging in the RRBI with RIRD or to appropriately engage with the item using DRV. The FITBI initially used repeated practice in discrete trial training format and then transitioned to embedded trials into play-based activities. Supplemental individualized behavior management plans were developed if needed. A single-case concurrent multiple baseline across behaviors (two for each child) design was employed to evaluate the effects of FITBI, and the authors reported substantial reductions in RRBIs for all five participants (Boyd et al., 2011).

Perhaps much of the literature surrounding RRBIs is covered within challenging behavior and self-injury studies, specifically behavior maintained by non-social consequences, as RRBIs are often hypothesized to be self-stimulatory, or that the reinforcement for the behavior is not mediated by another person. Many procedures have been shown to be effective in reducing such behaviors such as differential reinforcement (e.g. Azrin, Besalel, Jammer, & Caputa, 1988), environmental enrichment strategies (e.g. Piazza, Adelinis, Hanley, Goh, & Delai, 2000), visual and verbal cues (e.g. Horner, Carr, Strain, Todd, & Reed, 2002). What seems to be missing from the current literature is the inclusion of these procedures within comprehensive treatment models for young children with ASD [e.g. Early Intensive Behavioral Intervention (EIBI), Early Start Denver Model (ESDM)]. A randomized control trial of 48 infants (Dawson et al., 2010) found significant improvements in adaptive behavior and IQ for the ESDM group; however, this intervention did not yield specific change in RRBIs as measured by the Repetitive Behavior Scale (Bodfish, Symons, Parker, & Lewis, 1999) (Leekam, Prior, & Uljarevic, 2011). Sallows and Graupner (2005) compared two applied behavior analysis (ABA) programs, one was clinic-based EIBI, and the other group was parent-implemented ABA. The parent-implemented ABA group performed as well as the clinic-based group including significant improvements on RRBIs as measured by the Autism Diagnostic Inventory—Revised (ADI-R; Lord, Rutter, & Le Couteur, 1994) for children described as "rapid learners" (Leekam et al., 2011). More research is needed investigating educating and coaching parents to address RRBIs in young children with or at risk for ASD using focused interventions and embedding them into existing, effective comprehensive treatment models.

Challenging Behaviors

Challenging behaviors such as tantrums, self-injury, and aggression are common among children with ASD (Durand, Hieneman, Clarke, Wang, & Rinaldi, 2013; Einfeld & Tonge, 1996; Emerson et al., 2001; Hemmeter, Ostrosky, & Fox, 2006) and often develop as a result of environmental issues, lack of reinforcement for desirable behaviors, and communication impairment for both the child and parent (Harrower, Fox, Dunlap, & Kincaid, 2000). Such challenging behaviors can cause direct harm to themselves or other people, and interfere with efforts to help these individuals live more independently by disrupting educational and vocational efforts as well as home life (Emerson, 1995; Fox, Vaughn, Wyatte, & Dunlap, 2002).

Additionally, managing challenging behavior, the most commonly reported parenting difficulty (Bromley, Hare, Davison, & Emerson, 2004), is a significant source of parental stress and impacts the quality of life of children with ASD and their families. Whether identified and described as behavioral deficits (e.g. a lack of socially appropriate communication skills) or behavioral excesses (e.g. repetitive and disruptive behaviors), persistent behavioral challenges, presented by a child with developmental delays can negatively impact the family unit (Baker et al., 2003). It is important to equip parents with the necessary tools to create a desirable family environment (Meadan et al., 2009). For example, Dunlap et al. (2006) taught two mothers to use functional communication training (FCT) during home routines to address serious challenging behaviors of their toddlers. The study procedures included (a) selecting home routines deemed especially problematic by the children's mothers, (b) conducting a functional behavior assessment, (c) training the mothers to use FCT, and (d) having the mothers implement the procedures in the home in accordance with a single-case concurrent multiple baseline across routines design. The FCT training was 1-h in length and conducted in the home. The individualized instruction consisted of (a) an explanation regarding the reasons for replacing the challenging behaviors with more appropriate replacement behaviors; (b) a review of the functional assessment information including the child's target behaviors, replacement communication behaviors, and selected reinforcers; (c) modeling by the researchers on how to prompt the child to use the replacement behavior to prevent the challenging behavior from occurring; (d) reminders that developing replacement behaviors also involves withholding reinforcers for challenging behavior; and (e) an opportunity for the mothers to ask questions regarding implementation of the FCT procedures. The mothers were also given a written script specific to their child as a guide and reference for how to implement the specific FCT procedures, which could be used as a prompt and referred to before intervention sessions. The results showed that the mothers were able to use the procedures correctly and interventions produced reductions in the children's challenging behaviors and increases in their use of communicative replacement skills.

In another example, Sears et al. (2013) examined the use of the family-centered prevent-teach-reinforce (PTR) model with families of children with ASD to decrease challenging behavior. The PTR model includes five steps aligned with the problem-solving process. It is a collaborative team driven process facilitated by a consultant who has expertise in behavioral principles and guides the team through five steps: Step 1: teaming (i.e. establishes membership and an agreement on how the team will function); Step 2: goal setting (i.e. focuses on identifying and defining the social, behavioral, and academic targets); Step 3: PTR assessment (i.e. functional assessment includes direct and indirect observations covering three categories relating to antecedent variables (Prevent), function and replacement variables (Teach), and consequence variables (Reinforce)); Step 4: intervention (i.e. team selects interventions and develops a plan for training and coaching adults to implement the strategies as intended); and Step 5: evaluation (i.e. uses targeted behavior change data to make decisions about the plan's effectiveness and next steps) (see Dunlap et al., 2010 for the model's manual). The initial team meeting was 2-h in length and covered Step 1 and 2. The second meeting was held after baseline to conduct the functional behavior assessment (Step 3) and develop the behavior intervention plan (Step 4) which was 3-h in length for each routine. The parents were then provided with a task analysis of each strategy and 30-min of training on the implementation steps using verbal and written instructions, modeling, rehearsal, and feedback. Results indicated that the parents were able to implement the behavior intervention plan with fidelity and successfully use the PTR process for a novel routine. The PTR intervention was associated with reduction in child challenging behavior and increases in alternative behavior in both target and non-target routines.

Pre-Academic Skills

Parents of children with ASD are increasingly encouraged to become active participants in their children's early education by applying behavioral intervention at home, often using Discrete Trial Teaching (DTT) (Crockett et al., 2007; Eikeseth, 2011; Sturmey & Fitzer, 2007). For example, Lafasakis and Sturmey (2007) taught three parents using behavioral skills training to implement DTT with their children with developmental disabilities. Behavioral skills training included giving the parent a typed list of definitions of the ten components of DTT, modeling three DTT trials with the child, and then having the parent perform the same three DTT trails with their child. Immediate performance feedback (i.e. positive comments on components performed correctly and corrective feedback on components that needed practice) was provided by the coach to the parent following the performance. Three additional discrete trials were modeled by the coach that included the specific components that were previously implemented incorrectly. The rehearsal and modeling procedure was repeated until 10 min elapsed. All three parents learned to implement DTT, parents were observed to use DTT with novel programs and children's correct responding increased.

In another study, Crockett et al. (2007) examined the effects of an intensive parent training program on the acquisition and generalization of DTT procedures with two parents of children with ASD. Each parent was individually trained and attended between 6 and 9, 2-h weekly training sessions. Parent training included a didactic lecture (i.e. definitions and examples of antecedents, consequences, intertrial intervals, and data collection), video demonstrations, role-play, and practice with feedback. Parents taught their children four different functional skills using DTT to assess generalization across stimulus exemplars. Both parents were able to acquire DTT for teaching their children with autism. Both parents improved their teaching across child skills before receiving training on all child skills, which supports generalization and the extent to which each parent extended their use of DTT procedures across untrained and topographically different child skills.

Functional Life Skills

Parents of children with ASD are often concerned about their ability to live safe, productive and independent lives (Shipley-Benamou et al., 2002), which makes teaching functional life skills an important target for intervention. The child's ability to perform functional life skills without assistance eases the burden placed on the parents, due to the time and energy needed to perform these tasks (Batu, 2014; Shipley-Benamou et al., 2002). Functional life skills include behaviors that allow the child to live more independently, such as preparing simple meals, performing household chores, and getting dressed. Several teaching strategies have been used to teach functional life skills, including backward and forward chaining procedures (Cooper, Heron, & Heward, 2007), task analysis (Test, Spooner, Keul, & Grossi, 1990), simultaneous prompting (Fetko, Schuster, Harley, & Collins, 1999), least-to-most and most-to-least prompting (Taber, Alberto, Seltzer, & Hughes, 2003), and in-vivo and video modeling (Ayres, Maguire, & McClimon, 2009; Goodson, Sigafoos, O'Reilly, Cannella, & Lancioni, 2007; Shipley-Benamou et al., 2002). In one study, Shipley-Benamou et al. (2002) used instructional video modeling to teach functional life skills to three children with autism (ages 5–6 years). They used a single-case research multiple-probe design across five different tasks (i.e. making orange juice, preparing a letter to mail, putting a letter in the mailbox, feeding a pet, cleaning a fishbowl, and setting a table) to examine the efficacy of the video modeling strategies. Their findings suggest that video modeling was effective in promoting acquisition of functional life skills for all three participants. Results were maintained during a no-video phase and at 3-month follow-up.

In another study, Batu (2014) examined the effectiveness of teaching parents to use simultaneous prompting through visual supports to increase functional life skills (i.e. eating pudding and hand washing) in preschool-aged children with developmental delay. A single-case research multiple-probe design across three participants was used to determine the efficacy of the intervention. Results of the study suggest that mothers were able to learn the procedure and children were able to acquire skills, which maintained at 2-week follow-up and generalized to new skills. The authors suggest that both parent and child were able to generalize the acquired skills.

Discussion and Future Research

Parent training has emerged over the past 40 years as an important target for interventions regarding children with developmental disabilities (Kaminski et al., 2008; Maughan et al., 2005). Parents are recognized as the best intervention agents because of the amount of time they spend with their child as well as the variety of settings they have the chance to teach skills in (Sears, 2010). Research also indicates that parent training is time- and cost-effective and leads to better generalization and maintenance than therapist-implemented intervention models (Brookman-Frazee, Vismara, Drahota et al., 2009). BPT literature also suggests that parents typically find training acceptability, especially when compared to pharmacological intervention (e.g. Waschbusch, Cunningham, Pelham et al., 2011). However, there are several gaps in the literature that suggest several future research directions. Parent training in the ASD literature has not reached the level of treatment packages seen for typically developing children with compliance problems (Matson, Mahan & LoVullo, 2009; Matson, Mahan & Matson, 2009). Future research is needed to determine the best treatment package for ASD symptom severity, but also to identify essential intervention components, and to determine comparative effectiveness between intervention approaches. Parent education programs often use multiple intervention strategies (e.g. didactic instruction including lecture with video modeling and role play followed by practice with child with immediate performance feedback in natural setting) making difficult the extent to which we can identify the active ingredients of the intervention. Certainly the amount and type of parent education and coaching will vary across targeted skills and parent-child dyads, but the current literature base does not inform this type of clinical decision making. Identifying the essential components of a packaged parent education intervention given the target parent and child skills and parent-child demographic variables (e.g. age of child, severity of ASD symptoms, educational background of parent) could yield several benefits including decreasing response effort and time commitment for the parent and clinician, improving treatment fidelity and the amount of time it takes to reach a criterion level of performance supporting behavioral change, and maximizing clinical time so that more families can be served in a shorter amount of time or more intensive parent education and coaching can be delivered to those families whose situations warrant it. Research informing the individualization and intensity of parent education programs would also further theoretical models of tiered intervention for families (see Stepping Stones Triple P-Positive Parenting Program; Tellegen & Sanders, 2013; McIntyre & Phaneuf, 2007). Several research teams have suggested the need to conduct multi-component analysis of parent education interventions to determine which intervention components, training formats (group versus one to one), and dosage yield the most effect on parent and child outcomes (Lang et al., 2009; Patterson et al., 2012; Roberts & Kaiser, 2011; Strauss et al., 2013). Single-case research designs offer an efficient and flexible way to conduct multi-component analyses (Lerman, Swiezy, Perkins-Parks, & Roane, 2000; Moore & Fisher, 2007; Ward-Horner & Sturmey, 2010). Future research should conduct multi-component analyses of parent education programs with the goal of better understanding the active ingredients of parent education programs, dosage related issues, and how interventions are best adapted for individual parent-child dyads or populations.

Relatedly, parent education and training studies are complicated in their "study within a study" design (Meadan et al., 2009). That is, the logic model of any parent-implemented intervention involves cascading logic where (a) a parent education program is implemented to effect change on parent behavior, and (b) the trained parent subsequently implements intervention with his/her child. However, the majority of parent-implemented intervention studies do not take baseline data on parent use of targeted strategies. Therefore, it is impossible to say a functional relation exists between the parent education training and change in parent behavior. We acknowledge two possible reasons for this oversight: (a) the worry that providing parents with any training prior to baseline will not constitute baseline performance, and (b) the difficult inherent in obtaining a baseline of parent behavior when the intervention is based on child assessment (e.g. parent implemented function based intervention for challenging behavior). In our own work, we have been successful in obtaining stable baseline data on parent performance by conducting assessment before the start of the study and providing parents with limited instruction (e.g. reading or lecture and task analysis of behavior intervention plan) prior to baseline. This also allows us to evaluate whether a functional relation exists between a single component of parent education and intervention (e.g. performance feedback) and change in parent behavior. Future research on parent-implemented interventions should include baseline measures of parent use of targeted strategies wherever possible.

In addition, although cultural and socioeconomic variables are widely acknowledged to be important when designing parent education programs (e.g. Mueller, Singer, & Grace, 2004), we currently lack sufficient evidence of effectiveness and social validity for use of parent education and training programs supporting parents' implementation of EI for ASD for diverse populations (Lang et al., 2009; Magaña, Lopez, & Machalicek, in press; Patterson et al., 2012; Roberts & Kaiser, 2011; Strauss et al., 2013). Moreover, there is a current focus on the involvement of mothers and middle-class families (and parents who have agreed to participate in study) (Meadan et al., 2009). For those families facing the double disadvantage of a child with a developmental disability and stressful life situations (e.g. incarceration of family members, teen parents, parents with IDD, poverty), evidence-based parent education and training programs will likely require some degree of adaptation. Two obvious barriers to conducting research with diverse populations is recruiting and maintaining such families in research studies and the absence of available templates for culturally adapting EIBI and focused interventions. Researchers may find helpful literature in other fields on cultural adaptation of interventions (Davidson et al., 2013) and the recruitment and retention of diverse families (UyBico, Pavel, & Gross, 2007). Despite the barriers to conducting research with diverse populations, to assure the effectiveness and ecological validity of currently available parent education and training programs for all types of families, future research must be conducted with fathers and other family members from diverse cultural, linguistic, socio economic backgrounds.

Finally, there is a relative lack of research evaluating the bidirectional relationship between parent and child outcomes. Understandably, research on parent-implemented EI/EIBI is primarily concerned with measuring the impact of the intervention on child outcomes. However, parental well-being has been correlated with a range of child outcomes in cognitive, behavioral, and psychological development (Brand & Brennan, 2009). Parent and child variables may have a mutually escalating effect on each other (Baker et al., 2003; Neece, Green, & Baker, 2012). For example, high levels of child challenging behavior exacerbate parental stress over time, while high levels of parental stress can lead to increased child challenging behavior. In addition, parental mental health outcomes may contribute to less positive outcomes of behavioral interventions (Osborne et al., 2008), including failure to engage with services, less effective parenting, less developmental progress, and higher incidences of behavioral problems (Brinker, Seifer, & Sameroff, 1994). Due to the strong link between parental and child outcomes, it is important that future research both directly target and measure parental outcomes in behavioral interventions with children with ASD (for a review and proposed intervention model see Karst & Van Hecke, 2012).

Suggestions for Practice

Based on the extant literature and concerns discussed in this chapter, the following suggestions for practice in EI for ASD are made:

1. Pre-service and in-service training programs for EI professionals working with families of children with ASD must ensure coverage of applied behavior analysis principles and evidence-based assessment and intervention, but should also cover family-systems theory and best practices in working with families of young children including capacity-building interventions, helpgiving interventions and family and professional collaboration. The Council for Exceptional Children Division for Early Childhood (2014) offers a free download of DEC Recommended Practices in Early Intervention/Early Childhood Special Education that includes coverage of family-centered practices at (see www.dec-sped.org/recommendedpractices).
2. EI professionals should gain competency in using BPT with diverse parents and children through direct instruction and supervision by professionals competent in BPT with high needs populations.
3. EIBI and focused intervention programs for children with ASD should develop programs that include parent participation as an interventionist, but do not entirely rely on parent-implemented intervention. We know that EIBI program are more effective than less intensive EIBI (Reichow & Wolery, 2009) and less intensive EIBI is more effective than eclectic treatment (Strauss et al., 2013), but findings are mixed if parent implemented EIBI programs are as effective as center-directed programs with some research suggesting effects are equal (Sallows & Graupner, 2005) and other research suggesting clinical programs have superior outcomes on intelligence, visual-spatial skills, language and academics when compared to parent-implemented programs (Smith, Groen, & Wynn, 2000).
4. Intensive parent training yields better outcomes and there is some evidence that children may benefit more from parent implemented when they have basic skill prerequisites (Strauss et al., 2013).
5. EI programs should guarantee that parent education and training offerings prioritize the core symptoms of ASD and related comorbidities, but also deliver trainings on commonly experienced difficulties in early childhood such as feeding and sleep issues, and toilet training.
6. For maximal positive parent and child outcomes, parent education and training programs require ongoing measures of treatment fidelity or integrity (i.e. the degree to which an intervention is implemented as intended (usually an observer is present; Gresham, Gansle, & Noell, 1993)) of both the implementation of the education and training program and parent implementation of the intervention.
7. Professionals should program for and assess the maintenance of parent training effects (i.e. parent continues to implement intervention in the absence of clinician) to improve the longevity of treatment effects on child skills/behavior. A statewide survey of parents of children with autism suggests that adherence to

prescribed behavioral and medical interventions to be very low (approximately 24 % and 16 %, respectively; Moore & Symons, 2009). Parent education programs and the interventions we ask parents to implement with their children should be routines-based so that they fit into the daily context of life and we should routinely assess the contextual fit of interventions for families by asking parents to rate the social validity of goals, procedures, and expected/obtained outcomes at beginning, middle, and end of intervention (Meadan et al., 2009).

8. Professionals using telecommunication technology to increase parent access to education and training programs should develop protocols to ensure confidentiality, parental choice of delivery options, and effective training (Lee et al., 2015).

Conclusion

Encouraging findings in the parent-implemented EI literature include a wide range of parent and child skills and behaviors targeted by interventions and the effectiveness of parent-implemented interventions to address the social communication delays and challenging behavior common to young children with ASD. As the literature base grows, professionals can look forward to gaining clarity on the comparative effectiveness of different approaches and dosages of parent education and training programs for children with differing ASD severity.

References

Alvero, A., Bucklin, B., & Austin, J. (2001). An objective review of recent research on carers supporting people with intellectual disabilities and challenging behaviour. *Journal of Intellectual Disability Research, 43*, 325–339.

American Psychiatric Association. (2013). *Diagnostic and statistical manual of mental disorders* (5th ed.). Arlington, VA: American Psychiatric Publishing.

American Speech-Language-Hearing Association. (2005). *Speech-Language Pathologists Providing Clinical Services via Telepractice: Position Statement* [Position Statement]. Retrieved from www.asha.org/policy. Doi: 10.1044/policy.PS2005-00116.

Arnott, B., McConachie, H., Meins, E., Fernyhough, C., Le Couter, A., Turner, M., … Leerkam, S. (2010). The frequency of restricted and repetitive behaviors in a community sample of 15-month-old infants. *Journal of Developmental and Behavioral Pediatrics, 3*, 223–229.

Artiles, A. J., Trent, S. C., & Kuan, L. (1997). Learning disabilities empirical research on ethnic minority students: An analysis of 22 years of studies published in selected refereed journals. *Learning Disabilities Research and Practice, 12*, 82–91.

Autism Speaks (2015, July 30). *FAQS: Autism Insurance Reform Laws*. Retrieved from https://www.autismspeaks.org/advocacy/insurance/faqs-state-autism-insurance-reform-laws.

Ayres, K. M., Maguire, A., & McClimon, D. (2009). Acquisition and generalization of chained tasks taught with computer based video instruction to children with autism. *Education and Training in Developmental Disabilities, 44*, 493–508.

Azrin, N. H., Besalel, V., Jammer, J. P., & Caputa, J. N. (1988). Comparative study of behavioral methods of treating severe self-injury. *Behavior Resident Treatment, 3*, 119–152.

Babbit, R., Hoch, T. A., Coe, D., Cataldo, M., Kelly, K., Stackhouse, C., et al. (1994). Behavioral assessment and treatment of pediatric feeding disorders. *Journal of Developmental and Behavioral Pediatrics, 15*, 278–291.

Bagner, D. M., & Graziano, P. A. (2012). Barriers to success in parent training for young children with developmental delay: The role of cumulative risk. *Behavior Modification, 37*, 356–377.

Baharav, E., & Reiser, C. (2010). Using telepractice in parent training in early autism. *Telemedicine and e-Health, 16*, 727–731.

Bailey, D. B., Raspa, M., & Fox, L. C. (2012). What is the future of family outcomes and family-centered services? *Topics in Early Childhood Special Education, 31*, 216–223.

Baker, B. L., McIntyre, L. L., Blacher, J., Crnic, K. A., Edelbrock, C., & Low, C. (2003). Preschool children with and without developmental delay: Behaviour problems and parenting stress over time. *Journal of Intellectual Disability Research, 47*, 217–230.

Baker-Ericzèn, M. J., Brookman-Frazee, L., & Stahmer, A. (2005). Stress levels and adaptability in parents of toddlers with and without autism spectrum disorders. *Research and Practice for Persons with Severe Disabilities, 30*, 194–204.

Barretto, A., Wacker, D. P., Harding, J., Lee, J., & Berg, W. K. (2006). Using telemedicine to conduct behavioral assessments. *Journal of Applied Behavior Analysis, 39*, 333–340.

Barton, E. E., & Fettig, A. (2013). Parent-implemented interventions for young children with disabilities: A review of fidelity features. *Journal of Early Intervention, 35*(2), 194–219.

Batu, S. (2014). Effects of teaching simultaneous prompting through visual supports to parents of children with developmental disabilities. *Education and Training in Autism and Developmental Disabilities, 49*, 505–516.

Beckman, P. J., & Bristol, M. M. (1991). Issues in developing the IFSP: A framework for establishing family outcomes. *Topics in Early Childhood Special Education, 11*, 19–31.

Benson, P. R. (2006). The impact of child symptom severity on depressed mood among parents of children with ASD: The mediating role of stress proliferation. *Journal of Autism and Developmental Disorders, 36*, 685–695.

Benzies, K. M., Magill-Evans, J. E., Hayden, K. A., & Ballantyne, M. (2013). Key components of early intervention programs for preterm infants and their parents: A systematic review and meta-analysis. *BMC Pregnancy and Childbirth, 13*(Suppl 1), 1–15.

Biglan, A. (1995). Translating what we know about the context of antisocial behavior into a lower prevalence of such behavior. *Journal of Applied Behavior Analysis, 28*, 479–492.

Binnendyk, L., & Lucyshyn, J. M. (2009). A family-centered positive behavior approach to the amelioration of food refusal behavior. *Journal of Positive Behavior Interventions, 11*, 47–62.

Blackledge, J. T., & Hayes, S. (2006). Using acceptance and commitment training in the support of parents of children diagnosed with autism. *Child and Family Behavior Therapy, 28*, 1–18.

Bodfish, J. W., Symons, F. J., Parker, D. E., & Lewis, M. H. (1999). *The repetitive behavior scale*. Morgantown, NC: Western Carolina Center Research Reports.

Boyd, B. A., McDonough, S. G., Rupp, B., Khan, F., & Bodfish, J. W. (2011). Effects of a family-implemented treatment on the repetitive behaviors of children with autism. *Journal of Autism and Developmental Disorders, 41*, 1330–1341.

Boyd, B. A., McDonough, S. G., & Bodfish, J. W. (2012). Evidence-based behavioral interventions for repetitive behaviors in autism. *Journal of Developmental Disorders, 42*, 1236–1248.

Brand, S. R., & Brennan, P. A. (2009). Impact of antenatal and postpartum maternal mental illness: How are the children? *Clinical Obstetrics and Gynecology, 52*, 441–455.

Briesmeister, J. M., & Schaefer, C. E. (1998). *Handbook of parent training*. New York, NY: John Wiley & Sons.

Brinker, R. P., Seifer, R., & Sameroff, A. J. (1994). Relations among maternal stress, cognitive development, and early intervention in middle- and low-SES infants with developmental disabilities. *American Journal on Mental Retardation, 98*, 463–480.

Brofenbrenner, U. (1986). Ecology of the family as a context for human development: Research perspective. *Developmental Psychology, 22*, 723–742.

Bromley, J., Hare, D. J., Davison, K., & Emerson, E. (2004). Mothers supporting children with autism spectrum disorders: Social support, mental health status, and satisfaction with services. *Autism: The International Journal of Research and Practice, 8*, 409–423.

Brookman-Frazee, L., Stahmer, A., Baker-Ericzèn, M. J., & Tsai, K. (2006). Parenting interventions for children with autism spectrum and disruptive behavior disorders: Opportunities for cross fertilization. *Clinical Child and Family Psychology Review, 9*, 181–200.

Brookman-Frazee, L., Vismara, L., Drahota, A., et al. (2009). Parent training interventions for children with autism spectrum disorders. In J. Matson (Ed.), *Applied behavior analysis for children with autism spectrum disorders: A handbook* (pp. 237–257). New York, NY: Springer Science & Business Media.

Bruder, M. B. (2000). The Individual Family Service Plan (IFSP). ERIC Digest #E605.

Butter, E. M. (2007). Parent training for children with pervasive developmental disorders: A multi-site feasibility trial. *Behavioral Interventions, 22*, 179–199.

Cachia, R. L., Anderson, A., & Moore, D. W. (2015). Mindfulness, stress, and well-being in parents of children with autism spectrum disorder: A systematic review. *Journal of Child and Family Studies, 25*, 1–14.

Coolican, J., Smith, I. M., & Bryson, S. E. (2010). Brief parent training in pivotal response treatment for preschoolers with autism. *Journal of Child Psychology and Psychiatry, 51*, 1321–1330.

Cooper, J. O., Heron, T. E., & Heward, W. L. (2007). *Applied behavior analysis* (2nd ed.). Upper Saddle River, NJ: Pearson Education.

Crockett, J. L., Fleming, R. K., Doepke, K. J., & Stevens, J. S. (2007). Parent training: Acquisition and generalization of discrete trials teaching skills with parents of children with autism. *Research in Developmental Disabilities, 28*, 23–36.

Dabrowski, A., & Pisula, E. (2010). Parenting stress and coping styles in mothers and fathers of pre-school children with autism and Down syndrome. *Journal of Intellectual Disability Research, 54*, 266–280.

Davidson, E. M., Liu, J. J., Bhopal, R., White, M., Johnson, M. R., Netto, G., … Sheikh, A. (2013). Behavior change interventions to improve the health of racial and ethnic minority populations: A tool kit of adaptation approaches. *The Milbank Quarterly, 91*, 811–851.

Davis, N. O., & Carter, A. S. (2008). Parenting stress in mothers and fathers of toddlers with autism spectrum disorders: Associations with child characteristics. *Journal of Autism and Developmental Disorders, 38*, 1278–1291.

Dawson, G., Jones, E. J. H., Merkle, K., Venema, K., Lowy, R., Faja, S., … Webb, S. J. (2012). Early behavioral intervention is associated with normalized brain activity in young children with autism. *Journal of the American Academy of Child and Adolescent Psychiatry, 51*, 1150–1159.

Dawson, G., Rogers, S., Munson, K., Smith, M., Winter, J., Greenson, J., Donaldson, A., & Varley, J. (2010). Randomized, controlled trial of an intervention for toddlers with autism: The early start denver model. *Pediatrics, 125*, e17–e23.

Diggle, T., McConachie, H. R., & Randle, V. R. L. (2002). Parent-mediated early intervention for young children with autism spectrum disorder. *The Cochrane Database of Systematic Reviews, 2*, (Art. No.: CD003496).

Division for Early Childhood. (2014). DEC recommended practices in early intervention/early childhood special education 2014. Retrieved from http://www.decsped.org/recommendedpractices.

Dunlap, G., Ester, T., Langhans, S., & Fox, L. (2006). Functional communication training with toddlers in home environments. *Journal of Early Intervention, 29*, 81–97.

Dunlap, G., Iovannone, R., Kincaid, D., Wilson, K., Christiansen, K., Strain, P., & English, C. (2010). *Prevent-teach-reinforce: A school based model of positive behavior support*. Baltimore, MD: Paul H. Brookes.

Dunst, C. J., Bruder, M., & Espe-Sherwindt, M. (2014). Family capacity-building in early childhood intervention: Do context and setting matter? *School Community Journal, 24*, 37–48.

Dunst, C. J., Trivette, C. M., Humphries, T., Raab, M., & Roper, N. (2001). Contrasting approaches to natural learning environment interventions. *Infants and Young Children, 14*, 48–63.

Dunst, C. J., Trivette, C. M., & Hamby, D. W. (2006). *Family support program quality and parent, family and child benefits*. Asheville, NC: Winterberry Press.

Dunst, C. J., Trivette, C. M., & Hamby, D. W. (2007). Meta-analysis of family-centered helpgiving practices research. *Mental Retardation and Developmental Disabilities Research Reviews, 13*, 370–378.

Dunst, C. J., Trivette, C. M., & Hamby, D. W. (2008). *Research synthesis and meta-analysis of studies of family centered practices*. Asheville, NC: Winterberry Press.

Durand, V. M., Hieneman, M., Clarke, S., Wang, M., & Rinaldi, M. L. (2013). Positive family intervention for severe challenging behavior I: A multisite randomized clinical trial. *Journal of Positive Behavior Interventions, 15*, 133–143.

Eikeseth, S. (2011). Intensive early intervention. In J. L. Matson & P. Sturmey (Eds.), *International handbook of autism and pervasive developmental disorders* (pp. 321–338). New York, NY: Springer.

Einfeld, S. E., & Tonge, B. J. (1996). Population prevalence of psychopathology in children and adolescents with mental retardation: II Epidemiological findings. *Journal of Intellectual Disability Research, 40*, 99–109.

Elder, J. H., Valcante, G., Won, D., & Zylis, R. (2003). Effects of in-home training for culturally diverse fathers of children with autism. *Issues in Mental Health Nursing, 24*, 273–295.

Emerson, E. (1995). *Challenging behaviour: Analysis and intervention in people with severe intellectual disabilities*. Cambridge: Cambridge University Press.

Emerson, E., Kiernan, C., Alborz, A., Reeves, D., Mason, H., Swarbrick, R., … Hatton, C. (2001). Predicting the persistence of severe self-injurious behavior. *Research in Developmental Disabilities, 22*, 67–75.

Espe-Sherwindt, M. (2008). Family-centered practice: Collaboration, competence and evidence. *Support for Learning, 23*, 136–143.

Evans, D. W., Leckman, J. F., Carter, A., Reznick, J. S., Henshaw, D., King, R. A., & Pauls, D. (1997). Ritual, habit, and perfectionism: The prevalence and development of compulsive-like behavior in normal young children. *Child Development, 68*, 58–68.

Fabiano, G. A. (2007). Father participation in behavioral parent training for ADHD: Review and recommendations for increasing inclusion and engagement. *Journal of Family Psychology, 21*, 683–693.

Falk, N. H., Norris, K., & Quinn, M. G. (2014). The factors predicting stress, anxiety and depression in the parents of children with autism. *Journal of Autism and Developmental Disorders, 44*, 3185–3203.

Fetko, K. S., Schuster, J. W., Harley, D. A., & Collins, B. C. (1999). Using simultaneous prompting to teach a chained vocational task to young adults with severe intellectual disabilities. *Education and Training in Mental Retardation and Developmental Disabilities, 34*, 318–329.

Fettig, A., & Barton, E. E. (2014). Parent implementation of function-based intervention to reduce children's challenging behavior: A literature review. *Topics in Early Childhood Special Education, 34*, 49–61.

Flippin, M., & Crais, E. R. (2011). The need for more effective father involvement in early autism intervention. *Journal of Early Intervention, 33*, 24–50.

Fox, L., Vaughn, B. J., Wyatte, M. L., & Dunlap, G. (2002). "We can't expect other people to understand": Family perspectives on problem behavior. *Exceptional Children, 68*, 437.

Friend, A. C., Summers, J. A., & Turnbull, A. P. (2009). Impacts of family support in early childhood intervention research. *Education and Training in Developmental Disabilities, 44*, 453.

Frost, M. S., & Bondy, A. (2002). *The picture exchange communication system training manual* (2nd ed.). Newark, DE: Pyramid Educational Consultants.

Goodson, J., Sigafoos, J., O'Reilly, M., Cannella, H., & Lancioni, G. E. (2007). Evaluation of a video-based error correction procedure for teaching a domestic skill to individuals with developmental disabilities. *Research in Developmental Disabilities, 28*, 458–467.

Graeff-Martins, A. S., Flament, M. F., Fayyad, J., Tyano, S., Jensen, P., & Rohde, L. A. (2008). Diffusion of efficacious interventions for children and adolescents with mental health problems. *Journal of Child Psychology and Psychiatry, 49*, 335–352.

Gresham, F. M., Gansle, K. A., & Noell, G. H. (1993). Treatment integrity in applied behavior analysis with children. *Journal of Applied Behavior Analysis, 26*, 257–263.

Guralnick, M. J. (2011). Why early intervention works: A systems perspective. *Infants and Young Children, 24*, 6–28.

Harrower, J. K., Fox, L., Dunlap, G., & Kincaid, D. (2000). Functional assessment and comprehensive early intervention. *Exceptionality, 8*, 189–204.
Hastings, R., & Beck, A. (2004). Practitioner review: Stress intervention for parents of children with intellectual disabilities. *Journal of Child Psychology and Psychiatry, 45*(8), 1338–1349.
Hastings, R., Robertson, J., & Yasamy, M. (2012). Interventions for children with pervasive developmental disorders in low and middle income countries. *Journal of Applied Research in Intellectual Disabilities, 25*, 119–134.
Hattie, J., & Timperley, H. (2007). The power of feedback. *Review of Educational Research, 77*, 81–112.
Hemmeter, M. L., Ostrosky, M., & Fox, L. (2006). Social and emotional foundations for early learning: A conceptual model for intervention. *School Psychology Review, 35*, 583–601.
Hodge, N., & Runswick-Cole, K. (2008). Problematising parent-professional partnerships in education. *Disability and Society, 23*, 637–647.
Horner, R. H., Carr, E. G., Strain, P. S., Todd, A. W., & Reed, H. K. (2002). Problem behavior interventions for young children with autism: A research synthesis. *Journal of Autism and Developmental Disorders, 32*, 423–446.
Howlin, P., Magiati, I., & Charman, T. (2009). Systematic review of early intensive behavioral interventions for children with autism. *American Association on Intellectual and Developmental Disabilities, 114*, 23–41.
Ingersoll, B., & Gergans, S. (2007). The effect of a parent-implemented imitation intervention on spontaneous imitation skills in young children with autism. *Research in Developmental Disabilities, 28*, 163–175.
Kabat-Zinn, M., & Kabat-Zinn, J. (1997). *Everyday blessings: The inner work of mindful parenting*. New York, NY: Hachette Books.
Kaiser, A. P., & Hancock, T. B. (2003). Teaching parents new skills to support their young children's development. *Infants and Young Children, 16*, 9–21.
Kaiser, A. P., Hancock, T. B., & Nietfeld, J. P. (2000). The effects of parent-implemented enhanced milieu teaching on the social communication of children who have autism. *Early Education and Development, 11*, 423–446.
Kaiser, A. P., & Roberts, M. Y. (2013). Parent implemented enhanced milieu teaching with preschool children who have intellectual disabilities. *Journal of Speech, Language, and Hearing Research, 56*, 295–309.
Kaminski, J. W., Valle, L. A., Filene, J. H., & Boyle, C. L. (2008). A meta-analytic review of components associated with parent training program effectiveness. *Journal of Abnormal Child Psychology, 36*, 567–589.
Karst, J. S., & Van Hecke, A. V. (2012). Parent and family impact of autism spectrum disorders: A review and proposed model for intervention evaluation. *Clinical Child and Family Psychology Review, 15*, 247–277.
Kasari, C., Gulsrud, A., Paparella, T., Hellemann, G., & Berry, K. (2015). Randomized comparative efficacy study of parent-mediated interventions for toddlers with autism. *Journal of Consulting and Clinical Psychology, 83*, 554–563.
Kasari, C., Lawton, K., Shih, W., et al. (2014). Caregiver-mediated intervention for low-resourced preschoolers with autism: An RCT. *Pediatrics, 134*, 72–79.
Kashinath, S., Woods, J., & Goldstein, H. (2006). Enhancing generalized teaching strategy use in daily routines by parents of children with autism. *Journal of Speech, Language, and Hearing Research, 49*, 466–485.
Kim, S. H., & Lord, C. (2010). Restricted and repetitive behaviors in toddlers and preschoolers with autism spectrum disorders based on the Autism Diagnostic Observation Schedule (ADOS). *Autism Research, 3*, 162–173.
Koegel, R. L., Schreibman, L., Good, A., Cerniglia, L., Murphy, C., & Koegel, L. K. (1989). *How to teach pivotal behaviors to children with autism: A training manual*. Santa Barbara, CA: University of California.
Kroeger, K., & Sorensen, R. (2010). A parent training model for toilet training children with autism. *Journal of Intellectual Disability Research, 54*, 556–567.

Lafasakis, M., & Sturmey, P. (2007). Training parent implementation of discrete-trial teaching: Effects on generalization of parent teaching and child correct responding. *Journal of Applied Behavior Analysis, 40*, 685–689.

Lang, R., Machalicek, W., Rispoli, M., & Regester, A. (2009). Training parents to implement communication interventions for children with autism spectrum disorders (ASD): A systematic review. *Evidence-based Communication Assessment and Intervention, 3*, 174–190.

Leaf, R. B., Taubman, M. T., McEachin, J. J., Leaf, J. B., & Tsuji, K. H. (2011). A program description of a community-based intensive behavioral intervention program for individuals with autism spectrum disorders. *Education and Treatment of Children, 34*, 259–285.

Lee, J. F., Schieltz, K. M., Suess, A. N., Wacker, D. P., Romani, P. W., Lindgren, S. D., … Padilla Dalmau, Y. C. (2015). Guidelines for developing telehealth services and troubleshooting problems with telehealth technology when coaching parents to conduct functional analyses and functional communication training in their homes. *Behavior Analysis in Practice, 8*, 190

Leekam, S. R., Prior, M. R., & Uljarevic, M. (2011). Restricted and repetitive behaviors in autism spectrum disorders: A review of research in the last decade. *Psychological Bulletin, 137*, 562–593.

Lerman, D. C., Swiezy, N., Perkins-Parks, S., & Roane, H. S. (2000). Skill acquisition in parents of children with developmental disabilities: Interaction between skill type and instructional format. *Research in Developmental Disabilities, 21*, 183–196.

Lord, C., Rutter, M., & Le Couteur, A. (1994). Autism diagnostic interview-revised: A revised version of a diagnostic interview for caregivers of individuals with possible pervasive developmental disorders. *Journal of Autism and Developmental Disorders, 24*, 659–685.

Lovaas, O. I., Ackerman, A., Alexander, D., Firestone, P., Perkins, M., & Young, D. B. (1981). *Teaching developmentally disabled children: The ME book.* Austin, TX: Pro-Ed.

Lucyshyn, J. M., Albin, R. W., Horner, R. H., Mann, J. C., Mann, J. A., & Wadsworth, G. (2007). Family implementation of positive behavior support for a child with autism: Longitudinal, single-case, experimental, and descriptive replication and extension. *Journal of Positive Behavior Interventions, 9*, 131–150.

Machalicek, W., Knowles, C., Raulston, T., Ruppert, T., Carnett, A., & Alresheed, F. (2016). Challenging behavior. In J. Matson (Ed.), *Comorbid conditions among children with autism spectrum disorders*. New York, NY: Springer.

Machalicek, W., Lang, R., Knowles, C., Raulston, T., Ruppert, T., & Gerow, S. (2014, July). *Parent involvement in interventions for children with intellectual and developmental disabilities: A review of reviews*. Oral presentation at American Association for Individuals with Intellectual and Developmental Disabilities. Orlando, FL.

Machalicek, W., LeQuia, J., Pinkelman, S., Knowles, C., Raulston, T., Davis, T., & Alresheed, F. (in press). Behavioral telehealth consultation with families of children with autism spectrum disorder. *Behavioral Interventions*.

Machalicek, W., O'Reilly, M. F., Rispoli, M., Davis, T., Lang, R., Franco, J. H., & Chan, J. M. (2010). Training teachers to assess the challenging behaviors of students with autism using video teleconferencing. *Education and Training in Autism and Developmental Disability, 45*, 203–215.

Magaña, S., Lopez, K., & Machalicek, W. (in press). Parents taking action: A psycho-educational intervention for Latino parents of children with autism spectrum disorder. *Family Process*.

Mahoney, G., Kaiser, A., Girolametto, L., MacDonald, J., Robinson, C., Safford, P., & Spiker, D. (1999). Parent education in early intervention: A call for a renewed focus. *Topics in Early Childhood Special Education, 19*(3), 131–140.

Mahoney, G., & Perales, F. (2005). Relationship-focused early intervention with children with pervasive developmental disorders and other disabilities: A comparative study. *Developmental and Behavioral Pediatrics, 26*(2), 77–85.

Makrygianni, M. K., & Reed, P. (2010). A meta-analytic review of the effectiveness of behavioural early intervention programs for children with autistic spectrum disorders. *Research in Autism Spectrum Disorders, 4*, 577–593.

Malow, B. A., Adkins, K. W., Reynolds, A., Weiss, S. K., Loh, A., Fawkes, D., … Clemons, T. (2014). Parent-based sleep education for children with autism spectrum disorders. *Journal of Autism and Developmental Disabilities, 44*, 216–228.

Martinez, C. K., & Betz, A. M. (2013). Response interruption and redirection: Current research trends and clinical application. *Journal of Applied Behavior Analysis, 46*, 1–6.

Matson, J. L., & Konst, M. J. (2013). What is the evidence for long term effects of early autism interventions? *Research in Autism Spectrum Disorders, 7*, 475–479.

Matson, J. L., Mahan, S., & LoVullo, S. V. (2009). Parent training: A review of methods for children with developmental disabilities. *Research in Developmental Disabilities, 30*, 961–968.

Matson, M. L., Mahan, S., & Matson, J. L. (2009). Parent training: A review of methods for children with autism spectrum disorders. *Research in Autism Spectrum Disorders, 3*, 868–875.

Maughan, D. R., Christiansen, E., Jenson, W. R., Olympia, D., & Clark, E. (2005). Behavioral parent training as a treatment for externalizing behaviors and disruptive behavior disorders: A meta-analysis. *School Psychology Review, 34*, 267–286.

Mayer, G. R., Sulzer-Azaroff, B., & Wallace, M. (2014). *Behavior analysis for lasting change* (3rd ed.). Cornwall-on-Hudson, NY: Sloan Publishing.

McConachie, H., & Diggle, T. (2006). Parent implemented early intervention for young children with autism spectrum disorder: A systematic review. *Journal of Evaluation in Clinical Practice, 13*, 120–129.

McDuffie, A., Bullard, L., Nelson, S., Machalicek, W., & Abbeduto, L. (in press). A spoken language intervention for school-aged boys with fragile X syndrome. *American Journal on Intellectual and Developmental Disabilities.*

McDuffie, A., Machalicek, W., Oakes, A., Haebig, E., Weismer, S. E., & Abbeduto, L. (2013). Distance video-teleconferencing in early intervention: Pilot study of a naturalistic parent implemented language intervention. *Topics in Early Childhood Special Education, 33*, 172–185.

McIntyre, L. L., & Phaneuf, L. K. (2007). A Three-Tier Model of Parent Education in Early Childhood Applying a Problem-Solving Model. *Topics in Early Childhood Special Education, 27*, 214–222.

Meadan, H., Ostrosky, M. M., Zaghlawan, H., & Yu, S. Y. (2009). Promoting the social and communicative behavior of young children with autism spectrum disorders: A review of parent-implemented intervention studies. *Topics in Early Childhood Special Education, 29*, 90–104.

Moes, D. R., & Frea, W. D. (2002). Contextualized behavioral support in early intervention for children with autism and their families. *Journal of Autism and Developmental Disorders, 32*, 519–533.

Moore, J. W., & Fisher, W. W. (2007). The effects of videotape modeling on staff acquisition of functional analysis methodology. *Journal of Applied Behavior Analysis, 40*, 197–202.

Moore, T. R., & Symons, F. J. (2009). Adherence to behavioral and medical treatment recommendations by parents of children with autism spectrum disorders. *Journal of Autism and Developmental Disorders, 39*, 1173–1184.

Mueller, T. G., Singer, G. H. S., & Grace, E. J. (2004). The individuals with disabilities education act and California's proposition 227: Implications for English language learners with special needs. *Bilingual Research Journal: The Journal of the National Association for Bilingual Education, 28*, 231–251.

Najdowski, A. C., Wallace, M. D., Reagon, K., Penrod, B., Higbee, T. S., & Tarbox, J. (2010). Utilizing a homebased parent training approach in the treatment of food selectivity. *Behavioral Interventions, 25*, 89–107.

National Institute of Mental Health. (1998). *Priorities for prevention research at NIMH: A report by the national advisory mental health council workgroup on mental disorders prevention research* (NIH Publication No. 98-4321). Washington, DC: U. S. Government Printing Office.

Neece, C. L. (2014). Mindfulness-based stress reduction for parents of young children with developmental delays: Implications for parental mental health and child behavior problems. *Journal of Applied Research in Intellectual Disabilities, 27*, 174–186.

Neece, C. L., Green, S. A., & Baker, B. L. (2012). Parenting stress and child behavior problems: A transactional relationship across time. *American Journal on Intellectual and Developmental Disabilities, 117*, 48–66.

Nefdt, N., Koegel, R., Singer, G., & Gerber, M. (2010). The use of a self-directed learning program to provide introductory training in pivotal response treatment to parents of children with autism. *Journal of Positive Behavior Interventions, 12*, 23–32.

Noyes-Grosser, D. M., Rosas, S. R., Goldman, A., Elbaum, B., Romanczyk, R., & Callahan, E. H. (2014). Conceptualizing child and family outcomes of early intervention services for children with ASD and their families. *Journal of Early Intervention, 35*, 332.

O'Reilly, M., Renzaglia, A., Hutchins, M., Koterbra- Buss, L., Clayton, M., Halle, J. W., & Izen, C. (1992). Teaching systematic instruction competencies to special education student teachers: An applied behavioral supervision model. *Journal of the Association for the Severely Handicapped, 17*, 104–111.

Oono, I. P., Honey, E. J., & McConachie, H. (2013). Parent-mediated early intervention for young children with autism spectrum disorders (ASD). The Cochrane Collaboration. Hoboken, NJ: John Wiley & Sons, Ltd.

Osborne, L. A., McHugh, L., Saunders, J., & Reed, P. (2008). Parenting stress reduces the effectiveness of early teaching interventions for autistic spectrum disorders. *Journal of Autism and Developmental Disorders, 38*, 1092–1103.

Park, J. H., Alber-Morgan, S. R., & Cannella-Malone, H. (2011). Effects of mother-implemented Picture Exchange Communication System (PECS) training on independent communicative behaviors of young children with autism spectrum disorders. *Topics in Early Childhood Special Education, 31*, 37–47.

Parsons, M. B., & Reid, D. H. (1995). Training residential supervisors to provide feedback for maintaining staff teaching skills with people who have severe disabilities. *Journal of Applied Behavior Analysis, 28*, 317–322.

Patterson, S. Y., Smith, V., & Jelen, M. (2010). Behavioural intervention practices for stereotypic and repetitive behavior in individuals with autism spectrum disorder: A systematic review. *Developmental Medicine and Child Neurology, 52*, 318–327.

Patterson, S. Y., Smith, V., & Mirenda, P. (2012). A systematic review of training programs for parents of children with autism spectrum disorders: Single subject contributions. *Autism, 16*, 498–522.

Peters-Scheffer, N., Didden, R., Korzilius, H., & Sturmey, P. (2011). A meta-analytic study on the effectiveness of comprehensive ABA-based early intervention programs for children with autism spectrum disorders. *Research in Autism Spectrum Disorders, 5*, 60–69.

Piazza, C. C., Adelinis, J. D., Hanley, G. P., Goh, H. L., & Delai, M. D. (2000). An evaluation of the effects of matched stimuli on behaviors maintained by automatic reinforcement. *Journal of Applied Behavior Analysis, 33*, 13–27.

Reichow, B., & Wolery, M. (2009). Comprehensive synthesis of early intensive behavioral interventions for young children with autism based on the UCLA young autism project model. *Journal of Autism and Developmental Disorders, 39*, 23–41.

Reid, M. J., Webster-Stratton, C., & Hammond, M. (2007). Enhancing a classroom social competence and problem-solving curriculum by offering parent training to families of moderate-to high-risk elementary school children. *Journal of Clinical Child and Adolescent Psychology, 36*, 605–620.

Richdale, A. L. (1999). Sleep problems in autism: Prevalence, cause, and intervention. *Developmental Medicine and Child Neurology, 41*, 60–66.

Richler, J., Biship, S. L., Kleinke, J. R., & Lord, C. (2007). Restricted and repetitive behaviors in young children with autism spectrum disorders. *Journal of Autism and Developmental Disorders, 35*, 73–85.

Rickards, A. K., Walstab, J. E., Wright-Rossi, R. A., Simpson, J., & Reddihough, D. S. (2009). One-year follow-up of the outcome of a randomized controlled trial of a home-based intervention programme for children with autism and developmental delay and their families. *Child: Care, Health and Development, 35*, 593–602.

Rinald, K., & Mirenda, P. (2012). Effectiveness of a modified rapid toilet training workshop for parents of children with developmental disabilities. *Research in Developmental Disabilities, 33*, 933–943.

Roberts, M., & Kaiser, A. (2011). The effectiveness of parent-implemented language interventions: A meta-analysis. *American Journal of Speech-Language Pathology, 20*, 180–199.

Rocha, M. L., Schreibman, L., & Stahmer, A. C. (2007). Effectiveness of training parents to teach joint attention in children with autism. *Journal of Early Intervention, 29*, 154–172.

Rogers, S. J., Estes, A., Lord, C., Vismara, L., Winter, J., Fitzpatrick, A., & Dawson, G. (2012). Effects of a brief Early Start Denver Model (ESDM)-based parent intervention on toddlers at risk for autism spectrum disorders: A randomized controlled trial. *Journal of the American Academy of Child & Adolescent Psychiatry, 51*, 1052–1065.

Rosenberg, S. A., & Robinson, C. (1988). Interactions of parents with their young handicapped children. In S. Odom & M. Karnes (Eds.), *Early intervention for infants and children with handicaps: An empirical base* (pp. 159–178). Baltimore, MD: Brookes.

Sallows, G. O., & Graupner, T. (2005). Intensive behavioral treatment for children with autism: Four-year outcome and predictors. *American Journal on Mental Retardation, 110*, 417–438.

Sanders, M. R. (1999). Triple P-Positive Parenting Program: Towards an empirically validated multilevel parenting and family support strategy for the prevention of behavior and emotional problems in children. *Clinical Child and Family Psychology Review, 2*, 71–90.

Sanders, M. R., Cann, W., & Markie-Dadds, C. (2003). The Triple P-Positive Parenting Programme: A universal population-level approach to the prevention of child abuse. *Child Abuse Review, 12*, 155–171.

Schertz, H. H., Odom, S. L., Baggett, K. M., & Sideris, J. H. (2013). Effects of joint attention mediated learning for toddlers with autism spectrum disorders: An initial randomized controlled study. *Early Childhood Research Quarterly, 28*, 249–258.

Sears, K. M. (2010). *Using the prevent-teach-reinforce model with families of children with autism* (Doctoral dissertation, University of South Florida).

Sears, K. M., Blair, K., Iovannone, R., & Crosland, K. (2013). Using the prevent-teach-reinforce model with families of young children with ASD. *Journal of Autism and Developmental Disorders, 43*, 1005–1016.

Serketich, W. J., & Dumas, J. E. (1996). The effectiveness of behavioral parent training to modify antisocial behavior in children: A meta-analysis. *Behavior Therapy, 27*, 171–186.

Shaffer, A., Kotchick, B. A., Dorsey, S., & Forehand, R. (2004). Parenting antisocial children and adolescents. In M. Hoghughi & N. Long (Eds.), *Handbook of parenting* (pp. 256–275). London: Sage.

Shipley-Benamou, R., Lutzker, J. R., & Taubman, M. (2002). Teaching daily living skills to children with autism through instructional video modeling. *Journal of Positive Behavior Interventions, 4*, 166–177.

Singer, G. H. S. (2006). Meta-analysis of comparative studies of depression in mothers of children with and without developmental disabilities. *American Journal of Mental Retardation, 111*, 155–169.

Singer, G. H. S., Ethridge, B. L., & Aldana, S. L. (2007). Primary and secondary effects of parenting and stress management interventions for parents of children with developmental disabilities: A meta-analysis. *Mental Retardation and Developmental Disabilities Research Reviews, 13*, 357–369.

Singh, N. N., Lancioni, G. E., Winton, A. S. W., Singh, J., Curtis, W. J., Wahler, R. G., & McAleavey, K. M. (2007). Mindful parenting decreases aggression and increases social behavior in children with developmental disabilities. *Behavior Modification, 31*, 749–771.

Smith, T. (2001). Discrete trial training in the treatment of autism. *Focus on Autism and Other Developmental Disabilities, 16*, 86–92.

Smith, T., Groen, A. D., & Wynn, J. W. (2000). Randomized trial of intensive early intervention for children with pervasive developmental disorder. *American Journal of Mental Retardation, 105*, 269–285.

Smith, I. M., Koegel, R. L., Koegel, L. K., Openden, D. A., Fossum, K. L., & Bryson, S. E. (2010). Effectiveness of a novel community-based early intervention model for children with autistic spectrum disorder. *American Journal of Intellectual and Developmental Disability, 115*, 504–523.

Sprick, R., Knight, J., Reinke, W., Skyles, T., & Barnes, L. (2010). *Coaching classroom management: Strategies and tools for administrators and coaches*. Eugene, OR: Pacific Northwest Publishing.

Stokes, J. V., & Luiselli, J. K. (2008). In-home parent training of functional analysis skills. *International Journal of Behavioral Consultation and Therapy, 4*, 259–263.

Strauss, K., Mancini, F., the SPC Group, & Fava, L. (2013). Parent inclusion in early intensive behavior interventions for young children with ASD: A synthesis of meta-analyses from 2009-2011. *Research in Developmental Disabilities, 34*, 2967–2985.

Strauss, K., Vicari, S., Valeri, G., D'Elia, L., Arima, S., & Fava, L. (2012). Parent inclusion in Early Intensive Behavioral Intervention: The influence of parental stress, parent treatment fidelity and parent-mediated generalization of behavior targets on child outcomes. *Research in Developmental Disabilities, 33*, 688–703.

Stronach, S., & Weatherby, A. M. (2014). Examining restricted and repetitive behaviors in young children with autism spectrum disorder during tow observational contexts. *Autism, 18*, 127–136.

Sturmey, P., & Fitzer, A. (Eds.). (2007). *Autism spectrum disorders: Applied behavior analysis, evidence and practice*. Austin, TX: Pro-Ed.

Suess, A. N., Romani, P. W., Wacker, D. P., Dyson, S. M., Kuhle, J. L., Lee, J. F., … Waldron, D. B. (2014). Evaluating the treatment fidelity of parents who conduct in-home functional communication training with coaching via telehealth. *Journal of Behavioral Education, 23*, 34–59.

Sy, S., Gottfried, A. W., & Gottfried, A. E. (2013). A transactional model of parent involvement and children's achievement from early childhood through adolescence. *Parenting: Science and Practice, 13*, 133–152.

Taber, T. A., Alberto, P. A., Seltzer, A., & Hughes, M. (2003). Obtaining assistance when lost in the community using cell phones. *Research and Practice for Persons with Severe Disabilities, 28*, 105–116.

Tellegen, C. L., & Sanders, M. R. (2013). Stepping Stones Triple P-Positive Parenting Program for children with disability: A systematic review and meta-analysis. *Research in Developmental Disabilities, 34*, 1556–1571.

Test, D. W., Spooner, F., Keul, P. K., & Grossi, T. (1990). Teaching adolescents with severe disability to use the public telephone. *Behavior Modification, 14*, 157–171.

The Individuals with Disabilities Act Amendments of 1997. (1997). Pub. L. No. 17-105, § 101, 111 Stat. 37.

The Individuals with Disabilities Education Act of 1990. (1990). 20 U.S.C. §§ 1400 et seq. The Individuals with Disabilities Education Improvement Act of 2004. (2004). Pub. L. No. 108-446, 101,118 Stat. 2647.

Thomas, R., & Zimmer-Gembeck, M. J. (2007). Behavioral outcomes of parent-child interaction therapy and Triple P—Positive Parenting Program: A review and meta-analysis. *Journal of Abnormal Child Psychology, 35*, 475–495.

Tiano, J. D., & McNeil, C. B. (2005). The inclusion of fathers in behavioral parent training: A critical evaluation. *Child & Family Behavior Therapy, 27*, 1–28.

Tonge, B., Brereton, A., Kiomall, M., Mackinnon, A., King, N., & Rinehart, N. (2006). Effects on parental mental health of an education and skills training program for parents of young children with autism: A randomized controlled trial. *Journal of the American Academy of Child and Adolescent Psychiatry, 45*(5), 561–569.

Turnbull, A. P., & Turnbull, H. R. (1990). *Families, professionals, and exceptionality: A special partnership* (2nd ed.). Columbus, OH: Merrill.

UyBico, S. J., Pavel, S., & Gross, C. P. (2007). Recruiting vulnerable populations into research: A systematic review of recruitment interventions. *Journal of General Internal Medicine, 22*, 852–863.

Van Camp, C. M., Vollmer, T. R., Goh, H. L., Whitehouse, C. M., Reyes, J., Montgomery, J. L., & Borrero, J. C. (2008). Behavioral parent training in child welfare: Evaluations of skills acquisition. *Research on Social Work Practice, 18*, 377–391.

Vasquez, E. III, Lopez, A., Straub, C., Powell, S., McKinney, T., Walker, Z., … Bedesem, P. L. (2011). Empirical research on ethnic minority students: 1995-2009. *Learning Disabilities Research and Practice, 26*, 84–93.

Vismara, L. A., & Rogers, S. J. (2008). The Early Start Denver Model a case study of an innovative practice. *Journal of Early Intervention, 31*, 91–108.

Vismara, L. A., Young, G. S., Stahmer, A. C., Griffith, E. M., & Rogers, S. J. (2009). Dissemination of evidence-based practice: Can we train therapists from a distance? *Journal of Autism and Developmental Disorders, 39*, 1636–1651.

Vismara, L. A., Young, G. S., & Rogers, S. J. (2012). Telehealth for expanding the reach of early autism training to parents. *Autism Research and Treatment, 47*, 1–12.

Wacker, D. P., Lee, J. F., Dalmau, Y. C. P., Kopelman, T. G., Lindgren, S. D., Kuhle, J., … Waldron, D. B. (2013a). Conducting functional analyses of problem behavior via telehealth. *Journal of Applied Behavior Analysis, 46*, 31–46.

Wacker, D. P., Lee, J. F., Dalmau, Y. C. P., Kopelman, T. G., Lindgren, S. D., Kuhle, J., … Waldron, D. B. (2013b). Conducting functional communication training via telehealth to reduce the problem behavior of young children with autism. *Journal of Developmental and Physical Disabilities, 25*, 35–48.

Wallace, K. S., & Rogers, S. J. (2010). Intervening in infancy: Implications for autism spectrum disorders. *Journal of Child Psychology and Psychiatry, 51*, 1300–1320.

Ward-Horner, J., & Sturmey, P. (2010). Component analysis using single-subject experimental designs: A review. *Journal of Applied Behavior Analysis, 43*, 685–704.

Warren, Z., McPheeters, M. L., Sathe, N., Foss-Feig, J. H., Glasser, A., & Veenstra-VanderWeele, J. (2011). A systematic review of early intensive intervention for autism spectrum disorders. *Pediatrics, 127*, 1303–1311.

Waschbusch, D. A., Cunningham, C. E., Pelham, W. E., et al. (2011). A discrete choice conjoint experiment to evaluate parent preferences for treatment of young, medication naïve children with ADHD. *Journal of Clinical Child and Adolescent Psychology, 40*, 546–561.

Webster-Stratton, C. (1984). Randomized trial of two parent-training programs for families with conduct-disordered children. *Journal of Consulting and Clinical Psychology, 52*, 666–678.

Webster-Stratton, C. (2001). The Incredible Years: Parents, teachers, and children training series. *Residential Treatment for Children & Youth, 18*, 31–45.

Webster-Stratton, C., & Hammond, M. (1997). Treating children with early-onset conduct problems: A comparison of child and parent training interventions. *Journal of Consulting and Clinical Psychology, 65*, 93–109.

Webster-Stratton, C., Hollinsworth, T., & Kolpacoff, M. (1989). The long-term effectiveness and clinical significance of three cost-effective training programs for families with conduct problem children. *Journal of Consulting and Clinical Psychology, 57*, 550–553.

Webster-Stratton, C., Kolpacoff, M., & Hollinsworth, T. (1988). Self-administered videotape therapy for families with conduct-problem children: Comparison with two cost-effective treatments and a control group. *Journal of Consulting and Clinical Psychology, 56*, 558–566.

Webster-Stratton, C., Reid, M. J., & Hammond, M. (2004). Treating children with early-onset conduct problems: Intervention outcomes for parent, child, and teacher training. *Journal of Clinical Child and Adolescent Psychology, 33*, 105–124.

Weiskop, S., Richdale, A., & Matthews, J. (2005). Behavioural treatment to reduce sleep problems in children with autism or fragile X syndrome. *Developmental Medicine and Child Neurology, 47*, 94–104.

White, P. J., O'Reilly, M., Streusand, W., Levine, A., Sigafoos, J., Lancioni, G. E., … Aguilar, J. (2011). Best practices for teaching joint attention: A systematic review of the intervention literature. *Research in Autism Spectrum Disorders, 5*, 1283–1295.

Williams White, S., Koenig, K., & Scahill, L. (2007). Social skills development in children with autism spectrum disorders: A review of the intervention research. *Journal of Autism and Developmental Disorders, 37*, 1858–1868.

Wolff, J. J., Botteron, K. N., Dager, S. R., Elison, J. T., Estes, A. M., Gu, H., … The IBIS Network. (2014). Longitudinal patterns of repetitive behavior in toddlers with autism. *Journal of Child Psychology and Psychiatry*, 55, 954–953.

Woods, J., Kashinath, S., & Goldstein, H. (2004). Effects of embedding caregiver-implemented teaching strategies in daily routines on children's communication outcomes. *Journal of Early Intervention, 26*, 175–193.

World Health Organization. (2007). Global resources for persons with intellectual disabilities. Available online at: http://www.who.int/mental_health/evidence/atlas_id_2007.pdf, accessed 24 August 2014.

Chapter 9
Fad, Pseudoscientific, and Controversial Interventions

Jason C. Travers, Kevin Ayers, Richard L. Simpson, and Stephen Crutchfield

Introduction

Special education and related professions are noteworthy for attracting and accepting unsubstantiated interventions (Metz, Mulick, & Butter, 2016). Professionals, families, and other stakeholders affected by ASD have especially been duped into believing in faddish "cures" and unconventional treatment methods. This problem historically has obstructed the progression of understanding and reliable application of effective methods for learners with ASD. The tendency toward unproven and disproven treatments has had harmful, dangerous, and sometimes fatal outcomes. The nefarious legacy and recent resurgence of facilitated communication (FC) perhaps best exemplifies how pseudoscience impinges on special education practice. Alternatively, scientific values and methodology are useful for preventing the spread of worthless and harmful interventions and establishing a repository of interventions supported by verifiable explanations. This special education scientific movement reflects intentions to positively influence how professionals support and educate learners with ASD. In many respects this important prophylactic role parallels the Hippocratic Oath: "First do no harm."

J.C. Travers (✉) • R.L. Simpson
Department of Special Education, University of Kansas,
1122 West Campus Road, Lawrence, KS 66045, USA
e-mail: jason.travers@ku.edu

K. Ayers
Department of Communication Sciences and Special Education,
University of Georgia, Athens, GA, USA

S. Crutchfield
Special Education, California Polytechnic State University,
444 Minnesota Avenue #300, Kansas City, KS, USA

R. Lang et al. (eds.), *Early Intervention for Young Children with Autism Spectrum Disorder*, Evidence-Based Practices in Behavioral Health,
DOI 10.1007/978-3-319-30925-5_9

However, advancing scientific methods, values, and thought has proven insufficient for preventing the proliferation of nonsense within the ASD community. Vyse (2005) explained that simply pointing out fad, disproven, and unproven interventions does not prevent them from spreading. In contrast developing and improving consumer's ability to evaluate interventions is indispensable. We wholeheartedly agree. Although this textbook provides clarity about intervention models most likely to be effective, mere identification will not ensure implementation nor sufficiently deter adoption of fad, pseudoscientific, and controversial interventions. Similarly, providing a list of historical and contemporary examples of fads and pseudoscientific interventions in ASD also is insufficient; such interventions evolve with astounding speed and are easily repackaged. Rather, understanding fundamental scientific principles and rules of argumentation presented alongside characteristics of pseudoscience will best ensure prudent and objective evaluation of educational interventions in ASD.

The intervention models described in previous chapters were derived from scientific investigation. Each represents the accumulation of knowledge acquired during decades of meticulous work. This chapter is in response to the ongoing need to understand why people affected by ASD continue toward unsupported, refuted, or sometimes bizarre treatments. The aim of this chapter is to support professionals and other stakeholders to avoid fad, controversial, and pseudoscientific interventions in ASD by outlaying the tools of science and pseudoscience in ways that support critical analysis of claims about interventions for learners with ASD. Specific attention is dedicated to contrasting science with pseudoscience as well as some related psychological phenomenon and errors in thinking that stimulate irrational thought and behavior. Various historical and contemporary examples also are reviewed to illustrate the characteristics, dangers, and persistence of fads and pseudoscience in ASD. Implications for professionals and families also are discussed.

The Rise in Popularity of Fad, Pseudoscientific, and Controversial Treatment

Much attention and has been dedicated to investigating fad and controversial treatments in ASD. Journal articles (e.g., Mudford et al., 2000; Simpson & Myles, 1995; Todd, 2012; Tostanoski, Lang, Raulston, Carnett, & Davis, 2014; Travers, Tincani, & Lang, 2014) textbooks (e.g., Foxx & Mulick, 2016), and popular print (e.g., Offit, 2010) have dealt with a variety of unsubstantiated claims regarding various treatments. Despite advances in understanding ASD etiology, early identification, and treatment, many unfounded beliefs and pseudoscientific interventions continue to proliferate. The intervention models outlined in this book represent those that have objectively produced desired improvements. These hard-won advancements in knowledge are products of science and represent the state of the art in early intensive behavior intervention (EIBI). Despite these developments, unsubstantiated or inaccurate information about the causes of characteristics of ASD may lead unsuspecting or uniformed parents to adopt treatments and interventions that are fads, unproven, disproven, and potentially harmful. Several basic factors can be used to explain this problem.

Children with ASD experience an array of challenges effecting social, communicative, and behavioral development. The extent that these areas of development are impaired varies considerably and their causes remain only partially understood. Nevertheless, many children are severely impacted by their ASD and other legitimate comorbid conditions. The resultant turmoil and anguish experienced by parents, family members, and/or other individuals who care about the person with the ASD diagnosis, as well as feelings of love, devotion, and protection undoubtedly serve as motivation for seeking out interventions and treatments that purportedly improve functioning (Metz et al., 2016). Fear of regret for omitting potentially helpful treatments also may play a role in adopting unproven or disproven ASD treatments. Such emotions may compromise rational thinking and lead even highly educated parents to seek interventions that promise small but supposedly important gains (e.g., sensory integration training; SIT) to miraculous breakthroughs (e.g., FC) and warnings of deterioration in functioning if an unsupported method is abandoned (e.g., special diets).

The baffling contradiction of savant-like qualities of a few people with severe ASD, as well as the relatively more common splinter skills among others, also may contribute to adoption of unsupported interventions. This may be because assumptions of hidden potential are inferred based on idiosyncratic splinter skills. For example, children with ASD are characterized as having extensive support needs that are sometimes accompanied by precocious reading ability or advanced visual-spatial skills. Similarly, some parents have reported their children developed normally and suddenly lost communication and social skills, although insufficient evidence of regressive ASD substantiates this claim (Hansen et al., 2008). In rare cases, people with ASD also have savant skills in music (e.g., recite symphonies), mathematical computation (e.g., calendar calculation), artistic ability (e.g., drawing, painting), and/or other areas (Howlin, Goode, Hutton, & Rutter, 2009). Despite the rarity of savant skills, popular media often portray people with ASD as regularly fitting this stereotype. The apparent incongruence between ability and disability is perplexing, even among experts, and may contribute to unfounded beliefs that a person with ASD has normal or superior intellectual functioning, but somehow is trapped in an "autistic world" or an unresponsive body (Stubblefield, 2011). These phenomena may generate an aura of mysticism about ASD etiology that contributes to adoption of related unfounded treatments.

The prevalence of ASD has dramatically increased since 1990 (CDC 2007, 2009; Fombonne, 2007; Yeargin-Allsopp, Rice, Karapurkar, Doernberg, Boyle, & Murphy, 2003). During these decades, fears of an ASD epidemic became increasingly widespread (Fombonne, 2001). The estimated epidemiological prevalence at the time this chapter was written was 1 in 68 (CDC, 2014). Fears of an "ASD epidemic" remain endemic (Lilienfeld & Arkowitz, 2007). Despite increased prevalence, popular belief of an ASD epidemic appears to be inconsistent with the evidence (Gernsbacher, Dawson, & Goldsmith, 2005). The increase has been largely (but not entirely) attributed to (1) broadening of the diagnostic criteria for ASD, (2) addition of ASD as a special education eligibility category in the Individuals with Disabilities Education Act of 1990 and its subsequent reauthorizations, (3) increased awareness of and monitoring for ASD, and (4) improved assessment and identification methods (Fombonne, 2009; Presmanes, Zuckerman, & Fombonne, 2014). Nevertheless, the apparently sudden and dramatic increase is often national news and has contributed to widespread concerns that vaccines might play a role. This belief is tied to a single retracted paper that appears to have been financially motivated (Offit, 2010). The resulting irrational behavior stemming from this scam includes anti-vaccine rhetoric and likely has contributed to the adoption of duplicitous treatments with limited or no efficacy for treating ASD symptomology.

The limited availability of and costs associated with effective interventions also may send parents to search for alternative (i.e., unproven) interventions (Metz et al., 2016; Tuzikow & Holburn, 2011). While ASD prevalence increased, more Americans gained access to the Internet and information about various fads and alternative treatments became readily available. Some of these alternatives are more affordable, at least in the short term, and easier to administer (e.g., megavitamins) than established methods (e.g., Discrete Trial Training). Some interventions trended in popularity, quickly gaining and losing attention (e.g., secretin therapy); but others have endured (e.g., SIT; FC). Parents who were unable to access proven interventions (e.g., rural families; impoverished families) or simply could not afford them might have turned instead to more accessible but unproven interventions.

The perceived mystery of ASD coupled with the fears of an ASD epidemic and the limited availability of intervention services represented ideal conditions for quacks, confidence men, and crackpots. When infrastructure for online commerce gained consumer confidence, misleading information could be easily disseminated to create an exploitative industry of massive size and scope. False causes were manufactured in lockstep with "miraculous" and "breakthrough" treatments designed to address those causes. Today we witness an array of unsubstantiated claims connected to unproven (and often unregulated) treatments on the Internet, some of which are described later in this chapter. Professionals and parents likely have been exposed to, tempted by, or duped by some of these alternatives. Few are immune to such exploitation.

Characteristics of Fad, Pseudoscientific, and Controversial Interventions

Fad, controversial, and pseudoscientific interventions are terms used to describe distinctively different phenomenon, but each is intended to achieve niche or broad acceptance. The Oxford dictionary defines fad as "an intense and widely shared enthusiasm for something, especially one that is short-lived; a craze; an arbitrary like or dislike." Fads can be beneficial, benign, or harmful as well as expensive or affordable. Fads in diet and fitness may be beneficial if they increase the health of participants, but harmful if they distract from more effective approaches. Fads in special education are almost always costly and harmful. Education fads rarely confer benefit and waste time, opportunities to learn, effort, and money while sapping optimism for and attainment of better outcomes (Kozloff, 2005). Yet fads are disturbingly common in education. Mostert (2000) explained how the bandwagon effect contributes to fads by attaining a self-perpetuating status that frequently depends on simple but divisive ideology and proselytizing. The field has encountered numerous fads that rapidly gain and lose popularity, but some fads are maintained and become malignant problems that obstruct progress (Kozloff, 2005). In this way, education fads can become controversial practices, usually through the pseudoscientific mechanisms, and be sustained via educational practice and acceptance. This illustrates the power of the bandwagon effect.

> Bandwagons provide a communal sense of purpose, an energizing camaraderie, and a collective voice whose power exceeds its importance. Bandwagons are used to champion a cause, engage in sweeping yet attractive rhetoric, and generally promise far more than they ever have hope of delivering while simultaneously downplaying or ignoring the negative aspects of their edicts (Mostert, 2000, p. 124).

Ideas can be controversial for a variety of reasons. In some cases, controversy refers to differences of opinion. In other circumstances, controversy might refer to an ethical argument that conflicts with evidence. For example, there exists substantial evidence supporting the effectiveness of aversive interventions for modifying extremely dangerous self-injury (e.g., eye-gouging), but many behavior analysts may disagree with the practice. Putting those issues aside, our purpose is to focus on controversial interventions used despite evidence of their effectiveness (Metz et al., 2016; Silver, 1995). Controversial interventions might cause confusion because the available evidence of treatment effects is contradictory or because no confirming or refuting evidence is available. This confusion partly stems from a credulous disposition of accepting a claim as true or withholding doubts until a claim is disproven (or belief becomes untenable) and the misperception that evidence is a synonym for absolute proof. Importantly, evidence exists on a continuum and correlates with degrees of confidence about the validity of claim. Strong evidence typically is represented by multiple methodologically sound studies that result in similar outcomes. Confidence in the claim increases with the quantity and quality of empirical evidence supportive of (or refuting) the claim. A body of high-quality evidence leads to scientific consensus, but is never considered an indication of absolute certainty (i.e., proof); there are no absolutes in science. Chance, poor research design, or confounding factors may produce findings that contradict a larger body of evidence, but do not warrant dismissal of the prevailing evidence.

When the preponderance of evidence supports a claim, that claim is treated as more likely accurate than an alternative explanation supported by a small body of conflicting evidence. Importantly, contradictory minority findings typically are not sufficiently meritorious to justify rejection of scientific consensus. Thus, controversial treatments can be explained in two ways. First, an intervention used in the absence of sufficient supporting evidence is controversial when being used outside carefully controlled and protective boundaries of scientific experimentation. Second, controversial treatments also are those used in spite of scientific consensus. Proponents of controversial treatments often point to flawed research to support their position, especially when it conflicts with consensus. They also argue that controversy is "proof that it works for some people" and therefore "worth trying for yourself." This logic, in turn, gives way to other claims of conspiracy to suppress alternatives, accusations of "close-mindedness", and shifting the burden of proof from the claimant to the skeptic. Such fallacious reasoning colludes with credulity to convey a sense that "controversial" is a permissive rather than prohibitive label.

Pseudoscience obviates the corrective mechanisms of the scientific method in that it relies on seeking confirmation of an already accepted conclusion. When evidence refuting the claim is obtained, belief often is maintained by altering the explanation for the phenomenon; evidence against is distorted as questionable or favorable evidence (e.g., ad-hoc hypotheses; moving the goalpost fallacy). Society is rife with pseudoscience because it often is difficult to distinguish from authentic science and thrives where there exists little cultivation of analytic behavior. Consequently, pseudoscientific beliefs like astrology, homeopathy, anti-vaccination, SIT, megavitamins, intelligent design, dowsing, ghost hunting, 9–11 truthers, and so on are well-subscribed. We return later to pseudoscience to contrast it with science, but suffice to say that many popular beliefs, therapies, and treatments exist wholly on pseudoscientific ground because (1) they are deceptively cloaked as science and (2) many individuals do not, cannot, and probably should not be expected to evaluate all claims to ascertain validity.

Science, Anti-Science, and Pseudoscience

According to Merriam-Webster, science is defined as "knowledge about or study of the natural world based on facts learned through experiments and observation; a particular area of scientific study (such as biology, physics, or chemistry); a particular branch of science; a subject that is formally studied in a college, university, etc." The Oxford dictionary defines science as action by stating it is "the intellectual and practical activity encompassing the systematic study of the structure and behavior of the physical and natural world through observation and experiment." Generally, science and scientific behavior entails the accumulation of facts via deployment of experimental methods to examine the natural order of our environment. From a behavior analytic perspective, science is comprised of a repertoire of complex behavior reinforced by discovering facts about natural phenomenon.

Science is more than the application of a method. Ultimately, science is a set of attitudes that emphasizes a disposition toward facts rather than arbitrary respect for authority, acceptance of evidence even when it conflict with desires, and suspension of belief or advocacy for a position until sufficient evidence is available (Skinner, 1957). Accordingly, a scientific attitude is conservative in that it minimizes assumptions and instead emphasizes evidence. Science also values testability (i.e., falsifiability), reliability, accuracy, replication, and precision. By definition and design, the scientific process is geared to facilitate knowledge advancement, positive systems change, and innovation through a systematic and controlled course of action. Logical theories, models, and hypothetical constructs lead to cogent predictions and hypotheses. In turn, ensuing postulations are subjected to measured, organized, and systematic evaluation. Ultimately, empirical investigations in ASD serve as the foundation for knowledge of effective practice. Relative to expediting a conceptual and practical understanding of ASD and pointing the way toward maximally effective and efficient interventions, science ensures conceptual models and theoretical explanations are linked to objective and empirical evaluations of purported interventions. This process stands in sharp contrast to indiscriminate and credulous acceptance of unproven interventions derived from vague and/or peculiar suppositions derived from unsubstantiated anecdotes as the primary or exclusive kind of evidence.

Scientific thinking and methodology are needed to evaluate, refine and bring to fruition beneficial and utilitarian innovations. It is an irrefutable fact that a number of current promising interventions originated as classroom practices that had limited theoretical and empirical support. Because of the heterogeneity of ASD symptomology, practitioners are often required to calibrate interventions to best fit the characteristics of the students in their care. This calibration lends itself to extension, creativity, and innovation. Practitioners who work daily with learners with ASD have developed a host of interventions that we know little about (i.e., consequence maps, social scripting, power cards, cartooning, and so on). These interventions and others like them represent the very essence of what teachers of students with ASD should strive to be: Persistent, imaginative, and dynamic. Indeed special education is replete with examples of interventions for learners with ASD initially devoid of scientific support, but rooted in sound theory (e.g. behavior analysis) and widely used. Some of these methods were later found to have varying degrees of efficacy and utility (Lang, Koegel, et al. 2010; Lang, O'Reilly, et al. 2010).

Social narratives (Bledsoe, Smith, & Simpson, 2003; Crozier & Tincani, 2005; Ganz, Kaylor, Bourgeois, & Hadden, 2008; Kokina & Kern, 2010) and visual schedules (Duttlinger, Ayres, Bevill-Davis, & Douglas, 2013; Cihak, Wright, & Ayres, 2010; Waters, Lerman, & Hovanetz, 2009) are examples of current promising methods. The genesis of both of these interventions was in classrooms for students with ASD and both examples involved wide-scale adaptation of the methods by classroom professionals, independent of and prior to empirical validation via scientific scrutiny. Conversely, and on a far less positive note, myriad examples of intervention methods used by educators have been found to be ineffective and/or detrimental to learners with ASD. The thoroughly discredited FC method was widely used and adopted prior to scientific scrutiny that quickly revealed its destructive and disreputable nature (Palfreman, 1993; Wheeler, Jacobson, Paglieri, & Schwartz, 1993). Such problems highlight the important role of the scientific process as the most effective mechanism for identifying and vetting information about untested methods prior to dissemination. This vetting serves as an objective way of advancing potentially positive methods through a systematic process that enables professionals and other stakeholders to maximize attainment of desirable outcomes.

With only about 40 years of painstaking research, the field remains in early stages of intervention development. Some discoveries have been made and are outlined in previous chapters, but these are hardly satisfactory stopping points for self-congratulation. There remain numerous questions to be answered and our ignorance about various phenomena related to ASD vastly exceeds our collective knowledge. Accordingly, it would be foolish to not pursue refinements of existing repositories or pursue novel methods that enhance our understanding of how best to support persons with ASD. It is equally imprudent, however, to capriciously and impulsively pursue matters related to ASD according to whimsical, unsupported, and unreasoned assumptions and groundless claims. Such pursuits distract from promising research of legitimate interventions. Fad and pseudoscientific interventions claim to be the product of innovative, cutting edge research and discovery in response to (or defiance of) authentic progress portrayed as too slow, deliberate, methodical, and conservative. Yet this is precisely what pseudoscience does; stymies innovation by misdirecting intellectual, financial, and human capital from legitimate and promising investment to the pockets of ideologues and charlatans (e.g., Nancy Lurie Marks Foundation, John P. Hussman Foundation). This protective attitude is, ironically, distorted to persuade consumers that researchers are elitist, self-serving, protective, and conspiratorial.

Scientific illiteracy manifests in myriad ways ranging from superstition to gullibility and outright rejection of evidence (e.g., science denial). Scientific illiteracy is the absence of the basic understanding of the methods and philosophy of science (i.e., rationalism). Scientific illiteracy is perhaps more common, but science denial has become more popular among well- and less-educated individuals alike (Funk & Rainie, 2015). Although science is the best method ever devised for understanding the way the universe works, it remains an imperfect process. There can be no absolute certainties in science. Conclusions are always tentative and subject to scrutiny or disposal when new evidence becomes available. Accepted explanations are accompanied by caveats and differing degrees of confidence. The limitations of the scientific method are often misunderstood and misrepresented as reasons to dismiss scientific evidence, theory, and expertise. Criticism is a fundamental to the scientific method, but healthy criticism is starkly different from anti-science (Schiebinger, 2001). Wholesale rejection of science (Gross & Leavitt, 1997; Kavale & Mostert, 2003; Kozloff, 2005; Sasso, 2001) relies on poorly informed individuals who often confuse free speech with a right to be heard and respected. Treating all ideas with equal respect is intellectually dishonest and a dangerous proposition.

Scientists in fields related to ASD should be unapologetic critics of fads, hyperbolic claims, and treatment whims, but also equally strong advocates for responsible innovation. We argue for a reasoned course of action. First, rely on evidence-based interventions while simultaneously pursuing novel, rational, and plausible explanations along with innovative methods derived from prevailing theories of learning (i.e., operant, respondent, and observational). Second, include content in professional and parent training to aid the establishment of skills for evaluating claims for scientific (or pseudoscientific) merit. Discovery and validation of interventions via the scientific method will expedite productive research and development outcomes that, in turn, translate to improvements in the lives of the children with ASD and their families. This advancement is unlikely without consumers who readily recognize the ploys associated with pseudoscience.

Pseudoscience

Pseudoscientific interventions are those that do not adhere to scientific standards, but attempt to cloak themselves in the fabric of science. This deceptive tactic makes establishment of a clear demarcation between science and pseudoscience difficult. Indeed, "science probably differs from pseudoscience in degree rather than kind" (Lillienfeld, Lynn, & Lohr, 2003, p. 5). However, there exist clear indicators of pseudoscience that enhance differentiating between plausible and fantastic claims. Whereas science pursues knowledge by accumulating facts via observations to inform development of beliefs, pseudoscience *begins with a conclusion* rather than a hypothesis and seeks ways to confirm the suspicion rather than test it. In other words, whereas scientific thought requires suspension of belief until sufficient evidence is available, pseudoscience begins with unsupported conclusions followed by biased selection of information that conforms to preconceived belief. Science recognizes the potential impact of bias and has designed systems to limit human tendencies to confirm inaccurate but personally favorable or cherished beliefs. Pseudoscience relies on a preconceived agenda and pursues supportive findings while simultaneously (and often subconsciously) dismissing negating results. Lack of controls for the influential effects of this confirmation bias is a hallmark of pseudoscience.

Pseudoscience typically is associated with grandiose claims that are uncoupled from evidence. It also is dogmatic in the face of new and conflicting evidence. Arguments in support of pseudoscientific interventions appear rooted in scientific evidence or theory and thereby convey a sense of legitimacy. For example, learners with ASD often engage in repetitive behavior and sometimes those behaviors serve the purpose of self-stimulation. Sensory integration has attached itself to this phenomenon to give credence to "mentalistic" and unverified suppositions of causes of and treatments for stereotyped (and other) behaviors. When studies fail to find predicted effects, or when studies reporting positive findings do not meet minimal quality standards for methodological rigor, proponents rely on selective evidence and retreat to dogmatic and fallacious reasoning ("I've seen it for myself. It worked for my son."). Indeed, pseudoscience relies on testimonial rather than empirical data to advance the claim and protect belief. Inspirational anecdotes usually are provided to support extravagant claims of major breakthroughs (i.e., appeals to emotion) or quell criticism. In this way, it becomes clear how such thinking and behavior contributes to the proliferation of pseudoscience in ASD. Drawing conclusions without evidence about an intervention, defending those conclusions, and delivering interventions according to those beliefs beyond experimental conditions is potentially harmful.

A related defensive tactic of pseudoscientists is to demand that all ideas be treated as equally valid and deserving of respect. In this way, criticism of ideas is taken as an offensive attack on the person rather than their espoused beliefs. People may confuse their right to an opinion with a right to have their opinion heard and respected, perhaps because personal beliefs often are deeply intertwined with personal identity. This is especially common among uninformed or misinformed individuals who receive criticism from well-informed others. Indeed, "Anti-intellectualism has been a constant thread winding its way through our political and cultural life, nurtured by the false notion that democracy means that '*my ignorance is just as good as your knowledge*'" (Asimov, 1980, p. 19, italics in original). The posturing by purveyors of pseudoscience is conducive to ad-hominem attacks in defense of their wares. In a society that increasingly and rightly values cultural, ethnic, and linguistic diversity, a progressive attitude may sometimes lead to overly cautious treatment of bad ideas for fear of giving offense or being labeled a bigot. When questions or doubt arise, the skeptic is considered "close-minded." This political correctness run amok combined with attacks to suppress criticism promotes undue caution, thereby legitimizing unfounded beliefs and behavior. We should not confuse value for respecting people with respect for their ideas, especially when the ideas directly impact the lives of others.

Pseudoscience differs from science in that it often relies on ostentatious claims unsubstantiated by evidence. Claims of "miraculous", "amazing", and "breakthrough" treatments constitute red flags for pseudoscience. Pseudoscience makes claims of "proof" obtained from anecdotal and testimonial endorsement. Statements from actual or purported consumers who claim the treatment was effective are presented as evidence of the positive effects of a particular treatment. Conversely, science requires careful interpretation of findings in light of experimental limitations that, in turn, lead to conservative interpretation and tentative claims. To be clear, scientists should never claim to be absolutely certain of anything; caveats and hedges abound in accordance with available evidence. Science usually results in incremental change and revolutionary evidence is exceptionally rare. Credence is not granted to testimonial evidence because its susceptibility to a broad array of mistaken conclusions and errors in thinking. Thus, consumers should recognize that extraordinary claims should be carefully scrutinized both in terms of the reliability of the source and the ways the claim is being disseminated. Consumers should take pause when grandiose or seemingly legitimate claims derived from testimonials are promoted by popular media without peer review for publication in reputable scientific journals.

Peer review is a pillar of science because it provides a mechanism for filtering erroneous findings to provide increasing clarity about phenomena under investigation. Scientists engage in criticism of peer ideas and evidence while actively seeking criticism of their own. This community of scholarship serves as a mechanism for maintaining quality during the imperfect scientific process. Accordingly, scientists recognize that it is better to prove yourself wrong than be proven wrong by others. Conversely, pseudoscientists avoid peer review or, when their methods do not meet basic quality indicators of empirical research, claim conspiracy and seek alternative ways to disseminate their flawed findings (Lillienfeld et al., 2003). Pseudoscientists advance agendas that conflict with finding truth, though they may claim and genuinely believe to be seeking it. Quacks and con artists make no attempt (or are unable)

Table 9.1 Contrasted characteristics of science and pseudoscience

Science	Pseudoscience
Discovers evidence and uses it to inform belief; relies on entire body of evidence.	Forms belief and selects evidence to confirm; disqualifies or rejects disconfirming evidence.
Conservative claims that are tentative and based on evidence; changes in conjunction with evidence.	Grandiose claims uncoupled from evidence; dogmatic and unchanging when provided new/conflicting evidence.
Precise and measurable terminology conducive to understanding and replication.	Convoluted explanations with jargon to elude criticism, inhibit replication, and defend outstanding findings.
Knows, understands, and applies logic with body of evidence to defend position.	Relies on logical fallacy and selected evidence to advance a position.
Views critics as colleagues; seeks criticism and refutation.	Views critics as adversaries; avoids criticism and condemns dissent; works alone.

to critically examine the methods used to support their claims or develop alternative explanations for findings. When confronted with questions or refuting evidence, they revert to fallacious argument including conspiracy to suppress evidence, shifting the burden of proof, hypothesis saving, ad hominem attack, straw man fallacy, and so on. Table 9.1 provides a side-by-side contrast of distilled characteristics of science and pseudoscience to support consumer evaluation of any claim.

Skepticism and Credulity

Skepticism is "not a position; skepticism is an approach to claims, in the same way that science is not a subject but a method" (Shermer, 2002, p. xvii). Credulity, by contrast, is an almost complete willingness to trust claims and positions put forth by others as being true without evaluating their plausibility. We may, in social engagements, silently accept as true what someone tells us to avoid conflict or embarrassment. We sometimes may find ourselves at least tacitly agreeing with someone's position. For example, we may entertain flattery even when the logic is absurd (e.g. "You're a Scorpio so you must be very brave!") or attempt to carefully navigate social situations, but critical skepticism should guide most of our actions. This is especially important when making decisions that affect lives (i.e., treatment for a medical condition; addressing education needs). We may accept without thinking benign declarations, but the degree to which we accept a claim without evidence is proportionate to the plausibility of the claim, its convention, and its impact. Ordinary claims that are plausible, conventional, and of little impact are granted more credence and require little or no evidence (e.g., I have a pet dog). Extraordinary claims (e.g., I have a pet dragon.) are implausible, unconventional, and directly impact a worldview and therefore require much stronger evidence. The great science communicator Carl Sagan often quipped that extraordinary claims require extraordinary evidence.

Credulity exists on a continuum from extreme optimism (total credulity—accepting all claims without question) to complete pessimism (incredulity—rejecting all claims as false without examination). Credulity may be taken to mean gullible and incredulity may be mistaken for skepticism, but these terms refer to different approaches to a claim. The credulous, incredulous, and skeptical individual all make decisions about belief when presented with new information. Invoking some classical examples of this tension, if we situate Candide and Dr. Pangloss (characters from Voltaire's satire) discussing the latest fad in ASD treatment, we would witness two distinct approaches to a novel claim of treatment efficacy. As a classical optimist, Dr. Pangloss would assume that "all is for the best in the best of all possible worlds" and therefore a new nasal spray treatment for ASD must be effective; the spray was created to treat ASD so surely it must (i.e., credulity). Candide, on the other hand, would respect the nature of the claim but question its veracity until presented with supporting evidence (i.e., skepticism). A credulous person immediately accepts the claim as true irrespective of the (absent or conflicting) evidence. An incredulous person rejects the claim outright irrespective of the evidence. Candide (the skeptic) is the only person who evaluates the claim and remains open to either possibility. Skeptics suspend belief in a claim until sufficient evidence exists for either position. Similarly, the skeptic rejects a claim when evidence indicates it should be. The skeptic values evidence and therefore changes belief in accordance with the evidence. Conversely, the judging process of the incredulous individual parallels the credulous individual: Both make and adhere dogmatically to decisions irrespective of the evidence.

Skeptical behavior entails ongoing examination of evidence and reformation of belief. Likewise, science is a process involving testing hypotheses and the acknowledgement that conclusions derived from the scientific process are temporary. This illustrates the imperfection of science resultant of human proclivity for errors in thinking. Shermer (2002) highlights "the fallibility of science and the scientific method. But within this fallibility lies its greatest strength: self-correction" (p. 21). Dr. Panglos might self-correct, but this may occur as rapidly as the wind changes direction and on the basis of weak logic. Conversely, a scientist may change positions on an issue but only does so after careful consideration of evidence. This means science progresses with meticulous analysis of claims. This also means admitting that claims made via the scientific process progress from temporary to incontrovertible fact. Some claims hold sway for centuries (e.g. Newton's laws of motion) and become foundational fact, while others are short lived and abandoned (e.g., cold fusion). In either case, scientific claims inspire refutation and innovation via replication.

Skepticism is a repertoire of behavior that typically is developed gradually and in lockstep with scientific literacy. The concept alone is difficult to understand because many individuals have acculturated a credulous disposition and repertoire of superstitious behavior. Science fundamentally involves acquiring an understanding of problems or phenomena, gathering evidence through experimentation, followed by close analysis of that evidence. From a scientific perspective, the skeptic posits a testable statement about a phenomena and proceeds to evaluate evidence that may support or refute that position before ascribing belief.

Errors in Reason and Psychological Explanations Related to Unsupported Interventions

Pseudoscience and credulous thinking often are associated with shortcuts around critical thinking. Espousing or defending a position requires the organization of reasons consistent with sound and valid logic. Although science commands logical consistency, pseudoscience wins appeal with simple violations of the rules of critical thinking and debate. Importantly, a fully developed ability to detect fallacious arguments confers a wealth of benefits that extend beyond recognizing pseudoscience in ASD. However, an understanding of a handful of tactics often employed to defend fad, pseudoscientific, and controversial interventions in ASD may support professionals in avoiding them. Table 9.2 provides an overview of some common errors in thinking along brief explanations, examples, and problems associated with fad, controversial, and pseudoscientific interventions.

Fallacious Logic and Argument

An argument from ignorance fallacy is an attempt to support a position by asserting that a claim is or could be true and therefore should be treated as such until refuting evidence is available (e.g., "We don't know what causes autism, so it could be vaccines."). This fallacy often is packaged with anecdotal evidence (e.g., "Chelation worked for my child, so it might work for yours.") and shifting the burden of proof. Shifting the burden of proof is a fallacy in which the person making a claim requires the challenger to disprove it rather than offering evidence to support their assertion (e.g., "Prove to me chelation won't help my child."). Each of these fallacies operates from a credulous disposition in which credence in the claim is granted until evidence against it is available. However, at least two problems arise when subscribing to this logic. First, it discounts the influence of investment in an intervention/product. People are more likely to subconsciously perceive a positive effect when none exists if time, money, effort, emotion, and other resources are invested in a treatment. Second, fallacious reasoning welcomes an ocean of unproven interventions that hinge on claims impervious to refutation or confirmation through experimentation (e.g., telepathic claims made by some proponents of FC). Indeed, pseudoscience depends on untestable claims and fallacious logic. If all claims were to be treated as potentially valid until disproven, then effective interventions would have to contend with those proposed by individuals who unwittingly or intentionally violate the rules in the competition of ideas. The amount of nonsense alone would sufficiently bewilder consumers, obscure access to validated interventions, and stymie progress.

Purveyors of pseudoscience also may use appeal to authority and/or false authority fallacies. These fallacies distract from an argument by emphasizing the status of the person making the claim rather than the reasons behind it. The false authority is often used by self-proclaimed experts (e.g., holistic doctor; certified reiki practitioner). By asserting false authority, quacks and frauds claim that the person without the authority does not (and could not) adequately appreciate the claim to fairly criticize it.

Table 9.2 Common errors in thinking, brief explanations, examples, and problems associated with fad, controversial, and pseudoscientific interventions

Error	Brief explanation	Example	Problem
Argument from Ignorance Fallacy	Lack of evidence is treated as evidence in favor of a claim.	"We don't know if gluten-free diet will improve ASD symptoms, so we should try it."	Absence of data and potential harm using an unknown treatment or accepting unsupported claim.
Anecdotal Evidence	Testimonial from people who claim to have benefited.	"It worked for my child."	Anecdotes do not qualify as scientific evidence; no experimental control is provided.
Shifting the Burden of Proof Fallacy	Requiring the skeptic to refute unfounded claim	"Can you prove that sensory integration training won't work for my child?"	Claimant not required to support position with evidence; skeptic is expected to prove a negative.
Appeal to Authority Fallacy	Relying on status of the claimant to support the claim.	"That doctor said anti-fungal medication may help behavior, so why should we doubt it?"	Belief stems from person making claim; has nothing to do with evidence for claim.
False Authority Fallacy	Relying on purported expertise to refute argument.	"Only a homeopathic doctor can accurately comment on the efficacy of homeopathy."	Gives credence to claims made by quacks and frauds by discounting arguments from those without the credential.
Argument to Moderation Fallacy	Asserting the truth lies between two claims despite of amount or quality of evidence.	"Some say FC doesn't work at all, but others say it is a type of communication. It must work for some people or some of the time."	Position with or less/no evidence is perceived as valid as the position supported by more or most evidence. Concludes truth is somewhere between both positions.
Ad Hominem Fallacy	Attacking the person making the claim rather than their argument or the evidence presented.	"That guy is a rude jerk so anything he says shouldn't be trusted."	Ignores the opponent's argument and instead focuses on attacking their character.
Ad-hoc Fallacy	Adjusting claims to preserve belief in spite of contradictory evidence.	"Putting people in test conditions causes the intervention to stop working."	Refutation is always just beyond the realm of science. Claim is treated as too sensitive or complex for scientific evaluation; demands faith.
Straw Man Fallacy	Intentionally misrepresenting the opposing argument then attacking the misrepresentation as if suggested by the opponent.	"I don't believe in using negative reinforcement because it requires the child to want to escape discomfort. Wanting to make children uncomfortable just to get them to learn is unethical and immoral."	Intentionally avoids discussing the crux of the argument by replacing it with a position not espoused by the opponent and attacking it instead.
Confirmation Bias	Selecting and conforming evidence to maintain cherished beliefs.	"We started using hyperbaric oxygen therapy a few weeks ago and he really seems to be improving."	Ignores contradictory data and elevates positive data; discounts the influence of personal investment in outcome on perceptions.
Magical Thinking	Attributes causality to unfalsifiable phenomena.	"Disruptions in spiritual energy are causing his tantrums"	Outside the scientific process because it cannot be tested.

Similarly, authorities with more social status and respect (e.g., medical doctor; professor) may be used as an appeal to authority fallacy. In this way, people may argue that the authority made a claim and, given their status, the claim is more likely true than untrue (e.g., "She's a doctor, so she's probably basing her judgment on science."). To be clear, people with authority are often intentionally misrepresented and also are susceptible to conflicting values (e.g., money) that encourage endorsement of a product or practice. Consumers should recognize these fallacies as a likely reflection of inadequate evidence to support a claim.

If the proponent of an unsupported claim gives any ground, it is often via an argument to moderation fallacy. This fallacy relies on perspectives that two positions represent extremes on a continuum of possible truths and these extreme positions are always incorrect. The mistake stems from presumptions that an apparently less extreme position better approximates the truth. For example, one position in the FC "debate" is that the method is without merit and should be completely avoided. This position is entirely consistent with the prevailing evidence. The alternative (and unsupported position) is that FC works for "some individuals". The argument to moderation fallacy implies that FC should be *part of* a communication support system in which the person uses multiple means of communicating. Not surprisingly, this is precisely the position FC advocates espouse (ICI, n.d.). In this way, a harmful intervention can gain some legitimacy by appealing to moderation (i.e., "FC probably works for some people."). The fallacy is that an accurate position (FC is a farce) is treated as an extreme and therefore not likely factual. There can be no compromise when the evidence is unequivocal; to do so is to accept falsity. Further problematic is that the moderate position can then be presented as the new extreme in an attempt to compel agreement from the previously uncompromising perspective. Truth is conceded for regressive moderation.

Other fallacies commonly used to protect pseudoscience from criticism include ad hominem (e.g. "You think you know everything."), ad-hoc fallacy (i.e., adjusting evidence to accommodate belief), argument from personal incredulity (e.g., "I can't imagine how that could be true."), correlation fallacy (e.g., "He started talking after we gave him vitamins."), straw man (e.g., "ABA used punishment like electric shock. Why do you support inhumane treatment like electric shock?"). As stated, there are numerous fallacies commonly used to defend unproven interventions in ASD. Consumers would be wise to refine their ability to recognize them.

Confirmation Bias

"The first conclusion colors and brings into conformity with itself all that come after" (Bacon, 1620/1939, p. 36). Given the confluence of circumstances that give rise to spurious interventions, it is understandable that stakeholders might be convinced an intervention is responsible for some improvement when none exists. Improvements might be attributed to the questionable intervention when other known or unknown factors (e.g., other interventions, child learning, teacher skills, parent knowledge, maturation) are more likely the cause. The expectation of change when instituting a new treatment generates increased attention to specific behaviors that were previously less attended to (or ignored) and can result in perceived changes (i.e., increased awareness and attention explain noticed differences when no actual difference exists). Documentation by invested persons also may be skewed to provide further confirmation. This phenomenon is a main reason why double-blind randomized trials are highly valued; they control for confirmation and other biases that wreak havoc on the internal validity of experimental studies.

Confirmation bias usually is an implicit thought process in which an individual selects evidence and molds facts in order maintain alignment with personally favored beliefs (Nickerson, 1998). This flawed thinking acts as a protective boundary against potentially threatening evidence that contradicts cherished beliefs (Davies, 1993). Pseudoscience and confirmation bias often accompany each other because both emphasize attention to stimuli that support pre-conceived ideas, judgments, or expectations rather disconfirming stimuli. This tendency is complicated by the presence of denial when contradictory evidence is produced, causing a retreat to the original conclusion rather than acceptance of a more probable alternative (Garb & Boyle, 2003). Travers et al. (2014) described the role of confirmation bias in maintaining belief in and continued dissemination of FC, a widely debunked intervention responsible for a variety of traumatic and tragic outcomes (see, for example, Boynton, 2012; Flaherty, 2015; Green, 1994; Siegel, 1995). Increasingly bizarre trends associated with FC underscore the moral obligation to remain empirical (Todd, 2012) and the importance of developing a thorough understanding of the influence of confirmation bias in ASD intervention research and practice.

Magical Thinking

Magical thinking is the attribution of causality to some unverifiable phenomena and partly explains our human tendency to engage in superstitious behavior. People from various cultures have entertained fanciful (or frightening) ideas to explain phenomena that did not have easily observable causes (e.g., disease, famine, luck). Advances in our knowledge have eliminated many beliefs of our ancient ancestors, but superstitions still abound. Peculiar beliefs are commonly subscribed to and often serve to explain things in ways that prevent identification of actual causes. For example, teachers may believe that a full moon or the weather explains inappropriate behavior of children in school (Van Buskirk & Simpson, 2013). Teachers may simultaneously witness two distinct and unrelated phenomena and attribute the cause of one to the appearance of the other when, in fact, the two are entirely coincidental (e.g., child eats cheese and later has a tantrum; cheese is eliminated and child has a good day). Rather than explore as many potential causes for behavior, consultation of a lunar calendar or meteorologist absolves responsible agents from identifying actual (but less salient) causes for the phenomenon. Scientists tend to be inspired by their ignorance, while others may find not knowing terribly discomforting.

Humans have a desire for explanations for seemingly inexplicable events and therefore often rely on magical thinking (Shermer, 2002). We experience this in our daily interactions and witness it in the popular media. Lucky charms, rituals, cursed words, karma, forbidden foods, and etcetera are commonplace. Adherence to these beliefs may seem provincial, but they and others have been reinforced by cultures and are cherished to various degrees. For example, popular tropes like lunar explanations for classroom misbehavior are extensions of archaic attributions of inexplicable causes of various behavior to the lunar cycle. The term "lunatic" is rooted in astrology and was for nearly 2000 years commonly believed to be the cause of epilepsy and other diseases and disorders. In this way, these and countless other "self-evident truths" were passed on through the folklore of the culture. These explanations helped people cope with daily tragedies (e.g., disease, pain, famine) that often accompanied humankind's collective ignorance, but they anesthetized curiosity and inhibited searches for verifiable causes or explanations. Adopting an inaccurate explanation is more comforting than having no explanation, but science has taught us that knowledge, acquired through scientific method, confers unprecedented benefits to humankind. Nevertheless specious beliefs of all sorts apply the brakes to this advancing agenda in order to protect beloved but untenable beliefs. Advances in medicine, chemistry, biology, astronomy, physics, technology, education, and others have bestowed fantastic benefit. Each generation has been better off than the previous.

The misattribution of observations to unsupported causes is not a benign phenomenon. Given our limited knowledge about ASD, it is no surprise that many speculative and supernatural explanations and treatments exist. Divine communication, extrasensory perception, telepathic communication, spiritual medium, and others have been offered as having something to do with ASD. One child died during an exorcism to cast out demons alleged to be the cause of his ASD (Collins, 2003). Other, more earthly but unfounded explanations include vaccine injury, intestinal bacterial overgrowth, genetically modified foods, non-organic produce, hormones in beef, and unloving parents. Belief in these or other groundless causes and treatments lead parents to tragic outcomes. For example, children with ASD have died from chelation therapy, a medical procedure to remove metals mistakenly thought to cause ASD from the body (e.g., Baxter & Krenzelok, 2008; Davis et al., 2013).

Well-intentioned professionals, passionate about their work and dedicated to students with ASD and their families, are not immune from similar folly. In an educational setting, similar scenarios run their course and entire schools or programs are shaped by a combination of a few anecdotes and a climate of confirmation bias. People see examples of "effective" intervention and ignore examples of the same intervention failing. This has the effect of allowing unfounded practices to proceed unchecked and opens the proverbial schoolhouse doors to exploitative charlatans. A stroll of many major education conference expositions reveals a buffet of baloney, pitched by brash swindlers bent on bamboozling benevolent professionals. Buyers beware!

Specific Fad, Controversial, and Pseudoscientific Interventions in ASD

It would be impossible to overview every present or historical fad, controversial, and pseudoscientific intervention associated with ASD. The intent of our discussion up to this point was illustrating some key indicators of potentially harmful treatment approaches in ASD. Red flags include grandiose claims that are contrary to mainstream scientific discovery, usually supported only by baseless assertions, testimonial anecdotes, and fallacious reasoning. We also outlined some reasons why disproven and unproven interventions become popular. Nevertheless, it seems pertinent to contextualize some ways these problems have manifested over the past 40 years. In the following sections, we discuss some communication, sensory, developmental, and biomedical interventions that have gained and lost (and sometimes recaptured) attention.

Communication-Based Interventions

Communication deficits are a core characteristic of ASD and often are central to EIBI programming. The progression of communication intervention research has been particularly slow, perhaps because of the complex topographical and functional features of communicative behavior. Learning essential and complex communication requires a technology of teaching that is both effective and efficient. Unfortunately practitioners have not consistently mastered this. The limited knowledge about promoting communication, the advanced technical skill required for teaching most communication skills, and limited resources are, as discussed previously, fertile conditions for fad, pseudoscientific, and controversial interventions. Indeed, quintessential fad and pseudoscientific interventions in ASD are directly related to communication.

Facilitated Communication

Facilitated communication (FC) is a method of physically prompting a person to use a keyboard or letter board to spell words that allegedly convey their thoughts (Biklen, 1992; Institute for Communication and Inclusion, n.d.). The underlying theory advanced by FC proponents is that the person with ASD has intact (and often untaught) reading and writing skills and FC taps into those skills. The method involves holding the person's finger, hand, wrist, arm, or shoulder to prompt the person to point to letters/type, give reminders to look at the letterboard/keyboard, and to pull the FC user's hand back from the keyboard between letters when typing. However, over time increasingly subtle prompts including touching the back, waist, or non-physical indicators (head movement, verbal prompts, and so on) can be used to manipulate the user to type words. Supplemental verbal prompts to begin or stop pointing are essential for ensuring the FC user looks at the keyboard as well clarifying questions from the facilitator to FC user (ICI). The ICI also emphasizes facilitator emotional support via development of a relationship for FC success.

Rosemary Crossley developed the method in Australia (Crossley & MacDonald, 1984) and Douglas Biklen brought it to the United States in the late 1980s (Biklen, 1990). The introduction initiated an unprecedented cult-like movement in special education and related fields. The dramatic results accompanied claims consistent with pseudoscience (i.e., miraculous, revolutionary, breakthrough treatment method) (Berger, 1991), but only were supported with testimonials disguised as qualitative research (Biklen, 1990; 1997). Researchers immediately responded and failed to validate claims made about FC (Hudson, Melita, & Arnold, 1993; Szempruch & Jacobson, 1993; Wheeler et al., 1993). Subsequently, study after study failed to demonstrate any authenticity of FC (Mostert, 2001; 2010; Simpson & Myles, 1995). It is widely accepted that messages obtained via FC are mere manifestations of the ideomotor response, the same phenomenon associated with the movement of the Ouija board planchette (Burgess et al., 1998). To date, no person has demonstrated the validity of FC under well-designed experimental conditions and, despite proclamations to the contrary, no person has become an independent author of thoughts due to FC. In sum, FC users indefinitely depend on the presence of a facilitator who can see the keyboard/letterboard to communicate.

The absence of supporting evidence and the wealth of refuting evidence has not stopped FC proponents from advancing the technique. Proponents appear to exploit hyperlexia, the authentic but rare phenomenon of precocious reading by some people with ASD, to argue in support of FC. Other absurd rationales also exist, including supernatural autistic telepathy (Haskew & Donnellan, 1993), divine inspiration (Bilu & Goodman, 1997) and ASD as a movement disorder (e.g., Biklen, 1993; Stubblefield, 2011). Travers et al. (2014) described how FC proponents have rebranded FC as "supported typing" and portray the technique with tablet computers, exploiting popular beliefs about the benefits of touch technology. Travers et al. also pointed out other rebranding and marketing tactics to advance FC including changing the FC Institute name to ICI, dishonestly referring to FC as a type augmentative and alternative communication, and promoting FC in popular media instead of traditional academic channels.

The FC crusade has brought unwarranted resurgence in FC's popularity, but this has come at deeply troubling costs. More parents have been unjustly accused and charged with sexual crimes via FC and families have been devastated (Braiser & Wisely, 2014). One mother killed her 8-year-old son after claiming he suggested via FC they both commit suicide (McKinley Jr, 2014; Sanchez & Remizowski, 2014). A university philosophy professor was convicted of two counts of sexual assault after she claimed she obtained consent for sex via FC from a man with a severe disability (Flaherty, 2015). Similarly, a caregiver pleaded guilty to sexual crimes after claiming her client consented via FC to various sexual acts with her (Sundstrum, 2014). These and numerous other but similar issues associated with FC overshadow larger concerns that FC usurps the voice of people with disabilities, treats them as puppets in their own lives, and attempts to diminish the very real effects of their disabling conditions. The long list of potential danger and actual damage associated with FC illustrates how well-intentioned people seek out, irrationally defend, and relentlessly promote interventions that have no tangible benefit and only cause harm.

Rapid Prompting Method™

Rapid Prompting Method (RPM) is a trademarked method in which a learner touches or points to letters on a board or tablet computer to spell out words, fragmented or full sentences, or entire paragraphs that reflect the thoughts of the learners. RPM™ users allegedly communicate very complex ideas, author books, and suggest radical change in the way ASD is understood. This explanation is similar to those provided for FC because the procedures and claims underpinning both methods are strikingly similar (Tostanoski et al., 2014). The mother of a child with ASD invented the method and claims "RPM is distinct from other methods as it is based upon how the brain works. The aim is to bring the student to maximum learning through the open learning channel and to elicit the best (not simply to test) out of the child to enable maximum output in that given time" (HALO, n.d.). Such claims are consistent with several qualities of pseudoscience.

The RPM™ appears to rely on the same ideomotor effect responsible for FC, but it differs in ways that may make it difficult for consumers to see the connection. A primary difference is that unlike FC, the RPM™ support-person holds the device (i.e., tablet computer) or letterboard instead of the person's finger, hand, wrist, arm, or shoulder. The letterboard is held under the hand of the pointing individual and each letter is announced as the person's finger touches the letter. As with FC, increasing subtle and non-physical cues are used to manipulate behavior that appears to emanate from the individual, including traditional handwriting, but there is no evidence to substantiate this claim. The dangerously persuasive power of RPM™ lies in its absence of physical touch to control the messages. The method has garnered widespread attention in the popular media, including features on 60 min II (Kohn, 2003), CNN (McEdwards, 2008), the New York Times (Blakeslee, 2002), and others. These sources portray RPM™ users in ways that eerily parallel FC in the early 1990s.

Only one experimental study has examined RPM, but the findings do not warrant application of RPM as an intervention method to support communication or any other skills. Chen, Yoder, Ganzel, Goodwin, & Belmonte, 2012 examined videotaped sessions of RPM sessions to evaluate effects on joint attention, repetitive behavior, open learning prompts (i.e., a concept of sensory integration treatment), response complexity, and relationship between types of prompt and accurate responding. Authorship authenticity was not evaluated. They reported decreases in repetitive behavior, but no significant differences in their analyses were found in relation to the other behaviors investigated. Despite this, the authors made positive and speculative claims that appeared to contradict their results. A value-added abstract and commentary of Chen et al. indicated numerous serious methodological problems and specious conclusions about RPM's effectiveness (Lang, Tostanoski, Travers, & Todd, 2014). Lang et al. strongly suggested that RPM appears similar to FC and concluded results obtained by Chen et al. more likely reflected prompt dependency than a dramatic breakthrough in ASD.

Sensory-Based and Neurological Interventions

Sensory Integration

Sensory integration (SI) interventions purport to assist learners to interpret and respond to sensory input. The conceptual foundation for SI is that sensory processing is the way the nervous system takes in and makes meaning of environmental stimuli and sensations (Hanft, Miller, & Lane, 2000; Kandel, Schwartz, & Jessell, 2000). Thus, it follows that SI interventions and supports can be applied to facilitate meaningful awareness of how the body and environment are linked to inform treatment for improving the ability of people to understand the contextual features of their bodies (Coren, Porac, & Ward, 1984).

It is well known and empirically accepted that individuals with ASD commonly experience sensory irregularities and differences (American Psychiatric Association, 2013). Children and youth with ASD are characterized by hyper- and/or hyposensitivity to environmental stimuli (e.g., find it difficult to tolerate certain clothing fabrics, are unusually sensitive to certain noises and other common environmental stimuli, appear to be unaware of cold weather conditions). It is thus logical and reasonable to generally assume and accept the underlying biological and neurological explanation for ASD. The conceptual leap that follows is the bridge to SI, specifically that SI interventions and supports provide therapeutic benefit to individuals with ASD.

A variety of SI methods are widely used in countless ways by both clinical and educational professionals. Moreover, in many settings, SI is a generally accepted treatment and support for children and youth with ASD-related disorders and judged by many professionals and parents as a necessary part of a comprehensive ASD program. In spite of this popularity and implicit acceptance the effective-practice credentials of specific SI practices are questionable (National ASD Center, 2009).

Unlike many fads and pseudoscientific interventions for learners with ASD, SI is seemingly underpinned by a foundation of biological science and physiology. It is well documented that individuals with ASD manifest atypical responses to environmental stimuli. Indeed, teachers, parents and other stakeholders accept these characteristics as common elements and features of ASD; based on this knowledge, they plan accordingly. For example prudent and informed teachers of students with ASD carefully plan for fire drills and similar events that involve loud sirens and irregular loud sounds. Teachers and parents are aware of students' food-texture preferences and they make necessary accommodations and take steps to expand students' tolerance for different foods. Adjustments are made to deal with unusual responses to particular types of clothing, and so forth. These are practical, logical, and necessary accommodations, albeit not necessarily SI treatments.

What places SI in the camp of "unproven" and "unsupported" methods is advancement of the notion that therapists and other caregivers are able to manipulate and modify an individual's sensory system via application of a variety of untested and non-validated "sensory intervention techniques." These so-called interventions, treatments, and supports purport to modify an individual's vestibular, visual, hearing, smelling, and tasting systems. The intent is to manipulate an individual's neurology to improve how they orient in space and time so as to help the child make better decisions about appropriate actions. A number of purported SI tools are applied without treatment fidelity and with little logical or scientific connection to human biological and neurological structures. Consider, for example, weighted vests and support garments, vestibular movement activities such as swinging, sensory rooms, and sensory activities such as giving children opportunities to play at a water table and with vibrating materials lack the scientific support needed for evidence-based status (Lang et al., 2012).

Auditory Integration Training

Auditory integration training (AIT) was developed by the French otolaryngologist Guy Berard (Berard, 1993). Berard's method was based on the work of Alfred Tomatis, his predecessor and colleague. AIT typically consists of 20 half-hour sessions of listening to specially filtered and modulated music over 10 to 20 days. AIT has been reported to result in positive outcomes for individuals with a variety of disorders, including ASD. In spite of these claims there is little in the way of supporting empirical evidence for AIT and the method has not met scientific standards for efficacy that justify its use as a treatment for any disorder.

Berard developed the AIT method in the late 1960s as a treatment for auditory sensitivity and processing problems in persons with ASD and other disorders. According to Berard (1993), middle ear abnormalities and acute hyperactivity of cochlear hair cells are the cause of auditory distortions and related difficulties that adversely affect behavior and learning. AIT purportedly mitigates and treats these problems via exposure to modulated and filtered sound.

AIT was popularized in the 1990s through Annabel Stehli's book, *The Sound of a Miracle* (1994). Stehli described how AIT allegedly produced significant improvements in her daughter, an individual with a diagnosis of ASD. The publicity resulting from the book led to wide scale use of AIT during the 1990s. There was initial anecdotal evidence and claims of positive outcomes for AIT based on a few poorly designed studies. However, closer scrutiny and vetting based on more robust and scientifically grounded research consistently revealed the method to have little efficacy or utility. In sum, there is insufficient evidence to justify using the method with individuals diagnosed with ASD or other conditions.

Irlen Lenses

A *google* search "Irlen Lenses" leads to the Irlen Lenses website and the following claim: "The Irlen Method helps individuals with Autism (sic) & Asperger syndrome who have perceptual problems, light sensitivity & sensory overload" (n.d.). Irlen Lenses purportedly treat a condition known as scotopic sensitivity syndrome (SSS), allegedly a common malady among individuals with ASD. SSS is supposedly a central nervous system condition wherein a person's eyes interact with light levels to create visual distortions. Irlen Lenses claim to treat this condition through colored lenses and overlays.

In a joint statement by The American Academy of Ophthalmology, American Academy of Pediatrics, American Association for Pediatric Ophthalmology and Strabismus and American Association of Certified Orthoptists, experts bluntly rejected the notion that lenses were a suitable or effective treatment for SSS (American Academy of Pediatrics, 2009). The basis for this judgment was an absence of supporting scientific evidence. We agree with this assessment, and consider this method to be a classic example of a commercial enterprise preying on vulnerable and desperate individuals in search of simple solutions for developmental disorders and disabilities.

Brain Gym

"Brain Gym" is the prototypical personification of a faddish and pseudoscience intervention. The organization that promotes Brain Gym claims that doing specified exercises result in improved academic performance and other positive outcomes, including improved spatial, listening, eye-hand coordination, and memory and related cognitive gains. Case studies and anecdotal reports are used to support Brain Gym, including professed positive outcomes of children with ASD who are involved in Brain Gym activities. According to information on the Brain Gym website, the program is used to: "promote play and the joy of learning; draw out and honor innate intelligence; build awareness regarding the value of movement in daily life; facilitate the ability to notice and respond to movement-based needs; encourage self-responsibility; leave each participant appreciated and valued; empower each participant to better take charge of his own learning; encourage creativity and self-expression; inspire an appreciation of music, physical education and the fine arts." One might conclude Brain Gym could also increase the approval rating of the U.S. Congress, if only given the chance.

There is a wealth of data to support the benefits of exercise and physical activity. These advantages also apply to individuals diagnosed with ASD (Lang, Koegel, et al., 2010; Lang, O'Reilly, et al., 2010). Indeed a healthy lifestyle, including exercise, bodes well for the physical and emotional well-being of every person. In spite of this general acceptance, there is no supporting evidence for Brain Gym as a valid intervention program for individuals with ASD. The behavioral science principles and educational theorists used to prop up Brain Gym are unquestionably genuine (e.g., Piaget, Gesell, Carl Rogers). However, except in the most general and vague fashion, these supporting elements lack any scientific link to Brain Gym. In his review of Brain Gym research, Hyatt (2007) concluded that the five studies supporting the method were poorly designed and that Brain Gym was linked to the discredited and dangerous Doman-Delacato theory of development, further raising questions as to its suitability for use with persons with ASD.

Psychomotor Patterning

In spite of consistent findings over several decades that it offers no positive outcomes and has all the markings of a classic pseudoscience method, psychomotor patterning interventions continue. Psychomotor patterning was first promoted and used as a treatment for individuals with intellectual impairments, learning disabilities and neurological impairment. It has more recently been promoted as an intervention for individuals with ASD. In all cases psychomotor patterning has failed to yield convincing and scientifically-supported positive outcomes.

The notion of patterning as a therapeutic treatment is credited to Glenn Doman and C. Delacato; thus often referred to as the Doman-Delacato technique (Doman, Spitz, Zucman, Delacato, & Doman, 1960). The theoretical underpinnings for psychomotor patterning are loosely based on theories of ontogeny (stages of development, beginning from a single cell stage to full maturity) and that an organism should develop through each of the adult stages of its evolutionary history. The assumption is that normal childhood neurodevelopmental stages of crawling, creeping, and the various phases of walking are a direct link to historical human development (i.e., amphibian, reptilian, and mammalian evolution). Doman and Delacato theorized that intellectual disability was a failure of the individual to develop through the proper evolutionary stages. Related to psychomotor patterning methodology, the treatment attempts to stimulate the proper sequential development of developmental stages. The purported therapeutic stimulation is known as "patterning."

Patterning takes the form of individuals repeatedly engaging in moving in accordance with various stages of development (e.g., crawling). Exercises are sometimes combined with other techniques, such as sensory stimulation, breathing exercises, and attempts to program and influence hemispheric dominance. In spite anecdotal and unsupported claims that the technique can lead to normal social, intellectual, physical and motor abilities, there is overwhelming evidence psychomotor patterning methodology is without merit. Moreover, because it preys on desperate parents and families and requires a heavy financial and emotional toll, we consider psychomotor patterning to be a potentially harmful method.

Neurofeedback and Mirror Neurons

A mirror neuron is a cell that supposedly processes and transmits information relative to performing an action and performing the same action of others. Thus, the neuron "mirrors" the behavior of the other, as though the observer were itself acting.

Mirror neurons have been directly observed in animals, especially related to imitative behaviors; and there is some neurological evidence suggesting the presence of some form of mirroring system consistent with the presence of mirror neurons in humans (Molenberghs, Cunnington, & Mattingley, 2009). The exact function, as well as the existence of the mirror system, is a subject of much conjecture and theory. Some researchers speculate the mirror neuron system is the neurological structure supporting the link between observations, perceptions, and actions. Thus mirror neurons are considered by some to be important in understanding the actions of others, learning new skills through imitation, and understanding others' actions and intentions. Relative to persons with ASD, mirror neurons are speculated to be the neurological mechanism responsible for imitative learning and cognitive difficulties and emotional and "theory of mind" impairments (Dapretto et al., 2006).

Studies of mirror neuron activity among individuals with ASD purport to show atypical neurological patterns. One indicator in particular is known as mu brainwave suppression; this mechanism is supposedly absent in individuals with ASD. Based on the theory individuals with ASD have deficient mirror neuron activity, neurofeedback training (NFT) is used to normalize mu suppression and therefore mirror neuron activity. Outcomes of this treatment purportedly result in improved learning ability, especially in imitation, as well as improvements in emotional, social and behavioral functioning (Oberman, Ramachandran, & Pineda, 2008). To date there are no credible scientific studies that have described how mirror neuron activity supports imitation learning and other cognitive and emotional functions (Murphy, Brady, Fitzgerald, & Troje, 2009). Thus, in spite of significant hype over the presence and impact of mirror neuron treatments, neurofeedback has yet to be supported by research and therefore is controversial outside of experimental conditions.

Developmental Treatment Models and ASD

One approach to early learning for students with autism is a developmental approach. Developmental learning encourages practitioners and caregivers to use typical developmental sequences as the foundation for interventions and assessments (Wagner, Wallace, & Rogers, 2014). These early intervention procedures primarily focus on adult-child attachment and social interactions within the context of natural environments, and are often intensive in nature (Wagner et al., 2014). Some developmental interventions target skills using principles and approaches consistent with applied behavior analysis (ABA), and have shown very promising results. However, other developmental interventions appear particularly concerned with improving and repairing the relationships and interpersonal connections of individuals with ASD. These interventions focus on increasing attachment, appropriate affect, and interpersonal bonds to indirectly improve social, communication, and other core ASD deficits (Heflin & Simpson, 1998). Common treatments of this variety include: *gentle teaching*, *holding therapy*, the *Son-Rise Program*, and *Floortime*.

Gentle Teaching

Gentle teaching (GT) is focused on establishment of a deep relationship with the child in order for the child to feel completely valued and respected. A secondary goal is to instill in therapists an appreciation for the individual with ASD and to respond with affection (Howlin, 1997). According to proponents, GT was developed in response to vehement and absurd claims that ABA used tactics consistent with torture (Jones & McCaughey, 1992). Given this emotional rather than empirical foundation, it is particularly concerning that vague procedures and unmeasurable outcomes (i.e., bonding, solidarity) are the primary focus (Bailey, 1992). Terms are used that borrow from ABA, such as errorless learning, task analysis, prompting, extinction, and feedback routines, but differ in that the procedural explanations are vague and accompanied with dramatic claims of improvement (Bailey, 1992). These qualities have made rigorous investigation of GT largely impossible and the evidence from initial investigations indicate it is both ineffective for improving targeted skills associated with ASD and developing relationships (Heflin & Simpson, 1998). GT is absent sound theoretical explanations, fails to describe clear procedures for replication in experimental or practical situations, does not emphasize verifiable outcomes of the method, and relies on emotional appeal and testimonial anecdotes as evidence. Thus, GT appears wholly pseudoscientific.

Holding Therapy

The holding therapy (HT) approach purportedly improves the attachment and bonding between caregivers and children with ASD and attachment disorders. It became popular in Europe in the 1980s (Tinbergen, Tinbergen, & Welch, 1983). HT proponents posit that lack of eye contact signifies a breakdown in the attachment between child and caregiver and that caregivers must maintain close physical contact (holding) and proximity, with breaks of no more than 2 h to restore this bond and improve social relatedness (Heflin & Simpson, 1998). This is an invasive treatment; it requires confrontation accompanied by physical restraint to rebuild the bond, but is void of any scientific support (Pignotti & Mercer, 2007). HT also has been implicated in several deaths (Shermer, 2004). Clearly HT is a controversial treatment for children with ASD and in our opinion it should be avoided.

Son-Rise Program™

Also called "Options" the Son Rise Program™ (SRP) is an intensive developmental treatment designed by Barry Neil Kauffman for his son who was diagnosed with autism at an early age (Kaufman, 1976). SRP utilizes high intensity intervention (i.e., 40 h per week) in play environments to improve social initiations and social responsiveness. While SRP uses some traditional practices found in other skill interventions (i.e., naturalistic feedback), it relies on some unique practices, including imitations of the child as a means of social bidding. A substantial component of the intervention protocol is to imitate the child's play, ritualistic, and stereotypic behavior in order to develop and sustain attention (Heflin & Simpson, 1998). Social reinforcement (e.g., praise, attention) is recommended after the child attends to the therapist (through eye gaze or vocalizations), but otherwise the therapist ignores the child (Houghton, Schuchard, Lewis, & Thompson, 2013). Pitched as a cure for ASD, SRP proponents have for decades relied exclusively on anecdotal claims of effectiveness. Only recently has an investigation of SRP effectiveness been published in a peer-reviewed journal (Houghton et al., 2013), more than three decades after its inception. Importantly, SRP is expensive, highly intensive for the child and caregiver, and has very little scientific evidence. As such, SRP appears pseudoscientific and can be considered at best a controversial intervention.

Floortime

The Developmental, Individual Difference, Relationship-Based Approach Model (Floortime) was created by Stanley Greenspan in the early 1990s. Floortime encourages adult structured and spontaneous play sessions to build relationship, social engagement, and complex thinking and problem solving in young children with ASD (Wieder & Greenspan, 2003). Like SRP, Floortime is a largely home-based, parent delivered, intensive treatment for individuals with ASD, focused on improving social engagement and interaction (Pajareya & Nopmaneejumruslers, 2011). The key components include reciprocal social interactions, called communication circles. These communication circles purportedly are designed to take advantage of naturally occurring motivators and activities. Floortime therapists take advantage of the intense interests of children with ASD to facilitate and maintain these interactions. They also create opportunities for interaction attempts by blocking access to preferred items/activities or intentionally misinterpreting the child (Heflin & Simpson, 1998). Some evidence has emerged (see Liao et al., 2014; Pajareya & Nopmaneejumruslers, 2011; Solomon, Necheles, Ferch, & Bruckman, 2007) to suggest Floortime may be increase social interactions and engagement of young children with ASD. Similar to the SRP model however, Floortime proponents have been advocating its use for over 20 years, albeit without scientific evidence of its effectiveness.

Although a developmental approach in some ways makes sense for young children with ASD (especially when packaged with ABA methods), the models we discuss here lack scientific support. These models call for many hours of therapy per week and are often expensive to implement and maintain. These interventions require families and practitioners to invest heavily in a system in which there is little scientific support for positive returns. Thus, Floortime must currently be classified as a controversial intervention method and in our opinion most suited for controlled scientific vettting.

Biomedical Treatments of ASD

These types of treatments attempt to adjust the neurological and physiological processes that result in ASD symptomology (Bodfish, 2004; Levy & Hyman, 2005). Clearly, there are traditional pharmacological approaches to addressing the parallel behavioral (i.e., aggression, anxiety) and medical (i.e., seizures) symptoms associated with the ASD spectrum that have been thoroughly vetted through systematic investigation (Bodfish, 2004). However, there exists a host of alternative treatments, often referred to as complementary and alternative medical treatments (CAM) that lack sufficient scientific evidence, yet are widely adopted and administered. Surveys of the prevalence of CAM treatments estimate that between 52 and 95 % of youth with ASD are being treated by at least one of these alternative procedures (Golnik & Ireland, 2009). It appears that questionable organizations like Talk About Curing Autism and Defeat Autism Now! (DAN!) have encouraged parents, medical professionals, and practitioners to adopt CAM treatments despite lack of evidence. Common CAM treatments include vitamin supplements, secretin, probiotics and other gastrointestinal treatment, gluten-free casein-free (GFCF) diets, chelation therapy (CT), and hyperbaric oxygen therapy (HBOT).

Vitamin Supplements

Vitamins are easily obtained without a prescription, often have few side effects, and are taken by increasing numbers of the population in spite of significant evidence to their ineffectiveness in preventing chronic illness (Guallar, Stranges, Mulrow, Appel, & Miller, 2013). Orthomolecular psychiatry (Pauling, 1968) advocates the use of concentrated vitamins and minerals to treat a variety of disorders (i.e., schizophrenia, ASD, ADHD; Pfeiffer, Norton, Nelson, & Shott, 1995). While largely rejected due to unproven claims and poor research methodology (Lipton et al., 1973), this approach has found traction in the treatment of ASD due in large part to the support from the Autism Research Institute (ARI) and DAN!. The most common forms of concentrated vitamin treatments for ASD include Vitamin C, Vitamin B6, Magnesium, and Vitamin B12 (Levy & Hyman, 2005).

Investigations of outcomes connected to these treatments have been plagued by small sample sizes, poor research methodology, and inconsistent results (Levy & Hyman, 2005; Pfeiffer et al., 1995). More importantly the dosage regimens recommended by advocates often far exceed the recommended daily dosages for these supplements, and while adverse side effects of vitamins are largely unknown or minimal, there has been documentation of negative side effects connected to high dosages of certain vitamins (Guallar et al., 2013; Levy & Hyman, 2005). Vitamin and mineral supplements as treatments for ASD generally are pseudoscientific or fads reflective of the way society at large views vitamin supplements.

Secretin

Secretin became an enticing superfad to treat the symptoms of ASD following three case studies (Horvath et al., 1997) and attention from broadcast journalists. A pancreatic peptide that stimulates the pancreas, secretin is most commonly used to test pancreatic function. In one television story, a young child was given secretin to treat chronic gastrointestinal trouble and was reported to have remarkably improved language and behavior (Perry & Bangaru, 1998). A swift and robust response from the scientific community ensued and secretin therapy is distinguished as one of the most investigated ASD treatments; several randomized controlled trials were conducted and all failed to demonstrate evidence of its effectiveness (Bodfish, 2004). This fad has waned, but illustrates how rigorous scientific investigation often must distract from promising work to respond to fads and pseudoscience.

Probiotics and Other Gastrointestinal Treatments

While secretin may have fallen out of fashion, other gastrointestinal treatments remain commonplace. Gastrointestinal issues (i.e., diarrhea, constipation, reflux, excess gas, bloating, food selectivity) have been widely described for individuals with ASD (Molloy & Manning-Courtney, 2003), however population studies indicate many of these symptoms do not occur at a higher rate than among non-ASD groups (Ibrahim, Voigt, Katusic, Weaver, & Barbaresi, 2009). The prevailing argument made by individuals supporting these treatments (Horvath, Papadimitriou, Rabsztyn, Drachenberg, & Tildon, 1999; Wakefield et al., 2000) is that individuals with ASD have a unique inflammation of the intestinal tract. This irritation impacts the permeability of the intestines and allows built up toxins and proteins to pass into the bloodstream and ultimately to the brain where they produce the neurobehavioral symptoms associates with ASD (Ibrahim et al., 2009). This "leaky gut syndrome" is controversial and unproven (Cass et al., 2008; Robertson et al., 2008). Nevertheless treatments to decrease inflammation, adjust levels of intestinal bacteria flora (probiotics, antifungals), and improve digestion and eliminate toxins (enzymes), are widespread. These treatments have demonstrated efficacy treating authentic gastrointestinal symptoms, however claims these conditions are ASD causal factors are unsupported and evidence regarding efficacy for treating ASD symptomology is controversial.

Gluten-Casein-Free Diet

Though utilizing the same rationale as the other gastrointestinal treatments, gluten-and-casein-free (GCF) diet is a particularly pervasive treatment. It has been estimated that as high as 70 % of cases have accessed this treatment option (Levy & Hyman, 2005; Marí-Bauset, Zazpe, Mari-Sanchis, Llopis-González, &

Morales-Suárez-Varela, 2014). As the name suggests, the treatment involves eliminating foods that contain gluten (found in grains) and casein (found in all dairy products). Proponents (e.g., Reichelt, Ekrem, & Scott, 1990) argue that these foods release proteins during digestion that can pass through permeable intestines (i.e., "leaky gut syndrome"), cross the blood-brain barrier, and negatively affect neurological functioning (Marí-Bauset et al., 2014). However, no scientific evidence supports GCF diet (Mulloy et al., 2010, 2011). Rigorous investigations (e.g., Hyman et al., 2010) have found no positive effects of GCF diet for ASD symptoms. Further, side effects of elimination diets include nutritional deficiencies, financial loss, and stress maintaining protocol (Mulloy et al., 2010).

Chelation Therapy

Chelation therapy, in our opinion, is a dangerous and persistent ASD treatment. Chelation is a complex medical procedure used to remove lead and other heavy metals from the bloodstream, and has been historically used with individuals who have heavy metal toxicity. Chelation Therapy (CT) involves injections of chelating agents into the bloodstream that bind metal ions so they can be carried out of the body through urine and feces (Crisponi et al., 2015). The prevailing theory that perpetuates CT as a treatment for ASD is connected to the mercury compound thimerosal, a vaccination preservative. The theory posits ASD etiology associated with thimerosal toxicity as a result of vaccination regimens (Bernard, Enayati, Redwood, Roger, & Binstock, 2001; Crisponi et al., 2015; Wakefield et al., 1998). This linkage has never been thoroughly investigated and never substantiated (CDC, 2014), with several high profile and rigorous investigations refuting the linkage between thimerosal-containing vaccinations and ASD diagnosis (Madsen et al., 2003; Price et al., 2010). Furthermore, studies investigating the CT for individuals with ASD have found no discernable positive effects (see Davis et al., 2013). Unfortunately this unsupported and controversial practice is not without consequences. The chemicals used as chelating agents can have serious side effects, including cardiac arrest and deaths of young children with ASD have been attributed to CT (Baxter & Krenzelok, 2008).

Hyperbaric Oxygen Therapy

Historically HBOT has been used to treat decompression sickness associated with deep sea diving, and astronautics. HBOT involves the application of gases into a confined chamber, ranging from normal levels of oxygen (21 %) to enhanced levels of oxygen (up to 100 %) under differing amounts of pressure (Granpeesheh et al., 2010). Exploratory findings have indicated that individuals with ASD have oxidative stress and nueroinflammation, both of which have been successfully limited in rat populations using HBOT (Granpeesheh et al., 2010). As with the other treatments discussed above, this approach is based on flawed or unproven theoretical underpinnings, however this has not prevented its wide usage. To date rigorous scientific research (Granpeesheh et al., 2010; Jepson et al., 2011) has indicated that HBOT does not result in improvements in ASD symptoms. This is another example of a controversial, expensive treatment based on unfounded ideas that is without supporting evidence.

Conclusion

Our aim was to shed light on some of the factors that give way to unproven treatment and advance skeptical scrutiny by professionals, parents, and organizations responsible preparing individuals to work with individuals with ASD. Fad, pseudoscientific, and controversial interventions for ASD proliferate for various reasons. They often are more affordable and easier to access than evidence-based interventions. Evidence-based interventions can be time intensive and difficult to procure, resulting in misinformation of desperate and dedicated parents and professionals. These factors alone do not explain adoption of all unsupported treatments. Indeed, as we have discussed, a confluence of idiosyncratic factors, each with varying degrees of influence, likely encourage embracement of interventions that ought to be entirely avoided until substantiated by evidence. Development of an understanding of science and scientific thought, including skepticism and rhetorical fallacies, are safeguards against exploitation and self-deception associated with pseudoscientific and fad interventions.

When professionals and families approach intervention decisions buoyed by emotion rather than reason, optimism rather than skepticism, and anecdote rather than data, they ultimately become victims of an industry preying on benevolent but desperate people behaving under duress. Mere knowledge of what has been disproven or is unproven is insufficient for preventing dissemination of new fad, pseudoscientific, and controversial interventions. Our advocacy for skepticism and a scientific attitude toward treatment decisions is necessary because the list of dubious treatments will continue to grow. Combatting pseudoscientific and fad treatments begins with service providers and families who make decisions. Researchers, professionals, and parents who are skilled at evaluating ASD treatment claims must assume leadership roles and support individuals unaccustomed to this important type of decision-making. Such an informed and active community is the best and likely only way to effectively prevent exploitation of individuals connected to people with ASD.

References

American Academy of Pediatrics. (2009). Joint statement—Learning disabilities, dyslexia, and vision. *Pediatrics, 124*, 837–844.

American Psychiatric Association. (2013). *Diagnostic and statistical manual of mental disorders* (5th ed.). Washington, DC: Author.

Asimov, I. (1980, January 21). A cult of ignorance. *Newsweek*, 19.
Bacon, F. (1939). Novum organum. In E. A. Burtt (Ed.), *The English philosophers from Bacon to Mill* (pp. 24–123). New York, NY: Random House (Original work published in 1620).
Bailey, J. S. (1992). Gentle teaching: Trying to win friends and influence people with euphemism, metaphor, smoke, and mirrors. *Journal of Applied Behavior Analysis, 25*, 879–883.
Baxter, A. J., & Krenzelok, E. P. (2008). Pediatric fatality secondary to EDTA chelation. *Clinical Toxicology, 46*, 1083–1084.
Berard, G. (1993). *Hearing equals behavior*. New Canaan, CT: Keats.
Berger, C. L. (1991). *Facilitated communication guide*. Eugene, OR: New Breakthroughs.
Bernard, S., Enayati, A., Redwood, L., Roger, H., & Binstock, T. (2001). Autism: A novel form of mercury poisoning. *Medical Hypotheses, 56*, 462–471.
Biklen, D. (1990). Communication unbound: Autism and praxis. *Harvard Educational Review, 60*, 291–315.
Biklen, D. (1992). Typing to Talk: Facilitated communication. *American Journal of Speech-Language Pathology, 1*, 15–17.
Biklen, D. (1993). *Communication unbound: How facilitated communication is challenging traditional views of autism and ability/disability*. New York, NY: Teachers College Press.
Biklen, D. (1997). Science, disability, and voice: A response to Danforth. *Mental Retardation, 35*, 383–387.
Bilu, Y., & Goodman, Y. C. (1997). What does the soul say?: Metaphysical uses of facilitated communication in the Jewish ultraorthodox community. *Ethos, 25*, 375–407.
Blakeslee, S. (2002). A boy, a mother and a rare map of autism's world. Retrieved November 12, 2014, from http://www.nytimes.com/2002/11/19/science/a-boy-a-mother-and-a-rare-map-of-autism-s-world.html.
Bledsoe, R., Smith, B., & Simpson, R. L. (2003). Use of a social story intervention to improve mealtime skills of an adolescent with Asperger syndrome. *Autism, 7*, 289–295.
Bodfish, J. W. (2004). Treating the core features of autism: Are we there yet? *Mental Retardation and Developmental Disabilities Research Reviews, 10*, 318–326.
Boynton, J. (2012). Facilitated communication—What harm it can do: Confessions of a former facilitator. *Evidence-Based Communication Assessment and Intervention, 6*, 3–13.
Braiser, L., & Wisely J. (2014, November 7). Jury awards $3M to Wendrows in wrongful prosecution case. Retrieved from http://www.freep.com/story/news/local/michigan/oakland/2014/11/06/jury-awards-wendrow-millions-oakland/18611789/.
Burgess, C. A., Kirsch, I., Shane, H., Niederauer, K. L., Graham, S. M., & Bacon, A. (1998). Facilitated communication as an ideomotor response. *Psychological Science, 9*(1), 71–74.
Cass, H., Gringras, P., March, J., McKendrick, I., O'Hare, A. E., Owen, L., & Pollin, C. (2008). Absence of urinary opioid peptides in children with autism. *Archives of Disease in Childhood, 93*, 745–750.
Centers for Disease Control (2007). Surveillance summaries. Morbidity & Mortality Weekly Report (MMWR) 56(SS-1): 1–28.
Centers for Disease Control and Prevention (CDC). (2014). ASD data and statistics. Retrieved from http://www.cdc.gov/ncbddd/autism/data.html.
Centers for Disease Control (2009). Prevalence of autism spectrum disorders: autism and developmental disabilities monitoring network, United States, 2006. MMWR Surveillance Summaries 58(10): 1–20.
Chen, G. M., Yoder, K. J., Ganzel, B. L., Goodwin, M. S., & Belmonte, M. K. (2012). Harnessing repetitive behaviours to engage attention and learning in a novel therapy for autism: An exploratory analysis. *Frontiers in Psychology, 12*(3), 1–16.
Cihak, D. F., Wright, R., & Ayres, K. M. (2010). Use of self-modeling static-picture prompts via a handheld computer to facilitate self-monitoring in the general education classroom. *Education and Training in Autism and Developmental Disabilities, 45*, 136–149.
Collins, D. (2003, August 25). *Autistic boy dies during exorcism.* Retrieved from http://www.cbsnews.com/news/autistic-boy-dies-during-exorcism/.
Coren, S., Porac, C., & Ward, L. (1984). *Sensation and perception* (2nd ed.). Orlando, FL: Academic.

Crisponi, G., Nurchi, V. M., Lachowicz, J. I., Crespo-Alonso, M., Zoroddu, M. A., & Peana, M. (2015). Kill or cure: Misuse of chelation therapy for human diseases. *Coordination Chemistry Reviews, 284*, 278.

Crossley, R., McDonald, A., & Molloy, S. P. A. (1984). *Annie's coming out* (revised ed.). London: Penguin

Crozier, S., & Tincani, M. (2005). Using a modified social story to decrease disruptive behavior of a child with autism. *Focus on Autism and Other Developmental Disabilities, 20*, 150–157.

Dapretto, M., Davies, M., Pfeifer, J., Scott, A., Sigman, M., Bookheimer, S., & Iacoboni, M. (2006). Understanding emotions in others: Mirror neuron dysfunction in children with autism spectrum disorders. *Nature Neuroscience, 9*, 28–30.

Davies, M. F. (1993). Dogmatism and the persistence of discredited beliefs. *Personality and Social Psychology Bulletin, 19*, 692–699.

Davis, T. N., O'Reilly, M., Kang, S., Lang, R., Rispoli, M., Sigafoos, J., … Mulloy, A. (2013). Chelation treatment for autism spectrum disorders: A systematic review. *Research in Autism Spectrum Disorders, 7*, 49–55.

Doman, R. J., Spitz, E. B., Zucman, E., Delacato, C. H., & Doman, G. (1960). Children with severe brain injuries: Neurologic organization in terms of mobility. *Journal of the American Medical Association, 174*, 257–262.

Duttlinger, C., Ayers, K. M., Bevill-Davis, A., & Douglas, K. H. (2013). The effects of a picture activity schedule for students with intellectual disability to complete a sequence of tasks following verbal directions. *Focus on Autism and Other Developmental Disabilities, 28*, 32–43.

Flaherty, C. (2015). When research becomes rape. Retrieved from https://www.insidehighered.com/news/2015/10/05/rutgers-professor-convicted-sexually-assaulting-disabled-man.

Fombonne, E. (2001). Is there an epidemic of autism? *Pediatrics, 107*(2), 411–412.

Fombonne, E. (2007). Epidemiological surveys of pervasive developmental disorders. *Autism and Pervasive Developmental Disorders, 2*, 33–68.

Fombonne, E. (2009). Epidemiology of pervasive developmental disorders. *Pediatric Research, 65*, 591–598.

Foxx, R. M. & Mulick, J. A. (2016). *Controversial therapies for developmental disabilities: Fad, fashion, and science in professional practice*. New York, NY: Routledge

Funk, C., & Rainie, L. (2015). Public and Scientists' Views on Science and Society, Pew Research Center.

Ganz, J. B., Kaylor, M., Bourgeois, B., & Hadden, K. (2008). The impact of social scripts and visual cues on verbal communication in three children with autism spectrum disorders. *Focus on Autism and Other Developmental Disabilities, 23*, 79–94.

Garb, H. N., & Boyle, P. A. (2003). *Understanding why some clinicians use pseudoscientific methods: Findings from research on clinical judgment*. New York, NY: Guilford Press.

Gernsbacher, M. A., Dawson, M., & Goldsmith, H. (2005). Three reasons not to believe in an autism epidemic. *Current Directions in Psychological Science, 14*, 55–58.

Golnik, A. E., & Ireland, M. (2009). Complementary alternative medicine for children with autism: A physician survey. *Journal of Autism and Developmental Disorders, 39*, 996–1005.

Granpeesheh, D., Tarbox, J., Dixon, D. R., Wilke, A. E., Allen, M. S., & Bradstreet, J. J. (2010). Randomized trial of hyperbaric oxygen therapy for children with autism. *Research in Autism Spectrum Disorders, 4*, 268–275.

Green, G. (1994). Facilitated communication: Mental miracle or sleight of hand? *Behavior and Social Issues, 4*, 69–85.

Gross, P. R., & Leavitt, N. (1997). *Higher superstition: The academic left and its quarrels with science*. Baltimore, MD: Johns Hopkins University Press.

Guallar, E., Stranges, S., Mulrow, C., Appel, L. J., & Miller, E. R. (2013). Enough is enough: Stop wasting money on vitamin and mineral supplements. *Annals of Internal Medicine, 159*, 850–851.

HALO (n.d.). Learning methodology – Methodology. Retrieved October 24, 2014, from http://www.halo-soma.org/learning_methodology.php?sess_id=1878ca5439ccebde563ed643596c108b.

Hanft, B., Miller, L., & Lane, S. (2000). Toward a consensus in terminology in sensory integration theory and practice: Part 3: Observable behaviors: Sensory integration dysfunction. *Sensory Integration Special Interest Section Quarterly, 23*, 1–4.

Hansen, R. L., Ozonoff, S., Krakowiak, P., Angkustsiri, K., Jones, C., Deprey, L. J., … Hertz-Picciotto, I. (2008). Regression in autism: Prevalence and associated factors in the CHARGE Study. *Ambulatory Pediatrics, 8*, 25–31.

Haskew, P., & Donnellan, A. M. (1993). *Emotional maturity and well-being: Psychological lessons of facilitated communication*. Madison, WI: DRI Press.

Heflin, L. J., & Simpson, R. L. (1998). Interventions for children and youth with autism prudent choices in a world of exaggerated claims and empty promises. Part I: Intervention and treatment option review. *Focus on Autism and Other Developmental Disabilities, 13*, 194–211.

Horvath, K., Papadimitriou, J. C., Rabsztyn, A., Drachenberg, C., & Tildon, J. T. (1999). Gastrointestinal abnormalities in children with autistic disorder. *The Journal of Pediatrics, 135*, 559–563.

Horvath, K., Stefanatos, G., Sokolski, K. N., Wachtel, R., Nabors, L., & Tildon, J. T. (1997). Improved social and language skills after secretin administration in patients with autistic spectrum disorders. *Journal of the Association for Academic Minority Physicians: The Official Publication of the Association for Academic Minority Physicians, 9*, 9–15.

Houghton, K., Schuchard, J., Lewis, C., & Thompson, C. K. (2013). Promoting child-initiated social-communication in children with autism: Son-Rise Program intervention effects. *Journal of Communication Disorders, 46*, 495–506.

Howlin, P. (1997). Prognosis in autism: Do specialist treatments affect long-term outcome? *European Child & Adolescent Psychiatry, 6*, 55–72.

Howlin, P., Goode, S., Hutton, J., & Rutter, M. (2009). Savant skills in autism: Psychometric approaches and parental reports. *Philosophical Transactions of the Royal Society of London. Series B, Biological Sciences, 364*(1522), 1359–1367.

Hudson, A., Melita, B., & Arnold, N. (1993). Brief report: A case study assessing the validity of facilitated communication. *Journal of Autism and Developmental Disorders, 23*, 165–173.

Hyatt, K. J. (2007). Brain Gym: Building stronger brains or wishful thinking. *Remedial and Special Education, 28*, 117–124.

Hyman, S., Stewart, P., Smith, T., Foley, J., Cain, U., & Peck, R. (2010). The gluten free and casein free (GFCF) diet: A double blind, placebo controlled challenge study. In *International Meeting for Autism Research*, Philadelphia, PA.

Ibrahim, S. H., Voigt, R. G., Katusic, S. K., Weaver, A. L., & Barbaresi, W. J. (2009). Incidence of gastrointestinal symptoms in children with autism: A population-based study. *Pediatrics, 124*, 680–686.

Institute for Communication and Inclusion (no date). *What is supported typing?* Retrieved from http://soe.syr.edu/centers_institutes/institute_communication_inclusion/what_is_supported_typing/default.aspx

Irlen Lenses. (n.d.). Who we help: Autism/Asperger Syndrome. Retrieved from http://irlen.com/about-irlen-institute/.

Jepson, B., Granpeesheh, D., Tarbox, J., Olive, M. L., Stott, C., Braud, S., ... & Allen, M. S. (2011). Controlled evaluation of the effects of hyperbaric oxygen therapy on the behavior of 16 children with autism spectrum disorders. *Journal of Autism and Developmental Disorders, 41*, 575–588.

Jones, R. S., & McCaughey, R. E. (1992). Gentle teaching and applied behavior analysis: A critical review. *Journal of Applied Behavior Analysis, 25*, 853–867.

Kandel, E., Schwartz, J., & Jessell, T. (2000). *Principles of neural science*. New York, NY: McGraw-Hill.

Kaufman, B. N. (1976). *Son-rise*. New York, NY: Harper & Row.

Kavale, K., & Mostert, M. (2003). River of ideology, islands of evidence. *Exceptionality, 11*, 191–208.

Kohn, D. (2003). Breaking the silence: One woman's drive to teach her autistic son. Retrieved from http://www.cbsnews.com/news/breaking-the-silence-14-01-2003/.

Kokina, A., & Kern, L. (2010). Social Story interventions for students with autism spectrum disorders: A meta-analysis. *Journal of Autism and Developmental Disorders, 40*, 812–826.

Kozloff, M. (2005). Fads in general education: Fad, fraud, and folly. In J. W. Jacobson, R. M. Foxx, & J. A. Mulick (Eds.), *Controversial therapies for developmental disabilities* (pp. 3–17). Mahwah, NJ: Lawrence Erlbaum.

Lang, R., Koegel, L., Ashbaugh, K., Regester, A., Ence, W., & Smith, W. (2010). Physical exercise and individuals with autism spectrum disorders: A systematic review. *Research in Autism Spectrum Disorders, 4*, 565–576.

Lang, R., O'Reilly, M., Healy, O., Rispoli, M., Lydon, H., Streusand, W., … Giesbers, S. (2012). Sensory integration therapy for autism spectrum disorders: A systematic review. *Research in Autism Spectrum Disorders, 6*, 1004–1018.

Lang, R., O'Reilly, M. F., Sigafoos, J., Machalicek, W., Rispoli, M., Shogren, K., … Hopkins, S. (2010). Review of teacher involvement in the applied intervention research for children with autism spectrum disorders. *Education and Training in Autism and Developmental Disability, 45*, 268–283.

Lang, R., Tostanoski, A. H., Travers, J., & Todd, J. (2014). The only study investigating the rapid prompting method has serious methodological flaws but data suggest the most likely outcome is prompt dependency. *Evidence-Based Communication Assessment and Intervention, 8*, 40–48.

Levy, S. E., & Hyman, S. L. (2005). Novel treatments for autistic spectrum disorders. *Mental Retardation and Developmental Disabilities Research Reviews, 11*, 131–142.

Liao, S. T., Hwang, Y. S., Chen, Y. J., Lee, P., Chen, S. J., & Lin, L. Y. (2014). Home-based DIR/Floortime™ intervention program for preschool children with autism spectrum disorders: Preliminary findings. *Physical & Occupational Therapy in Pediatrics, 34*, 356–357.

Lilienfeld, S. O., & Arkowitz, H. (2007). Is there really an autism epidemic? *Scientific American, 17*, 58–61.

Lillienfeld, S. O., Lynn, S. J., & Lohr, J. M. (2003). *Science and pseudoscience in clinical psychology*. New York City, NY: Guilford Press.

Lipton, M. A., Ban, T. A., Kane, F. J., Levine, J., Mosher, L. R., & Wittenborn, R. (1973). *Megavitamin and orthomolecular therapy in psychiatry*. Washington, DC: American Psychiatric Association.

Madsen, K. M., Lauritsen, M. B., Pedersen, C. B., Thorsen, P., Plesner, A. M., Andersen, P. H., & Mortensen, P. B. (2003). Thimerosal and the occurrence of autism: Negative ecological evidence from Danish population-based data. *Pediatrics, 112*, 604–606.

Marí-Bauset, S., Zazpe, I., Mari-Sanchis, A., Llopis-González, A., & Morales-Suárez-Varela, M. (2014). Evidence of the gluten-free and casein-free diet in autism spectrum disorders: A systematic review. *Journal of Child Neurology, 29*, 1718–1727.

McEdwards, C. (2008). Autistic poet gives rare glimpse into mysterious illness. Retrieved from http://www.cnn.com/2008/US/03/28/Tito.autism/index.html?_s=PM:US.

McKinley Jr., J.C. (2014, November 5). Gigi Jordan convicted of manslaughter, not murder, in son's killing. Retrieved from http://www.nytimes.com/2014/11/06/nyregion/gigi-jordan-found-guilty-of-manslaughter-in-death-of-autistic-son.html.

Metz, B., Mulick, J. A., & Butter, E. M. (2016). Autism: A late 20th century fad magnet. R. M. Foxx, & J. A. Mulick (Eds.), *Controversial therapies for developmental disabilities* (2nd ed.) (pp. 237–263). New York, NY: Routledge.

Molenberghs, P., Cunnington, R., & Mattingley, J. (2009). Is the minor neuron system involved in imitation? A short review and meta-analysis. *Neuroscience and Biobehavioral Reviews, 33*, 975–980.

Molloy, C. A., & Manning-Courtney, P. (2003). Prevalence of chronic gastrointestinal symptoms in children with autism and autistic spectrum disorders. *Autism, 7*, 165–171.

Mostert, M. P. (2000). A partial etiology of discriminative disability: Bandwagons and beliefs. *Exceptionality, 8*, 117–132.

Mostert, M. P. (2001). Facilitated communication since 1995: A review of published studies. *Journal of Autism and Developmental Disorders, 31*, 287–313.

Mostert, M. P. (2010). Facilitated communication and its legitimacy—Twenty-first century developments. *Exceptionality, 18*, 31–41.

Mudford, O. C., Cross, B. A., Breen, S., Cullen, C., Reeves, D., Gould, J., & Douglas, J. (2000). Auditory integration training for children with autism: No behavioral benefits detected. *American Journal Mental Retardation, 105*, 118–129.

Mulloy, A., Lang, R., O'Reilly, M., Sigafoos, J., Lancioni, G., & Rispoli, M. (2010). Gluten-free and casein-free diets in the treatment of autism spectrum disorders: A systematic review. *Research in Autism Spectrum Disorders, 4*, 328–339.

Mulloy, A., Lang, R., O'Reilly, M., Sigafoos, J., Lancioni, G., & Rispoli, M. (2011). Addendum to "Gluten-free and casein-free diets in the treatment of autism spectrum disorders: A systematic review". *Research in Autism Spectrum Disorders, 5*, 86–88.

Murphy, P., Brady, N., Fitzgerald, M., & Troje, N. (2009). No evidence for impaired perception of biological motion in adults with autistic spectrum disorders. *Neuropsychologia, 47*, 3225–3235.

National Autism Center. (2009). *National standards project*. Randolph, MA: Author.

Nickerson, R. S. (1998). Confirmation bias: A ubiquitous phenomenon in many guises. *Review of General Psychology, 2*, 175–220.

Oberman, L., Ramachandran, V., & Pineda, J. (2008). Modulation of mu suppression in children with autism spectrum disorders in response to familiar or unfamiliar stimuli: The mirror neuron hypothesis. *Neuropsychologia, 46*, 1558–1565.

Offit, P. A. (2010). *Autism's false prophets: Bad science, risky medicine, and the search for a cure*. Columbia, NY: Columbia University Press.

Pajareya, K., & Nopmaneejumruslers, K. (2011). A pilot randomized controlled trial of DIR/Floortime™ parent training intervention for pre-school children with autistic spectrum disorders. *Autism, 15*, 563–577.

Palfreman, J. (1993). *Frontline: Prisoners of silence*. Boston, MA: WGBH Public Television.

Pauling, L. (1968). Orthomolecular psychiatry. *Science, 160*, 265–271.

Perry, R., & Bangaru, B. S. (1998). Secretin in autism. *Journal of Child and Adolescent Psychopharmacology, 8*, 247–248.

Pfeiffer, S. I., Norton, J., Nelson, L., & Shott, S. (1995). Efficacy of vitamin B6 and magnesium in the treatment of autism: A methodology review and summary of outcomes. *Journal of Autism and Developmental Disorders, 25*, 481–493.

Pignotti, M., & Mercer, J. (2007). Holding therapy and dyadic developmental psychotherapy are not supported and acceptable social work interventions: A systematic research synthesis revisited. *Research on Social Work Practice, 17*, 513–519.

Presmanes, A., Zuckerman, K. E., & Fombonne, E. (2014). Epidemiology of autism spectrum disorders. In F. Volkmar, S. Roders, R. Paul, & K. Pelphrey (Eds.), *Handbook of autism and pervasive developmental disorders* (4th ed.). Hoboken, NJ: Wiley.

Price, C. S., Thompson, W. W., Goodson, B., Weintraub, E. S., Croen, L. A., Hinrichsen, V. L., … DeStefano, F. (2010). Prenatal and infant exposure to thimerosal from vaccines and immunoglobulins and risk of autism. *Pediatrics, 126*, 656–664.

Reichelt, K. L., Ekrem, J., & Scott, H. (1990). Gluten, milk proteins and autism: Dietary intervention effects on behavior and peptide secretion. *Journal of Applied Nutrition, 42*, 1–11.

Robertson, M. A., Sigalet, D. L., Holst, J. J., Meddings, J. B., Wood, J., & Sharkey, K. A. (2008). Intestinal permeability and glucagon-like peptide-2 in children with autism: A controlled pilot study. *Journal of Autism and Developmental Disorders, 38*, 1066–1071.

Sanchez, R., & Remizowski, L. (2014, November 5). New York businesswoman guilty of manslaughter in son's death. Retrieved from http://www.cnn.com/2014/11/05/justice/new-york-autistic-death-trial/.

Sasso, G. M. (2001). The retreat from inquiry and knowledge in special education. *The Journal of Special Education, 34*, 178–193.

Schiebinger, L. (2001). Has feminism changed science?. Harvard University Press.

Shermer, M. (2002). *Why people believe weird things: Pseudoscience, superstition, and other confusions of our time*. New York City, NY: Holt Paperbacks.

Shermer, M. (2004). Death by theory. *Scientific American, 290*(6), 48.

Siegel, B. (1995). Brief report: Assessing allegations of sexual molestation made through facilitated communication. *Journal of Autism and Developmental Disorders, 25*, 319–326.

Silver, L. B. (1995). Controversial therapies. *Journal of Child Neurology, 10*(1), 96–100.

Simpson, R., & Myles, B. (1995). Facilitated communication and disabilities: An enigma in search of a perspective. *Focus on Exceptional Children, 27*, 1–16.

Skinner, B. F. (1957). *Verbal behavior*. New York City, NY: Appleton.

Solomon, R., Necheles, J., Ferch, C., & Bruckman, D. (2007). Pilot study of a parent training program for young children with autism The PLAY Project Home Consultation program. *Autism, 11*, 205–224.

Stehli, A. (1994). *The sound of a miracle*. New York, NY: Doubleday.

Stubblefield, A. (2011). Sound and fury: When opposition to facilitated communication functions as hate speech. *Disability Studies Quarterly, 31*, 1–22.

Sundstrum, K (2014, October, 16). Mother's anger: Someone abusing my son was my greatest fear. Retrieved from http://www.sunshinecoastdaily.com.au/news/mother-angered-by-suspended-sentences/2422829/.

Szempruch, J., & Jacobson, J. W. (1993). Evaluating facilitated communications of people with developmental disabilities. *Research in Developmental Disabilities, 14*, 253–264.

Tinbergen, N., Tinbergen, E. A., & Welch, M. (1983). *Autistic children: New hope for a cure*. London: Allen & Unwin.

Todd, J. T. (2012). The moral obligation to be empirical: Comments on Boynton's "Facilitated Communication—What harm it can do: Confessions of a former facilitator". *Evidence-Based Communication Assessment and Intervention, 6*, 36–57.

Tostanoski, A., Lang, R., Raulston, T., Carnett, A., & Davis, T. (2014). Voices from the past: Comparing the rapid prompting method and facilitated communication. *Developmental Neurorehabilitation, 17*, 219–223.

Travers, J., Tincani, M., & Lang, R. (2014). Facilitated communication denies people with disabilities their voice. *Research and Practice for Persons with Severe Disabilities, 39*, 195.

Tuzikow, J. E., & Holburn, S. (2011). Identifying fad therapies for autism spectrum disorders and promoting effective treatment. In J. L. Matson & P. Sturmey (Eds.), *International handbook of autism and pervasive developmental disorders* (pp. 307–319). New York, NY: Springer.

Van Buskirk, S. E., & Simpson, R. L. (2013). Meteorological variables and behavior of learners with autism: An examination of possible relationships. *Focus on Autism and Other Developmental Disabilities, 28*(3), 131–137.

Vyse, S. (2005). Where do fads come from? In J. W. Jacobson, R. M. Foxx, & J. A. Mulick (Eds.), *Controversial therapies for developmental disabilities* (pp. 3–17). Mahwah, NJ: Lawrence Erlbaum.

Wagner, A. L., Wallace, K. S., & Rogers, S. J. (2014). Developmental treatment approaches for young children with autism spectrum disorders. In P. Sturmey, D. Dixon, J. Matson, & J. Tarbox (Eds.), *The Handbook of Early Intervention for Autism Spectrum Disorders: Research, Practice, and Policy*. New York, NY: Springer.

Wakefield, A. J., Anthony, A., Murch, S. H., Thomson, M., Montgomery, S. M., Davies, S., … Walker-Smith, J. A. (2000). Enterocolitis in children with developmental disorders. *The American Journal of Gastroenterology, 95*, 2285–2295.

Wakefield, A. J., Murch, S. H., Anthony, A., Linnell, J., Casson, D. M., Malik, M., … Walker-Smith, J. A. (1998). RETRACTED: Ileal-lymphoid-nodular hyperplasia, non-specific colitis, and pervasive developmental disorder in children. *The Lancet, 351*, 637–641.

Waters, M. B., Lerman, D. C., & Hovanetz, A. N. (2009). Separate and combined effects of visual schedule and extinction plus differential reinforcement on problem behavior occasioned by transitions. *Journal of Applied Behavior Analysis, 42*, 309–313.

Wheeler, D. L., Jacobson, J. W., Paglieri, R. A., & Schwartz, A. A. (1993). An experimental assessment of facilitated communication. *Mental Retardation, 31*, 49–59.

Wieder, S., & Greenspan, S. I. (2003). Climbing the symbolic ladder in the DIR model through floor time/interactive play. *Autism, 7*, 425–435.

Yeargin-Allsopp, M., Rice, C., Karapurkar, T., Doernberg, N., Boyle, C., & Murphy, C. (2003). Prevalence of autism in a US metropolitan area. *Journal of the American Medical Association, 289*, 49–55.

Index

R. Lang et al. (eds.), *Early Intervention for Young Children with Autism Spectrum Disorder*, Evidence-Based Practices in Behavioral Health,
DOI 10.1007/978-3-319-30925-5

R

S

CPSIA information can be obtained
at www.ICGtesting.com
Printed in the USA
LVHW02*1928261117
557621LV00005B/307/P